FIRST EXPOSURE TO

INTERNAL MEDICINE:

HOSPITAL MEDICINE

To my students, from whom I learn every day;
to my colleagues in internal medicine at the University of Kentucky,
it's a joy to work with you all;
to my fellow clerkship directors around the country,
you inspire me with your idealism and dedication;
and to my family, my foundation.

Charles H. Griffith III, MD, MSPH

FIRST EXPOSURE TO

INTERNAL MEDICINE:

HOSPITAL MEDICINE

Charles H. Griffith III, MD, MSPH
Inpatient Internal Medicine Clerkship Director
Division of General Internal Medicine
University of Kentucky
Lexington, Kentucky

Andrew R. Hoellein, MD, MS
Ambulatory Internal Medicine Clerkship Director
Division of General Internal Medicine
University of Kentucky
Lexington, Kentucky

Christopher A. Feddock, MD, MS
Med-Peds Residency Program Director
Division of General Internal Medicine
University of Kentucky
Lexington, Kentucky

Heather E. Harrell, MD
Medicine Clerkship Director
Director of the Fourth Year Program
University of Florida College of Medicine
Gainesville, Florida

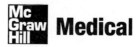

New York / Chicago / San Francisco / Lisbon / London / Madrid / Mexico City
Milan / New Delhi / San Juan / Seoul / Singapore / Sydney / Toronto

First Exposure to Internal Medicine: Hospital Medicine

Copyright © 2007 by the McGraw-Hill Companies, Inc. All rights reserved. Printed in the United States of America. Except as permitted under the United States Copyright Act of 1976, no part of this publication may be reproduced or distributed in any form or by any means, or stored in a data base or retrieval system, without prior written permission of the publisher.

1 2 3 4 5 6 7 8 9 0   DOC/DOC   9 8 7

ISBN-13: 978-0-07-145901-3
ISBN-10:   0-07-145901-4

This book was set in Palatino by International Typesetting and Composition.
The editors of this book were Jason Malley and Christie Naglieri.
The production supervisor was Sherri Souffrance.
Project management was handled by International Typesetting and Composition.
The indexer was Robert Swanson.
RR Donnelley was printer and binder.

This book is printed on acid-free paper.

Notice

Medicine is an ever-changing science. As new research and clinical experience broaden our knowledge, changes in treatment and drug therapy are required. The authors and the publisher of this work have checked with sources believed to be reliable in their efforts to provide information that is complete and generally in accord with the standards accepted at the time of publication. However, in view of the possibility of human error or changes in medical sciences, neither the authors nor the publisher nor any other party who has been involved in the preparation or publication of this work warrants that the information contained herein is in every respect accurate or complete, and they disclaim all responsibility for any errors or omissions or for the results obtained from use of the information contained in this work. Readers are encouraged to confirm the information contained herein with other sources. For example, and in particular, readers are advised to check the product information sheet included in the package of each drug they plan to administer to be certain that the information contained in this work is accurate and that changes have not been made in the recommended dose or in the contraindications for administration. This recommendation is of particular importance in connection with new or infrequently used drugs.

Library of Congress Cataloging-in-Publication Data

First exposure to internal medicine: hospital medicine / Charles H. Griffith III, Andrew R. Hoellein, Christopher A. Feddock, Heather Harrell.—1st ed.
    p. cm.
  Includes index.
  ISBN 0-07-145901-4 (alk.paper)
  1. Hospital care.   2. Internal medicine.   3. Clinical medicine.   I. Griffith, Charles H.
RA972.F57 2007
362.12—dc22   2006047349

C O N T E N T S

SECTION V   RENAL   245

CONTRIBUTORS

Eric Alper, MD
Medicine Clerkship Director
Associate Professor of Medicine
University of Massachusetts
   Medical School
Worcester, Massachusetts
Chapter 5

Lisa M. Antes, MD
Associate Professor of Medicine
Internal Medicine Assistant
   Inpatient Clerkship Director
Roy J. and Lucille A. Carver
   College of Medicine at
   The University of Iowa
Iowa City, Iowa
Chapters 33, 34, 37

Alison L. Bailey, MD
Fellow in Cardiovascular Medicine
University of Kentucky
Lexington, Kentucky
Chapter 6

Paula Bailey, MD, MHA
Assistant Professor of Medicine
University of Kentucky
Lexington, Kentucky
Chapter 18

Ashutosh J. Barve, MD, PhD
Fellow in Gastroenterology
University of Louisville
Louisville, Kentucky
Chapter 61

Pat F. Bass III, MD, MPH, MS
Assistant Professor of Internal
   Medicine and Pediatrics
LSUHSC—Shreveport
Shreveport, Louisiana
Chapter 8

Lisa Bellini, MD
Associate Dean for Graduate
   Medical Education
University of Pennsylvania
Philadelphia, Pennsylvania
Chapter 13

Eric Bensadoun, MD
Associate Professor of Medicine
University of Kentucky
Lexington, Kentucky
Chapter 21

Meriem Bensalem-Owen, MD
Assistant Professor of Neurology
University of Kentucky
Lexington, Kentucky
Chapter 57

Andrew Bernard, MD
Assistant Professor of Surgery
University of Kentucky
Lexington, Kentucky
Chapters 20, 49

Simrit Bhullar, DO
Fellow in Pulmonary and Critical
   Care Medicine
University of Kentucky
Lexington, Kentucky
Chapter 17

Anthony Bottiggi, MD
Fellow in Surgical Critical Care
University of Kentucky
Lexington, Kentucky
Chapter 20

Bernard R. Boulanger, MD, FACS
Associate Professor of Surgery
University of Kentucky
Lexington, Kentucky
Chapter 22

Ketan P. Buch, MBBS, FCCP
Assistant Professor of Medicine
University of Kentucky
Lexington, Kentucky
Chapter 4

Phillip K. Chang, MD
Assistant Professor of Surgery
University of Kentucky
Lexington, Kentucky
Chapter 30

Edward Cutolo, MD
Associate Professor of Medicine
University of South Florida
Tampa, Florida
Chapter 46

Susan Day, MD
Clinical Associate Professor of
   Medicine
University of Pennsylvania
Philadelphia, Pennsylvania
Chapter 59

Kristy S. Deep, MD
Fellow in Academic Internal Medicine
University of Kentucky
Lexington, Kentucky
Chapter 29

Steven Durning, MD, FACP
Associate Professor of Medicine
Uniformed Services University of
   the Health Sciences
Bethesda, Maryland
Chapter 40

Christopher A. Feddock, MD, MS, FAAP
Med-Peds Residency Program
   Director
Division of General Internal Medicine
University of Kentucky
Lexington, Kentucky
Chapters 10, 56, 60

Matthew Fitz, MD
Assistant Professor of Medicine
   and Pediatrics
Loyola University Medical Center
Maywood, Illinois
Chapters 35, 36

Erica Friedman, MD
Associate Dean for Undergraduate
   Medical Education
Associate Professor of Medicine
Mount Sinai School of Medicine
New York, New York
Chapter 55

Russell. C. Gilbert, MD
Assistant Professor of Medicine
Uniformed Services University of
   the Health Sciences
Bethesda, Maryland
Chapter 19

Misha Rhodes, MD
Assistant Professor of Medicine
University of Kentucky
Lexington, Kentucky
Chapter 24

D. Stephen Goggans, MD
Assistant Professor of Medicine
Medical College of Georgia
Augusta, Georgia
Chapter 7

Joel A. Gordon, MD
Professor and Vice Chair for
 Education
Internal Medicine Inpatient
 Clerkship Director
Roy J. and Lucille A. Carver
 College of Medicine at
 The University of Iowa
Iowa City, Iowa
Chapters 33, 34, 37

Sharon F. Green, MD, MA
Fellow in Academic Internal Medicine
University of Kentucky
Lexington, Kentucky
Chapter 51

Charles H. Griffith III, MD, MSPH
Inpatient Internal Medicine
 Clerkship Director
Division of General Internal Medicine
University of Kentucky
Lexington, Kentucky
Chapter 9

Heather E. Harrell, MD
Medicine Clerkship Director
Director of the Fourth Year Program
University of Florida College of
 Medicine
Gainesville, Florida
Chapter 1

Dan Henry, MD
Professor of Clinical Medicine
Course Director, Multidisciplinary
 Ambulatory Experiences and
 Advanced Clinical Experiences
University of Connecticut School
 of Medicine
Farmington, Connecticut
Chapters 12, 38

Paul Hering, MD
Professor of Medicine
Loyola University Medical Center
Maywood, Illinois
Chapter 35

Caridad A. Hernandez, MD
Assistant Professor and Chief,
 Hospitalist Section
University of Florida
Gainesville, Florida
Chapter 45

David M. Hiestand, MD, PhD
Assistant Professor of Medicine
University of Kentucky
Lexington, Kentucky
Chapter 14

Craig J. Hoesley, MD
Associate Professor of Medicine
University of Alabama at
 Birmingham
Birmingham, Alabama
Chapter 48

L. Chad Hood, MD
Adjunct Clinical Assistant
 Professor
University of Florida
Gainesville, Florida
Chapter 31

Bruce L. Houghton, MD
Associate Professor of Medicine
Creighton University
Omaha, Nebraska
Chapter 64

Deborah A. Humphrey, DO, FACP
Assistant Professor of Medicine
University of South Florida
Tampa, Florida
Chapter 47

M. Salik Jahania, MD
Assistant Professor of Surgery
University of Kentucky
Lexington, Kentucky
Chapter 58

Kanchan Kamath, MD
Assistant Professor of Medicine
University of South Florida
Tampa, Florida
Chapter 53

Paul Kearney, MD
Professor of Surgery
University of Kentucky
Lexington, Kentucky
Chapters 49, 63

Jennifer R. Kogan, MD
Assistant Professor of Medicine;
   Director of Undergraduate
   Education
University of Pennsylvania
Philadelphia, Pennsylvania
Chapter 59

Andrew J. Koon, MD
Assistant Professor of Medicine
University of South Florida
Tampa, Florida
Chapter 44

Ritu A. Kumar, MD
Fellow in Infectious Diseases
University of Alabama at
   Birmingham
Birmingham, Alabama
Chapter 48

Cynthia H. Ledford, MD
Assistant Clinical Professor of
   Medicine and Pediatrics
The Ohio State University
Columbus, Ohio
Chapter 2

Cortney Youens Lee, MD
Surgery Resident
University of Kentucky
Lexington, Kentucky
Chapter 63

James R. McCormick, MD, FCCP
Professor
Pulmonary/Critical Care Medicine
Associate Chief of Staff for
   Education
University of Kentucky and
   VA Medical Center
Lexington, Kentucky
Chapter 17

Malkanthie I. McCormick, MD
Associate Professor of Medicine
University of Kentucky
Lexington, Kentucky
Chapter 17

Robert T. Means, Jr., MD
Professor and Associate Chair for
   Research
University of Kentucky
Lexington, Kentucky
Chapter 51

R. Scott Morehead, MD
Associate Professor of Medicine
University of Kentucky
Lexington, Kentucky
Chapter 16

Janet N. Myers, MD, FACP, FCCP
Assistant Professor of Medicine
and Clerkship Director
Uniformed Services University of
the Health Sciences
Bethesda, Maryland
Chapter 19

Christopher S. Newell, MD
Assistant Professor of Medicine
University of Kentucky
Lexington, Kentucky
Chapter 39

Thomas D. Painter, MD
Professor of Internal Medicine
University of Pittsburgh
Pittsburgh, Pennsylvania
Chapter 15

John Poremba, MD
Staff Endocrinologist
Director, Introduction to
Clinical Medicine & Uniformed
Services
Assistant Professor of Medicine
University of the Health Sciences
Bethesda, Maryland
Chapter 40

Terri Postma, MD
Neurology Resident
University of Kentucky
Lexington, Kentucky
Chapter 41

Asha Ramsakal, DO, MBS
Assistant Clinical Professor of
Medicine
University of South Florida
Tampa, Florida
Chapter 50

Sushanth Reddy, MD
General Surgery Resident
University of Kentucky
Lexington, Kentucky
Chapter 22

Alexander I. Reiss, MD
Assistant Professor of Medicine
University of South Florida
Tampa, Florida
Chapter 28

Eric I. Rosenberg, MD, MSPH, FACP
Assistant Professor of Medicine
University of Florida
Gainesville, Florida
Chapter 65

Michelle L. Rossi, MD, FACP
Clinical Assistant Professor of
Medicine
University of Florida
Gainesville, Florida
Chapter 27

David W. Rudy, MD
Associate Professor of Medicine
University of Kentucky
Lexington, Kentucky
Chapter 32

Carabeth W. Russell, MD
Internal Medicine Resident
University of Kentucky
Lexington, Kentucky
Chapter 11

Sibu P. Saha, MD, MBA
Professor of Surgery
University of Kentucky
Lexington, Kentucky
Chapter 58

Lisbeth Selby, MD
Assistant Professor of Medicine
University of Kentucky
Lexington, Kentucky
Chapter 23

Carol D. Spears, MD
Clinical Instructor of Surgery
University of Kentucky
Lexington, Kentucky
Chapter 22

Winifred G. Teuteberg, MD
Assistant Professor of Medicine
University of Pittsburgh
Pittsburgh, Pennsylvania
Chapter 62

Christine Yasuko Todd, MD
Southern Illinois University
Springfield, Illinois
Chapters 25, 42

Deanna Todd Tzanetos, MD
Chief Resident, Internal Medicine
University of Kentucky
Lexington, Kentucky
Chapter 3

Douglas Bazil Tzanetos, MD
Chief Resident, Internal Medicine
University of Kentucky
Lexington, Kentucky
Chapter 26

Mark M. Udden, MD
Professor of Medicine
Baylor College of Medicine
Houston, Texas
Chapters 52, 54

Raymond Y. Wong, MD
Program Director
Student Education in Internal
  Medicine
Loma Linda University
Loma Linda, California
Chapter 43

PREFACE

One of the challenges of being a clerkship director of internal medicine is that there is no perfect textbook for one's course. More comprehensive textbooks often have all the information a student should have for their patient care needs, but the volume of information in these comprehensive textbooks is far too much for a student to read (much less reread, and study) in the few weeks of a medicine clerkship. Therefore, many students resort to purchasing one of the shorter textbooks, readable within the confines of a clerkship, but often not having the detail of information needed to understand in-depth the patient's problems (with that superficial knowledge inevitably exposed by attending-questioning on rounds!). To solve this dilemma, students often buy two text-books, one comprehensive, one more general; however, as the clerkship winds to an end, and final examinations loom, reading often defaults to the shorter textbook, resulting in less in-depth understanding of internal medicine.

This book, and its companion book *First Exposure to Internal Medicine: Ambulatory Medicine*, is an attempt to remedy this dilemma, with topics discussed in-depth enough for a student's patient care needs, and in-depth enough for deeper understanding, but presented in a brief enough fashion to be read in a short internal medicine clerkship. Why two textbooks, you may ask? After all, many medical conditions are encountered in both the ambulatory and inpatient settings (diabetes, asthma, anemia, and so forth), the only difference the severity of illness, why artificially assign a topic as inpatient versus ambulatory? Granted, this is true. However, most internal medicine clerkships are conducted in block fashion, with students rotating, for example, on a 4-week inpatient service, followed by a 4-week outpatient experience. In fact, in many schools, the outpatient experience occurs more often in a temporally separate rotation block than in the inpatient experience, such as in a "primary care" rotation. Therefore, the focus of student reading is often ambulatory topics during their ambulatory block, inpatient topics during their inpatient block. This textbook, the hospital medicine text, focuses on topics generally encountered on inpatient rotations. Some topics span both textbooks. For example, diabetes is encountered in both settings quite frequently. However, the focus of diabetes care is often different in the different settings. Therefore, the ambulatory text focuses on long-term complications of diabetes, and choice of maintenance medications. In contrast, the hospital text focuses on diabetic emergencies (ketoacidosis, hyperosmolar hyperglycemic state) and inpatient glycemic control. For students having both ambulatory and inpatient internal medicine rotations, these books can be read in tandem. However, for students with only an inpatient rotation, or only an ambulatory rotation, we hope you find these books self-contained enough that one book would suffice for that specific rotation's needs.

Chapter topics were chosen after much discussion and careful consideration, attempting to balance comprehensiveness with readability. In general, it was believed most chapters should be at least 4–5 pages in length for the desired degree of depth, but no longer than 8–10 pages, to promote readability (and rereading for study). The text itself was intentionally limited to about 400 pages in length, such that a student reading 8–10 pages a night could read the entire text in a 6- to 8-week internal medicine clerkship. Therefore, we aimed for about 65 chapters of text. Now, there are hundreds of topics one could encounter on an internal medicine clerkship; the discipline is that broad (consider what an internal medicine residency is: in contrast to some residencies where much of one's learning involves mastering various procedures or operations, an internal medicine residency is 3 more years trying to learn more internal medicine). However, if this textbook attempted to discuss all those myriad topics, the text would either become too unwieldy and unreadable in a short clerkship, or present topics so briefly as to sacrifice in-depth learning. Therefore, the student may encounter a patient with a condition not presented in this textbook, and for such occasional patients, one would need to consult another source for reading. One does not expect every student to master every topic in internal medicine, but there are some core topics in which every third year medical student should begin to becoming adept, as they form the knowledge base expected of any physician, regardless of specialty. To that end, in this text you will find all the hospital conditions in the Core Curriculum developed by the national organization of the Clerkship Directors of Internal Medicine (CDIM). In addition, realizing that this text could be very useful for fourth year students in their medicine subinternship, this text also includes all the conditions in the CDIM subinternship curriculum. Furthermore, we include chapters to help students in basic clinical skills they will encounter on the inpatient services, such as primers on ECG interpretation, reading chest x-rays, common inpatient procedures, and deciphering acid-base problems. We also devote chapters to evaluating various symptoms that may arise in patients on the inpatient setting, such as an approach to evaluating dyspnea, or fever, or nausea/vomiting. Realizing that some students will rotate in intensive care settings (or if they don't, many patients on the hospital wards will become critically ill, necessitating transfer to the ICU), we have included chapters on topics of intensive care, such as respiratory failure, sepsis syndrome, and ARDS. Other special topics include chapters on end-of-life discussions, on treating pain in hospitalized patients, and on nutrition. Finally, we have included several chapters generally not included in most student texts, yet commonly encountered on inpatient settings, such as issues of antibiotic choice, IV fluid choice, and transfusions.

The content of each chapter was guided by several principles. First, we strongly believe that a deeper and more lasting understanding of the conditions encountered in hospital settings relies on a strong understanding of the underlying pathophysiology, such a deeper understanding is one of the things that distinguishes a physician from other health care providers. Therefore, each chapter contains a brief review of the relevant pathophysiology. Student readers are strongly encouraged to read these sections carefully, as subsequent sections on diagnosis and management are grounded in these pathophysiologic principles. Second, the quality of chapter content is often only as good as the quality of the chapter author. Therefore, we have recruited master educators from across the country as contributors, many clerkship directors, many residency directors, all actively involved in medical student education. By doing this, we hope chapters are written at the appropriate student level, and that this textbook represents a truly national initiative. Third, each chapter was read carefully by myself and at least two other coeditors, for the inclusion of all the clinical "pearls" that may arise in discussions on rounds concerning these topics. Each of the editors has been the recipient of many teaching awards, and we hope we passed on some of our teaching expertise as we helped in the crafting of chapters.

We hope you enjoy the book. I have been clerkship director of internal medicine at the University of Kentucky since 1993, and have seen many internal medicine textbooks come and go, none in my view solving this tension of comprehensiveness versus readability. We are excited, a little nervous, but cautiously optimistic that perhaps this book and its companion text will begin to solve this conundrum.

Charles H. Griffith III, MD, MSPH

ACKNOWLEDGMENTS

We wish to acknowledge the critical assistance of Helen Garces at the University of Kentucky in helping to refine many of the textbook figures, any mistakes are ours, any laurels hers. We also appreciate the help of the folks at McGraw-Hill, including Jason Malley, Andrea Seils, and Christie Naglieri, thank you greatly.

Charles H. Griffith III, MD, MSPH
Andrew R. Hoellein, MD, MS
Christopher A. Feddock, MD, MS
Heather E. Harrell, MD

GENERAL

INTRODUCTION TO INPATIENT INTERNAL MEDICINE/GENERAL INPATIENT SKILLS

Heather E. Harrell

KEY POINTS

- Internal medicine is an intellectually stimulating field with rewarding patient contact, but it is frequently overwhelming as well.
- Active involvement in patient care is the best way to learn the subject.
- Internists are known for paying attention to details, this is the time to be very detail-oriented with your patient care.
- Understanding clinical reasoning (the "why" of your assessment and plan) is a priority of internal medicine training.

INTRODUCTION

The inpatient Internal Medicine rotation can be rather daunting as you consider the complexity of the patients, the breadth of diseases, and the frequently long hours. Yet, it is also routinely one of the highest rated experiences by medical students across the country. Most medical students enjoy the intellectual stimulation and direct patient care of inpatient internal medicine, and feeling like a valuable team member. At many schools, this may be one of the few opportunities you have to care for patients longitudinally and you will experience the rewards of patients looking to you as "their doctor." The time you have to spend with patients on a busy ward service is a valuable and necessary contribution to your team—remember this, particularly when you may be feeling insecure on rounds or overwhelmed preparing for an exam. Additional tips compiled by the Clerkship Directors in Internal Medicine may be found at: http://www.im.org/CDIM/primer.htm.

FIVE PRINCIPLES FOR SUCCESS

The following principles are adapted from Dr. James Lynch of the University of Florida and they will help you not only find success during your inpatient medicine rotation, but they can also be applied to any field in medicine. Reflect on the physicians you admire most. These are the qualities that set them apart as excellent, not just competent.

1. **Know everything about your patient**. Typically as a third-year student, you will only follow a couple of patients at a time. Therefore, you are held to a higher standard. Do not expect to formally present everything you know about your patient. But if you are asked about a lab value, medication, occupational history, or what the patient ate for breakfast, you better know. Housestaff are generally kind and will come to your rescue, but don't kid yourself, it will be "noted" by the team.
2. **Know why you're doing what you're doing**. It is frequently said that a good medical student is like a preschooler, always asking, "Why?" Certainly this is how learning occurs. But by following this principle you can also improve patient care as your constant querying may be the force that causes the team to reflect more carefully about why a patient is or is not on a certain medication, or why a certain test is being performed.
3. **Worry more about your patients than you do yourself**. This does not mean neglect your loved ones or your own basic needs. But, you are now caring for real patients who experience real suffering, are in their most vulnerable state, and trust you to help them. If you do not find yourself worrying at times whether Ms. Smith received her antibiotic or Mr. Jones' son was reached, it is time to step back and reassess your priorities. Your patients and team members can sense this and doing the right thing will also pay off in better evaluations.
4. **Pay attention to the details**. This is one of the hallmarks of internists. We pride ourselves on taking the most thorough histories, performing the most comprehensive exams, and leaving no stone unturned. With complex internal medicine patients, it can make all the difference.
5. **Work hard**. There is no substitute—enough said.

These principles may appear obvious or even unrealistic. Furthermore, and unfortunately, you have probably seen some doctors not follow these principles (although one can often learn as much from a negative role model—hopefully vowing to yourself to never behave similarly). But, the fact that you are reading this textbook (particularly this introductory chapter) implies that you want to excel, not merely pass the internal medicine clerkship. The remainder of this chapter will briefly review the general ward experience, structure, and common tasks you will be expected to perform. Since most clerkships provide detailed instructions about ward expectations, the daily schedule, and patient write-ups, this text will emphasize how to avoid common pitfalls.

ADMITTING A PATIENT: THE HISTORY AND PHYSICAL

You will be asked to "start seeing" or "get started on" a patient. This means you have a new patient to admit, often from the Emergency Department (ED). For your first admission, you should accompany your intern or resident if possible to see how the ED is structured and how they approach a new admission. **After that, however, always try to perform your history and physicals alone** even if this means waiting until the intern is finished. You will usually know the patients' chief complaint and this is a good time to read about the complaint or any of their known medical problems so your history will address all the pertinent information. In general, third-year medical students are expected to perform complete histories and physical examinations on inpatient services (this includes tracking down details about the past medical history (PMH) from old records and interviewing care givers). Finally, never decline to take an admission unless you can provide a very good reason. ("I've already picked up a patient with chest pain" or "I'm going off service tomorrow" are not good reasons.) Declining an admission is tantamount to being disinterested or lazy in the eyes of most house officers.

ADMITTING A PATIENT: WRITING ORDERS

Once you have collected the data from your history, physical examination, and initial blood tests and x-rays routinely performed in most EDs, you must decide what you think is wrong with the patient (the working diagnosis) as well other possibilities that could explain the presentation (differential diagnoses). This drives your order writing. Depending on how sick your patient is, diagnosis and treatment may need to occur simultaneously (e.g., beginning antibiotics in a patient with a fever while you are also thinking of the possible causes of the fever and ordering diagnostic tests). Interns are under great pressure to get orders written and patients transferred to the floor. This can make it difficult for you to write orders with your intern. One potential solution to give you more active involvement in order writing is to write your own set of orders (that will not go in the chart), compare them to what your intern wrote, and then discuss any differences.

ADMITTING A PATIENT: PRESENTING THE CASE

Giving a concise, pertinent, organized, and engaging presentation is a difficult skill that requires much **practice**. The oral presentation is never as detailed as the written presentation but the amount of details each physician wants to hear varies greatly. It is best to ask this up front and modify your presentations for each individual. In general, strive for a new patient presentation no longer than 5 minutes, as much longer will try the patience and attention spans of your often sleep-deprived audience. Also, if by chance you do not know some information you are asked, don't improvise, it's okay to say you do not know something rather than to mislead the team and potentially compromise patient care.

The traditional format of an oral presentation is as follows:

1. An opening statement that begins with the patient's **age** and **sex** and introduces the **chief complaint** and **reason for admission**.
2. The **history of present illness** (HPI) is presented in its entirety and should include any **PMH, family and social history**, and **review of systems** (ROS) that are pertinent to the chief complaint.
3. Present any PMH that will be relevant to the current admission (e.g., "diabetes" *not* "cataracts").
4. Present **medications** and **allergies** (ask whether doses should be reported).
5. ROS is not presented orally unless something potentially serious is uncovered that will need to be addressed during the admission that is unrelated to the chief complaint (as related symptoms would have already been presented in the HPI).
6. When presenting the physical examination, always **start with the vital signs and the patient's general appearance**. Beyond that, most people prefer only to hear about the pertinent aspects of the examination and any abnormal findings.
7. Pertinent laboratory, radiology, or other test results should be presented. (Ask whether your team wants to hear every lab value, and if so try not to read them off too fast.)
8. The **assessment** is by far the most difficult part of the presentation for students, but you should always try to present one rather than stopping after you present the data and waiting for the team to jump in. This can be accomplished by giving a one sentence summary of the patient's presentation, highlight any pertinent findings, and then state your working diagnosis. Stop at this point and move directly to the plan. (If someone

wants to hear a differential diagnosis or more discussion about your clinical reasoning, let him or her ask or read your written note.)
8. The **plan** should be specific (e.g., know the doses of any medications you plan to start) and will probably have been determined already by your intern or resident. But, you should always try to offer some plan of your own whenever possible and always make sure you understand the plan even if you didn't formulate it.

ADMITTING A PATIENT: THE WRITTEN PRESENTATION

Most schools and Clerkship Directors have specific guidelines about how they would like an admission write-up organized and you should read and follow any and all instructions offered at your program. This is the place where you fill in the details omitted from the oral presentation and make sure you are thorough. While you should always avoid redundancy, it is better for third-year medical students to err on the side of being too thorough rather than too concise. The assessment and plan in your written note may also be one of the few opportunities you have to clearly **show what you know and how you are thinking** (as rounds presentations frequently get cut off or interrupted by other team members). Your write-ups should show evidence that you are reading about your patient and applying it rather than parroting what your intern's or resident's note says.

THE DAILY WARD ROUTINE

Every program is structured a little differently but the basic routines are similar and involve prerounding, rounding, morning report, and trying to get notes and orders written and patients discharged in between conferences, new admissions, and clinics. As you can imagine it can get very hectic and it is important above all else that you be visible, asking to help, and reliably follow up on any assigned task.

The Daily Routine: Rounds
Prerounds. The time you spend seeing your patients on your own before the team meets to review all the patients. This typically involves checking vital signs and nursing notes to see if any events occurred overnight. The patients are woken up and asked how they are feeling followed by specific questions relevant to their main problem(s). A focused examination is performed that includes noting any tubes and infusions. New lab or other test results are recorded. Smart students record all this in the form of a progress note as they go along for efficiency and to help give a more organized oral presentation. You should allow 15–30 minutes per patient depending on your level of experience.

    Rounds. The time spent reviewing all the patients together as a team. This may be divided into work rounds and teaching rounds.

- **Work rounds.** These are typically run by the resident and every patient is briefly presented and seen so that plans can be made and orders written for the rest of the day. The key is brief. These rounds are typically fast paced and oral presentations should be very focused (1–3 minutes). Sometimes residents like to "card flip" or have "sit down rounds." This means you briefly present and discuss the patients without going to see them. (Faculty routinely frown on this practice, but it happens nonetheless.)
- **Teaching rounds.** This is a more formal round with the attending and typically only a few cases are reviewed. Some faculty like to do this at the bedside and it will likely be the only time you give a full presentation about your patient (refer to oral presentation guidelines above). Many times this is combined with returning to a workroom for more didactic teaching.
- **Combined work and teaching rounds.** This is the most common format you will experience. The attending will join the team for a more extended round during which all patients are seen, presentations are a bit more formal, and brief teaching points will be made as each patient is seen. Presentations by students and residents are generally in **SOAP** fashion (Subjective-Objective-Assessment-Plan) or perhaps SOAPP fashion (SOAP plus patient's perspective). Internal medicine patients are usually very complex, with multiple active problems. Many teams prefer you to present the assessment and plan by problem (i.e., assessment and plan for their heart failure, then for their diabetes, then for their pneumonia, and so forth) rather than mixing problems and their assessments.

The Daily Routine: Postrounds or "What Should I be Doing Now?"

The mornings are typically the structured portion of the day often culminating with a noon conference. The afternoons are the time spent more directly caring for your patients and admitting new patients. Since afternoons are less structured, it can be confusing for students to know what they should be doing. **First and foremost, take advantage of this opportunity to return to your patients' rooms and spend time with them**. One of the most valuable roles you can assume is that of "patient translator." After rounds, most patients are more confused or full of questions than ever. Because you are new to the medical field, you are often the team member best able to explain medical concepts in a way that patients can understand. Because you will follow fewer patients, you also have the luxury of more time to get to know your patients and their families making you a powerful advocate for them. These are just a few of the reasons patients often view a good medical student as "their doctor."

Direct patient care is the glamorous part of medicine, but there are also important but more mundane aspects of caring for patients that you should learn and to help you become a more helpful and integral team member. (It is a great sign when your teams don't want you to rotate off service.

Invariably this will be because you are so helpful, not because you are so knowledgeable and able to answer pimping questions correctly.) The following are common tasks that will help your intern and the care of the patient:

1. **Follow-up on any tests** that were ordered. This is not only getting results conveyed to your team but also includes making sure the blood was drawn, the patient made it down to radiology, the specimen made it to pathology, and so forth. (If you discover a problem, try to fix it yourself.)
2. Make sure all the plans discussed on rounds were ordered by looking at your order entry system. If something was missed this is your chance to practice writing an order, which is ALWAYS cosigned by a physician.
3. Review the patients' **medication administration records** (MAR), the list of medications used by nurses, to make sure the patients received important medications and that there are no mistakes. Given the number of medications a typical inpatient is receiving, unfortunately you are almost guaranteed to find something that you can help fix.
4. Calling consultations. It is controversial with some doctors whether it is appropriate for medical students to call consultations so check with your team first. If this is a practice at your school, call them as early as possible and identify yourself as the medical student. You will need the patient's name, medical record number, room number, and a very **clear and concise reason for the consult**. (What questions are you asking?) Let the consultant decide if they would like to know more about the history and be prepared to give a concise (1 minute) history.
5. **Discharge planning** typically involves a lot of paper work and phone calls to work out issues like placement, rides, and home health needs. Try to anticipate needs and begin filling out forms and making calls even days before the anticipated discharge. Many teams will have a social worker or patient care resource manager who will be your best help with this. Key considerations for preparing patients' discharges include whether they can eat, walk, be disconnected from IVs and tubes, and receive long-term treatments at home. Physical therapy, occupational therapy, and nutrition consultations may be appropriate to suggest. Also, always keep track of whether your patients can be disconnected from invasive monitors or tubes.

The Daily Routine: Going Home

You are not an intern and you have other responsibilities on your clerkship in addition to patient care (e.g., preparing for an exam and polishing patient write-ups). Thus, it is not appropriate for you to stay everyday until the last person leaves. In fact, you will frequently have your work completed before the interns with your lighter patient load. Yet, even the nicest house officer can forget this or confuse you with a fourth-year acting intern. The following are tried and true suggestions for making a graceful exit. Always "run" your patients by your intern, which means updating your intern about changes in the patients' progress, test results, and consultant recommendations (usually in the late afternoon). Ask if there is anything else you need to be doing for the patient. If not, ask if there is anything you can do to help him or her with other patients. If not, then find your resident and do the same. Typically, house officers will tell you to go home at this point. Take this at face value and leave. If they don't suggest you leave, then most students will remind the house officer of some of the other clerkship responsibilities they need to do and ask to leave. (For example, "If there is nothing more I can help you with, then I would really like to go home and read more about what could be causing Mr. X's renal failure.")

At Home

We wouldn't presume to really tell you what to do at home, but you will likely spend some of your time reading and studying. Given the amount you are expected to cover in internal medicine, daily reading is critical even if for only a few minutes. This textbook is designed to provide you with manageable chapters that will work well for nightly reading and help you cover the core topics of internal medicine at a level appropriate for your training. The more you can tie your reading directly to patient care, the better you will retain it. Study guides and practice questions can be very helpful and may have a role in your training, but be very careful of relying on them too heavily in internal medicine as they will not provide you with the depth you need to care for your patients (or to prepare for the subject exam used by many schools).

DIAGNOSTIC AND

THERAPEUTIC DECISION

MAKING

Cynthia H. Ledford

KEY POINTS

- There is a degree of uncertainty in every medical decision.
- The patient's clinical presentation determines the likelihood of disease.
- An estimate of pretest likelihood is essential to interpreting diagnostic test results.
- Sensitivity is the true positive rate.
- Specificity is the true negative rate.
- The likelihood of disease determines whether treatment is indicated.
- Treatment decisions are based on:
  - How likely the patient is to benefit?
  - The risk of treatment.

INTRODUCTION

Medicine is full of uncertainty and ambiguity. Medical science is incomplete, physicians do not know everything, and decisions must be made based on best knowledge at a point in time. Therefore, a physician must have the ability to assess degrees of uncertainty and apply this to his/her decision making. In practical terms, a physician must consider the panoply of a patient's signs and symptoms, bring his or her clinical expertise and experience to bear in considering the likelihood of disease in that situation, and depending on that assessment of likelihood of disease, decisions for further testing or treatment are made.

CLINICAL PRESENTATIONS

The path from the patient's clinical presentation to a physician's summarizing assessment requires clinical reasoning. Clinical **experts** often reason by **pattern recognition**, sometimes by thinking forward through a stepwise process, and less commonly through hypothesis testing. Experts are able to quickly recognize patterns of disease based on knowledge structured as "classic illness scripts":

- Who gets it (key epidemiology and risk factors)
- How it presents with respect to time (temporal pattern)
- Key clinical features (presenting syndromes)

Patients present with symptoms and physical signs and physicians automatically process this information into a uniform medical language. A patient complains of pain with deep breath; the physician notes pleuritic chest pain. A patient is short of breath, has dullness in the right lung base with decreased breath sounds and decreased fremitus; the physician notes right pleural effusion. Through this processing, physicians are able to be concise and precise, and they are better able to retrieve related knowledge. Physicians mentally prioritize and reduce the list of problems by eliminating redundancies, nonspecific details, and problems that are clearly due to other more specific problems. The physician focuses on the right pleural effusion, realizing that the pleuritic chest pain is due to the effusion.

A physician is able to conceptualize the patient's presentation concisely highlighting who this patient is as a host that makes him or her uniquely at risk for diseases that present similarly, how the patient presents with respect to time, and the key syndrome with which the patient presents. For example, "This is an elderly smoker who presents with chronic progressive right pleural effusion, pathologic regional lymphadenopathy and wasting." From this the pattern is quickly recognized as very likely primary lung carcinoma with pleural involvement. Alternatively, if the pattern had been sudden onset of pleuritic chest pain and shortness of breath in a patient with surgery the previous day, this pattern may have suggested pulmonary embolism rather than lung cancer.

In order to acquire more expert reasoning, medical students learn to

- Identify patient problems
  - Process problems into medical terminology
  - Prioritize problems
- Formulate a patient-specific synopsis (patient illness script), based on
  - Who is this (key epidemiology and risk factors)
  - How he/she presents with respect to time (temporal pattern)
  - Key clinical features (presenting syndrome)

- Compare and contrast the synopsis of the patient with classic diseases to identify which is most likely based on pattern match

The likelihood of a specific disease is determined by how well the patient's illness fits the pattern. In addition, keep in mind the medical version of William of Occam's razor, a single explanation for a constellation of symptoms is more likely to be true than multiple explanations. For example, if a patient presents with proteinuria, renal insufficiency, anemia, hypercalcemia, and lytic bone lesions, a unifying diagnosis such as multiple myeloma is much more likely than five separate diagnoses explaining these features.

EVALUATION

Diagnostic evaluation or testing follows clinical assessment. The decision whether to perform a diagnostic test is based on whether the patient's probability of disease exceeds the physician's threshold for performing the test. This takes into consideration the risk of the diagnostic test and the benefit of making the diagnosis. The physician's threshold for performing a test is appropriately lower if it is for a serious disease that he or she does not want to miss or if the test presents little risk to the patient and is inexpensive. The physician's threshold to perform a test is appropriately high if it is for a minor disease or if it poses great cost and risk to the patient.

Before a diagnostic test is performed, it is important to consider what the physician will do with the result. **Will the result of the test change the management of the patient?** In a patient with acute pharyngitis, will the positive streptococcal antigen test result in treatment with antibiotics, while a negative result will not? In a patient with acute pharyngitis whose children have confirmed streptococcal pharyngitis, the physician may choose to treat even if the tests were negative. If the result of the test does not change the physician's management, then the test should not be done. This principle also applies to intermediary tests, intermediary in that further tests may be done if this test is "positive." A classic example is the decision to perform an exercise stress test, to help in the diagnosis of coronary artery disease. In a younger patient with atypical chest pain, a "negative" stress test may reassure the physician to the point that further testing for heart disease (i.e., cardiac catheterization) would not be warranted. On the other hand, in an older patient with multiple cardiac risk factors and classic angina, one would proceed with cardiac catheterization if the stress test shows inducible ischemia ("positive"), but even if negative, the clinical suspicion may be so high that catheterization would occur despite a negative test. If the stress test will not change management, then it shouldn't be performed, one should proceed directly to catheterization in this situation.

The usefulness of a diagnostic test is measured by the sensitivity and specificity. The **sensitivity** is the proportion of patients with disease who test positive for disease (true positive rate). The **specificity** is the proportion of patients without disease who test negative for disease (true negative rate). The sensitivity and specificity are specific for the disease for which it tests.

Screening tests are designed to screen for disease in asymptomatic individuals. Screening tests are best if they are inexpensive and have a high sensitivity (detect most individuals with disease). Logically, it is most useful to screen for diseases that are common in the general population. If a disease is very rare, the positive test is more likely to be a false positive than a true positive. For the screening to be beneficial, patients who have disease detected earlier before symptoms develop should have significantly better treatment outcomes compared to patients who are diagnosed when symptoms begin. Examples of screening tests are mammography, colonoscopy, and PAP smears.

Confirmatory tests should have a high specificity to minimize false positive results. These tests are typically more costly than first-line tests. Examples of confirmatory tests are coronary angiography following abnormal stress test or biopsy of lung mass following lung computed tomography (CT). A positive confirming test confirms that the disease is present. A negative confirming test does not mean that the disease is not present, however. If the clinical suspicion is still high despite a negative "confirmatory" test, one should consider further testing. For example, if a patient postoperatively has sudden onset of shortness of breath, normal chest x-ray, unexplained hypoxia, and an elevated D-dimer level, but yet a CT scan with PE protocol shows no pulmonary embolism, the clinical suspicion of PE may still be so great that further testing is warranted (i.e., pulmonary angiogram).

Excluding tests have high sensitivities to minimize false negative results. These tests are useful to **rule out a diagnosis**. Examples of excluding tests are chest radiographs for pneumonia or alanine transaminase for hepatitis or antinuclear antibodies (ANA) for systemic lupus. A positive test does not rule out the disease, but does not confirm it either. A positive ANA does not confirm lupus, but a negative ANA does make lupus much less likely.

Interpreting Test Results

Never interpret a test result in isolation, always interpret the test in the context of the patient (i.e., no test is perfect). In addition to noting the performance characteristics of the test (sensitivity, specificity), one should also take into account the positive and negative predictive values of a test, and above all, the prevalence of the disease in the population tested. In plain terms:

- Sensitivity: people with the disease will have a positive test
- Specificity: people without the disease will have a negative test

- Positive predictive value: people with a positive test will have the disease
- Negative predictive value: people with a negative test will not have the disease

From these simple definitions, and knowing (or estimating) the prevalence of a disease or condition in the population like your patient, one can then interpret more readily the significance of a positive test. This can be done by constructing a 2 × 2 table, with disease (or gold standard) the top row, + and −, and the test performed in columns, + and −. For example, say a new screening test is developed for HIV infection which has a reported sensitivity of 99% and a specificity of 99%. This sounds like a great test, let's screen everybody, right? Well, say the prevalence of HIV in a screened population is 2 in a 1000. So given a sensitivity of 99%, for those 2 patients with the disease, 1.98 (or 2, to round off) will have a positive test. For a sensitivity of 99%, for the 998 people without the disease, 0.99 × 998, or about 990 will have negative test, with the other 8 having a positive test. Hence, the 2 × 2 table would be:

HIV

		+	−
Test	+	2	8
	−	0	990

Now, calculate the positive predictive value, the people with a positive test (represented by the first row of the table) who have the disease. Well, 10 people have positive tests, 2 have the disease, so the positive predictive value is 2/10, or 20%. Therefore, more positive tests will be false positives in this low prevalence population. So even if a test claims high sensitivity and specificity, the clinical significance of a positive test will be greatly attenuated if applied to the wrong, low-risk population.

MANAGEMENT

Whether to treat a patient depends on whether the probability of disease in this patient exceeds the physician's threshold for treatment. The consequences of disease if left untreated and the risk of treatment determine the physician's threshold for treatment. In a minor illness such as toenail fungus that may be treated by an oral medication that can permanently damage the liver, the treatment threshold may be very high. The consequence of disease is ugly toes. The risk of treatment is death or liver transplant. With this high threshold the physician would want to be very certain that the patient had toenail fungus and highly valued attractive toes before embarking on treatment. Alternatively, in a disease that has serious consequences if not identified immediately (such as myocardial infarction) but relatively low risk to treat (i.e., by admission to hospital on telemetry, aspirin, beta-blocker, and rest) the treatment threshold would be very low. A 15% probability of myocardial infarction would warrant treatment via admission.

PROCEDURES

Deanna Todd Tzanetos

INTRODUCTION

In the evaluation and management of patients, invasive procedures frequently need to be performed. Certain basic principles should be followed prior to every procedure. For all nonemergent procedures, informed consent must be obtained from the patient or the patient's next-of-kin or legal decision maker. The person providing consent (the performing physician) must understand the reasons for performing the procedure, the potential benefits, the possible risks, and any alternatives to the procedure. After this has been explained, the patient should feel free to ask questions and must agree to the procedure before it is performed. When the procedure is performed, sterile technique must be used. Although this varies with the invasiveness and risks of the procedure, handwashing should always occur before and after the procedure. Always prep the patient with antimicrobial soap and wear sterile gown, gloves, and mask as necessary. Drape the area with sterile towels or sterile drapes so that nothing used in the procedure comes in contact with a nonsterile area.

CENTRAL VENOUS LINE PLACEMENT

A central venous line is commonly placed when patients require fluids or medications and peripheral administration is either impossible or inappropriate. It also provides access for frequent blood draws and invasive monitoring.

Central venous lines are generally placed in three anatomic areas: the internal jugular vein, the subclavian vein, or the femoral vein. The internal jugular and the subclavian are the preferred sites, because they have lower risks of infection; however, both sites are also technically more difficult. The **internal jugular vein** lies below the anatomic triangle formed by the two heads of the sternocleidomastoid muscle and the clavicle (Fig. 3-1). To enter the vein, a needle should be inserted at the apex of the triangle (between the

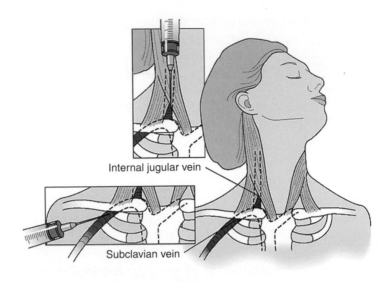

Figure 3-1 **Thoracic vein anatomy and insertion points for internal jugular and subclavian central venous catheterization.** (*Source:* Reproduced with permission from DeCherney AH, et al. *Current Obstetric & Gynecologic Diagnosis & Treatment*, 9th ed. New York: McGraw-Hill, 2003, Figure 58-1.)

heads of the sternocleidomastoid) and aimed toward the ipsilateral nipple. A common mistake is to puncture the carotid artery, so the carotid pulse located medially to the triangle should be palpated to avoid this complication. The **subclavian vein** lies directly below the clavicle, but veers toward the arm at the bend of the clavicle (midway between the suprasternal notch and acromion; Fig. 3-1). To find the subclavian vein, a needle should be inserted caudal to the distal third of the clavicle and directed toward the suprasternal notch. **Femoral vein** catheters should only be placed in an emergency or when all other options are exhausted. The femoral vein lies medial to the femoral artery. The femoral artery should be palpated and a needle inserted just medial to the artery.

Once the location is determined, the most common method for catheter placement is the Seldinger technique (Fig. 3-2). Occasionally, one may be unsure if the needle is in the vein or in an artery. In order to evaluate this, one can look for dark, nonpulsatile venous blood versus bright red, pulsatile arterial blood. Ultrasound guidance is being used more commonly to find the exact location of the vein, because it reduces the number of punctures to find the vein and complications. The most common complications of central venous lines are mechanical complications, such as arterial puncture, pneumothorax, or malposition. Thus, after any subclavian or internal jugular

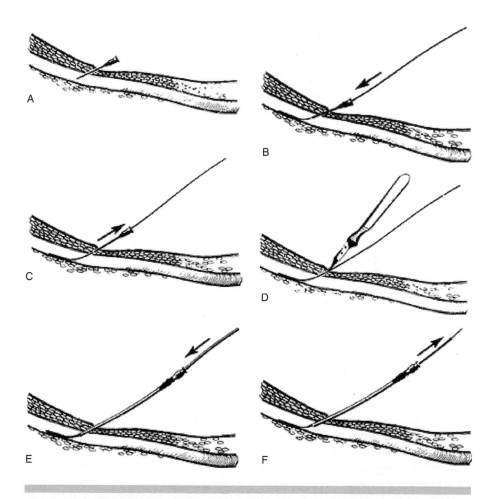

Figure 3-2 **Seldinger technique for placement of a central venous catheter. (A) Use a small needle to locate the vein; (B) once blood returns into the syringe, remove the syringe and thread the wire into the vein (never let go of the wire); (C) remove the needle, leaving the wire in the vein; (D) use a scalpel to make a small incision at the location where the wire enters the skin; (E) insert the dilator over the wire into the skin with a twisting motion; (F) remove the dilator leaving the wire in place. Finally, the catheter is placed over the wire and the wire can be removed.** (*Source:* Reproduced with permission from Conahan TJ III, Schwartz AJ, Geer RT. Percutaneous catheter introduction: the Seldinger technique. *JAMA* 1977;237:446.)

catheterization, a chest x-ray (CXR) should be obtained to evaluate for appropriate line placement and pneumothorax. Other complications include deep venous thrombosis and catheter line infections, both of which are most common with femoral vein catheters.

LUMBAR PUNCTURE

Lumbar puncture is performed to obtain cerebrospinal fluid (CSF) for evaluation of meningitis (fever with meningeal signs or mental status changes) and evaluation of central nervous system (CNS) disorders such as multiple sclerosis. Some important contraindications exist: soft tissue infection over the location of puncture, focal neurologic signs or papilledema, or bleeding disorders (e.g., international normalized ratio [INR] >1.5 or platelets <50,000). **Focal neurologic signs or papilledema** could reflect increased intracranial pressure or brain tumor, and a **computed tomography (CT)** scan of the head is necessary to guard against cerebral herniation.

Any location below the tip of the spinal cord is considered a safe location for lumbar puncture. Most patients have a spinal cord which ends at L2, but a small percentage have a spinal cord extending to L3. Because of this, the **L4-L5 intervertebral space** is preferred area, but the L3-L4 interspace is also acceptable. The L4-L5 space may be difficult to locate, but an imaginary line connecting the top of both iliac crests should intersect with the L4 vertebral body, so the space just caudal to this should be the site. A lumbar puncture can be performed with the patient seated or in lateral decubitus position. The decubitus position is generally preferred, because it allows the measurement of CSF pressure. When inserting the needle, a few general principles should be remembered. First, the bevel of the needle should be parallel to the spine to minimize injury to the longitudinal dural fibers. Second, in children the vertebral processes are directed perpendicular to the long axis of the body, so the needle should be inserted in a slight cephalad direction. With aging, osteophytes form and the vertebral bodies become more angulated, so the needle requires a greater cephalad angle, at times reaching almost 45°. Third, the needle must pass through skin, subcutaneous fat, dural fibers, and finally the ligamentum flavum to reach the subarachnoid space. Experienced operators will feel a "pop" when passing through the ligamentum flavum and into the subarachnoid space.

The most common complication is a "posttap **headache**," which occurs in 10–30% of patients, often attributed to the decrease in CSF pressure, and relieved by recumbency. As mentioned, cerebral herniation can occur if the patient has elevated intracranial pressure. Although damage to nerve tissues is often a concern, this is a very rare complication.

THORACENTESIS

The two most common indications for a thoracentesis are to evaluate a **new pleural effusion** or to remove pleural fluid for symptomatic relief in a patient with a chronic pleural effusion. No absolute contraindications exist; however, special attention should be made to patients at risk for respiratory complications (poor contralateral lung function) or patients with small or loculated effusions. Ultrasound can be useful to evaluate for loculation and to mark the exact location for thoracentesis if the effusion is small.

The general location for thoracentesis can be determined by percussing the extent of dullness (effusion) on the chest wall and using a site one to two interspaces below the top of the effusion. The usual site is either along the **posterior axillary line** or the midscapular line one intercostal space below the base of the scapula. The needle with syringe should be inserted into the intercostal space by aiming **just over the top of the rib**. The needle should always be inserted just superior to the rib to avoid the neurovascular bundle located inferior to all ribs (Fig. 3-3). Once you are able to draw back pleural fluid, stop advancing the needle to prevent parenchymal injury. For a diagnostic thoracentesis enough fluid should be obtained for all appropriate tests (see Chap. 18). If a therapeutic thoracentesis is performed, fluid removed should be limited to 1–1.5 L as exceeding this can lead to rebound pulmonary edema.

The most common complication is **pneumothorax** which occurs in ~10%. Many of these are minor, but approximately half will require chest tube thoracostomy. A CXR should always be obtained after the procedure to evaluate for pneumothorax. Most other complications are minor such as cough and pain at the puncture site.

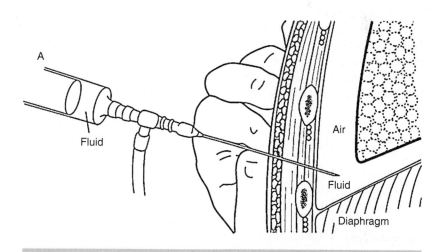

Figure 3-3 **Chest wall anatomy and proper technique for a thoracentesis.** (*Source:* Reproduced, with permission from Chesnutt MS, et al. *Office & Bedside Procedures.* Originally published by Appleton & Lange. New York: McGraw-Hill, 2002.)

PARACENTESIS

Paracentesis is performed to evaluate any patient with **new-onset ascites**, to diagnose **spontaneous bacterial peritonitis** in patients with suggestive symptoms and for symptomatic relief of patients with **tense ascites**. No absolute contraindications exist and coagulopathy is not necessarily a reason to delay paracentesis. Complications are not increased with an elevated INR unless associated with disseminated intravascular coagulation (DIC).

Patients should always be evaluated for ascites on physical examination first. With the patient lying supine, percuss the abdomen to determine the location of fluid (areas of dullness). If ascites is poorly localized on examination, an ultrasound should be obtained to quantify the fluid and mark an appropriate site for the procedure. The general location for paracentesis should be midway between the umbilicus and the anterior superior iliac spine. The midline is generally avoided because of large collateral veins located in this area. An Angiocath needle attached to a syringe is inserted while constantly aspirating until peritoneal fluid is returned. A "Z" track technique should be used to prevent postprocedure leakage of peritoneal fluid. Once the flow of peritoneal fluid is established, the needle should be removed leaving the Angiocath in place. This will limit any potential damage to bowel that may occur from the needle. If a diagnostic tap is being performed, a syringe can be used to draw off the amount of fluid needed. If removing a large volume, vacuum containers can be attached for faster removal of fluid.

The most common complications of paracentesis are local mechanical problems such as **persistent leak** of peritoneal fluid and abdominal wall hematoma. Although bowel perforation is a feared complication, it is uncommon and most heal without intervention. Patients with cirrhosis can have dramatic fluid shifts with large volume paracentesis causing systemic complications (see Chap. 27).

ARTERIAL PUNCTURE

Arterial blood is necessary for **blood gas** determination. Few contraindications to arterial puncture exist, but special consideration should be given to patients receiving thrombolytic therapy, because bleeding from an arterial site may be very difficult to stop. One important consideration for a radial arterial puncture is to ensure that the patient has sufficient blood flow through the ulnar artery (15–20% have inadequate collateral circulation). If the radial artery becomes thrombosed, arterial insufficiency will occur if the ulnar artery is nonviable. The **Allen test** is used to confirm patency—have the patient make a tight fist, occlude both the radial and ulnar arteries with your hand, have the patient open his or her fist, and release the ulnar artery.

Adequate blood supply is present if the palm returns pink and it is safe to perform an arterial puncture of the radial artery.

The most essential step is palpation and localization of the radial artery. This can be facilitated by having the patient hyperextend his or her wrist which will bring the radial artery closer to the surface. The needle with a syringe should be inserted bevel up at a 30–60° angle. After obtaining the specimen, pressure should be held at the site for at least 5 minutes to prevent postprocedure bleeding (the most common complication). Thrombosis although uncommon is another potential complication, so the Allen test should be repeated after the procedure to ensure patency of the radial artery.

NASOGASTRIC TUBE PLACEMENT

Gastrointestinal (GI) tubes are commonly used in medicine and have multiple indications. The most common reasons for placement are for **GI decompression** (paralytic ileus, bowel obstruction), gastric lavage for **GI bleeding**, or for administration of tube feeding or medicine in a patient unable to swallow. The only contraindications are patients with facial or basilar skull fractures (may cause additional trauma) or esophageal stricture (will be unable to pass).

When placing a nasogastric tube (NGT) it is important to know the length of tube necessary which can be estimated by measuring the distance from the corner of the mouth to the tragus to xiphoid process. This measurement provides the length of tubing which must be inserted to place the NGT into the stomach. The use of a water-soluble gel (K-Y Jelly or 2% lidocaine) will allow the tube to gently pass through the nasopharynx. Having the patient swallow while applying gentle but firm pressure once he or she feels the tube touching the back of the throat will also facilitate esophageal intubation (and not tracheal). The tube should be inserted to the previously measured depth. Prior to using the tube, proper placement is confirmed by either aspirating stomach contents or auscultating gurgling over the stomach when air is injecting into the NGT. The most serious complication is inadvertent placement into the trachea, so placement must always be confirmed. (A CXR is a reliable means to confirm proper placement.) Other complications include local irritation of the nose, pharynx, or stomach and a predisposition to sinusitis, because of sinus ostia blockage.

ENDOTRACHEAL INTUBATION

The main indications include cardiac arrest, hypoxemic respiratory failure, ventilatory failure, and to protect the airway in patients with high risk of aspiration. Endotracheal intubation should not be performed in patients with severe facial trauma or cervical spinal cord injury. These patients most frequently require either nasotracheal or fiberoptic intubation.

The most essential and often neglected step in intubation is proper position of the patient. Patients should be placed in the "sniffing position," flexion of the neck and slight extension of the head (Fig. 3-4). This position aligns the pharyngeal and laryngeal axes to allow optimum visualization of the glottic opening and relieves any obstruction to airflow (thus it improves the efficacy of bag-mask ventilation). A general rule is that a patient in proper position will have the tragus and sternum in the same horizontal plane. If the patient is not in proper position, the operator often must lift the head off the bed in order to obtain adequate visualization of glottic structures. The next step is to ensure the proper equipment is in place. Most adults require a 7.0–8.5 cuffed endotracheal tube (ETT) with a stylet inserted into the tube, because the tube itself is often too floppy to insert. A laryngoscope with a functional light and a blade should also be obtained. Two blades are commonly used, the Miller (straight) and the MacIntosh (curved) blade. The Miller blade retracts the epiglottis out of the way, whereas the MacIntosh is

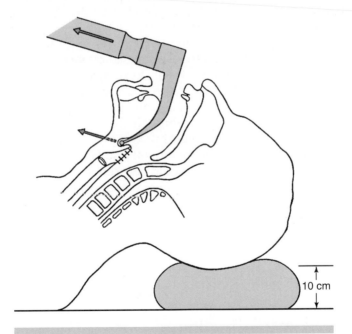

Figure 3-4 **Proper tracheal intubation technique with a Macintosh blade of a patient in the "sniffing position."** (*Source:* Modified and reproduced with permission from Dorsch JA, Dorsch SE. *Understanding Anesthesia Equipment: Construction, Care, and Complications.* Philadelphia, PA: Lippincott Williams & Wilkins, 1991.)

inserted into the vallecula (space anterior and superior to the epiglottis) which will cause the epiglottis to open. Some clinicians sedate the patient to aid in intubation. However, **no patient should be paralyzed without experienced airway assistance available**. When the laryngoscope is inserted, it should always be pulled at a 45° angle toward the patient's feet (Fig. 3-4), as this will provide maximum visualization and prevent damage to the teeth. Once the ETT is inserted between the vocal cords, several steps to confirm placement must be performed. Auscultation of lung sounds with ventilation through the ETT and placement of a carbon dioxide detector (proper placement is indicated by a color change from purple to yellow) can be used immediately to confirm proper placement. A CXR should be obtained immediately to evaluate tube location and proper placement (end of the tube should be ~2 cm above the carina).

Endotracheal intubation can be associated with several complications. Improper tube placement is the most common problem, including intubation of the esophagus or of the right mainstem bronchus. Trauma to the oropharynx, trachea, or epiglottis may occur, particularly with poor technique. Prolonged attempts at intubation commonly cause gastric distention (from continued bag-mask ventilation), but may also result in ischemic damage to the brain or cardiac arrest.

INTENSIVE CARE

MEDICINE

Ketan P. Buch

KEY POINTS

- A critically ill patient may have involvement of multiple organs at a given time.
- If the goal of managing critically ill patients can be summarized in one sentence, one can say that it is to optimize oxygen delivery (DO_2) to the tissues.
- Rapidly stabilizing respiratory and hemodynamic status of a critically ill patient improves survival and reduces morbidity.
- It is equally important to withhold and withdraw ineffective or futile therapy as it is to pursue aggressive treatments directed toward cure.

INTRODUCTION

Intensive care medicine, as the name suggests, involves employment of extraordinary diagnostic and therapeutic strategies to care for critically ill patients. If such critically ill patients are not promptly managed in intensive care units (ICUs) they face unacceptably high morbidity and mortality. Obviously, a number of diseases can progress to such life-threatening severity necessitating care in the ICU. Additionally, patients in the ICU are subject to iatrogenic diseases and complications as they are more frequently exposed to invasive procedures, indwelling devices, and potentially toxic therapies such as heavy analgesia and sedation.

Patient management in the ICU is characterized by:

1. Multidisciplinary team approach to patient care.
2. Ability to provide mechanical ventilation and other forms of respiratory support.

3. Availability of continuous noninvasive and invasive hemodynamic monitoring.
4. Ability to give medications by continuous infusions.
5. Higher nurse:patient ratio.
6. Ready access to physicians and other health care providers.
7. In many situations, the necessity to provide compassionate end-of-life care.

The vast majority of patients who require admission to an ICU share one common physiologic derangement—they have threatened or established tissue hypoxia. Adequate oxygen delivery to the tissues is essential for normal functioning and any interruption in this can lead to organ dysfunction which, if severe, can lead to death. If the **goal of managing critically ill patients** can be summarized in one sentence, one can say that it **is to optimize oxygen delivery (DO_2) to the tissues.**

As one can see from the accompanying diagram Fig. 4-1, a patient may end up in the ICU because of respiratory failure resulting in decreased SaO_2, decreased hemoglobin level from gastrointestinal (GI) hemorrhage, or because they have decreased cardiac output (CO) resulting from decreased left ventricular ejection fraction or decreased preload. Table 4-1 lists some of the common conditions that require admission to an ICU. Of these, **respiratory failure and shock are unique to and are the most common reasons for admission to the ICU.**

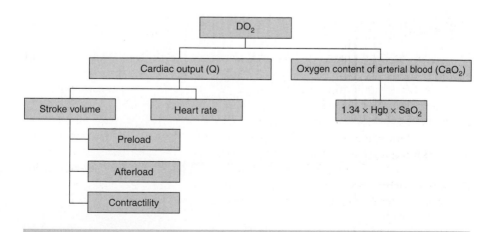

Figure 4-1 **Algorithm: Results of a patient ending up in the ICU because of respiratory failure.**

Table 4-1 **Common Reasons for ICU Admission**

1. Respiratory failure
   a. Acute respiratory distress syndrome (ARDS)
   b. Pneumonia
   c. Exacerbation of chronic lung disease (chronic obstructive pulmonary disease [COPD], asthma, bronchiectasis)
   d. Pulmonary embolism (PE)
2. Shock
   a. Hypovolemic (e.g., GI bleed and diarrhea)
   b. Cardiogenic (e.g., acute MI)
   c. Distributive (e.g., sepsis and anaphylaxis)
   d. Obstructive (e.g., massive PE and cardiac tamponade)
3. Cardiac disease
   a. Acute MI
   b. Decompensated heart failure
   c. Valvular heart disease
   d. Arrhythmia with hemodynamic instability
4. Trauma—massive, involving multiple organs
5. Burns
6. CNS injury
   a. Stroke
   b. Closed head injury
   c. Intracranial hemorrhage
   d. Status epilepticus
7. Infections
   a. Septic shock
   b. Toxic shock syndrome
   c. Meningitis
   d. Neutropenic fever
8. Metabolic derangements
   a. Acute renal failure/uremia
   b. Diabetic ketoacidosis
   c. Severe hypo- or hypernatremia
   d. Severe hypo- or hyperkalemia
   e. Severe hypophosphatemia
   f. Intentional or accidental poisoning
9. GI diseases
   a. GI hemorrhage
   b. Acute liver failure

Table 4-1 **Common Reasons for ICU Admission (Continued)**

10. Hematologic disease
    a. Severe anemia/thrombocytopenia
    b. Hemolytic uremic syndrome (HUS)/thrombotic thrombocytopenic purpura (TTP)
    c. Disseminated intravascular coagulation (DIC)
11. Psychiatric diseases
    a. Suicide attempt
    b. Neuroleptic malignant syndrome (NMS)

CLINICAL PRESENTATION

Patients present with features of underlying illness. Often these patients are unable to give a history as they are in extremis with altered consciousness or are intubated and mechanically ventilated. Frequently, patients present with severe hemodynamic or respiratory collapse or after having survived a cardiopulmonary arrest at home or elsewhere in the hospital. History may have to be obtained from family members, onlookers, or a review of available medical records AFTER the patient has been stabilized and there is no imminent threat of death.

As with history, initial physical examination is comprehensive and focuses on the ABCs (**A**irway, **B**reathing, and **C**irculation). Once the patient has stabilized, a complete physical examination must be performed with emphasis on diagnosing cardiopulmonary failure and impaired organ perfusion (e.g., altered consciousness, weak and thready peripheral pulses, and cold clammy extremities).

EVALUATION

Laboratory and radiologic tests are an integral part of managing critically ill patients. These tests usually complement the information obtained from history and physical examination but are often essential for making a diagnosis, for example, toxicology screen to diagnose poisoning in an unconscious patient. Additionally, data obtained from invasive and noninvasive monitoring at the bedside (e.g., continuous blood pressure monitoring with an arterial line, hemodynamic parameters from a pulmonary artery catheter, continuous electrocardiogram [ECG], electroencephalogram [EEG], and pulse oximetry) help in the management of patients in the ICU.

Frequent monitoring of arterial blood gas guides the ventilator management of patients with respiratory failure. Since relatively minor abnormalities in electrolytes and renal function can have significant impact in critically ill patients, these are monitored routinely. Monitoring blood glucose and maintaining euglycemia in ICU patients also helps reduce morbidity and mortality. Serum prealbumin gives a reliable estimate of the patient's nutrition status. Serum and urine toxicology studies should be readily considered in patients with altered sensorium and unexplained clinical presentations. The anteroposterior chest radiograph not only provides information about the lung parenchyma but also helps monitor placement of endotracheal tubes and intravascular catheters. Computed tomography (CT) scans are frequently used in the ICU setting to overcome the limitations of portable radiographs. Echocardiogram and endoscopic procedures are routinely employed in the ICU.

Swan-Ganz Catheter Monitoring

A properly placed and calibrated pulmonary artery catheter allows the clinician to estimate such parameters as pulmonary artery pressure (PAP), right atrial pressure (central venous pressure [CVP]), pulmonary capillary wedge pressure (PCWP), pulmonary vascular resistance (PVR), CO, and systemic vascular resistance (SVR). The usefulness of Swan-Ganz catheter in management of critically ill patients is often debated and it has been reported to be associated with increased morbidity and mortality. However, one must remember that it is a diagnostic tool and data obtained from it must be critically evaluated for accuracy and interpreted in the context of clinical presentation. It is the appropriate use of data obtained from pulmonary artery catheter that dictates outcome, not its mere placement.

The Swan-Ganz catheter is inserted into a central vein (jugular, subclavian, femoral, or brachial) and is sequentially directed to the right atrium, right ventricle, and pulmonary artery, with each compartment identified by characteristic waveforms relayed from the pressure transducer on the tip of the catheter. Waveform pressures can also be measured as the catheter "floats" downstream. As the catheter enters the pulmonary artery, the balloon on the end of the catheter is inflated, and "wedges" into a distal pulmonary artery, with pressure measured there. Left ventricular end-diastolic volume (LVEDV; preload) is under most circumstances directly proportional to left ventricular end-diastolic pressure (LVEDP), which is essentially the same as left atrial pressure in diastole, pulmonary venous pressure, and therefore the **PCWP**, which is used to predict preload. This assumption doesn't hold true in all situations, such as mitral stenosis or regurgitation, abnormal myocardial compliance, or in the setting of high intraparenchymal lung pressures, hence the need for experienced persons interpreting these measurements. The chapter on shock (see Chap. 12) will discuss these measures more, but in general, volume overload states such as congestive heart failure will have high PCWP, while volume depleted states will have low PCWP. In addition, CO can be measured directly through the pulmonary artery catheter, through a thermodilution technique. The **cardiac index** is the CO divided by the patient's body surface area in meters squared, to adjust CO for different size patients. **SVR** is the mean arterial pressure (diastolic pressure + 1/3 pulse pressure) minus right atrial pressure, with this value divided by the CO. In situations where there is massive vasodilation, such as septic shock, SVR will be low; conversely, SVR will be high in cardiogenic shock. Finally, **mixed venous 02 saturation** can be measured from blood obtained through the pulmonary artery catheter. This is a measure of global tissue perfusion, and will be low in situations such as an inadequate CO, reduced hemoglobin concentration, and/or a reduced arterial 02 saturation.

Mechanical Ventilation

Indications for mechanical ventilation are discussed in Chap. 14. Details of ventilator modes, settings, and weaning strategies are beyond the scope of this textbook and beyond what would be expected of a medical student. Nevertheless, many students will participate in the care of patients in the ICU, so it is useful to have a general understanding of terms used on ICU rounds when referring to patients on a ventilator.

Major settings on the ventilator include the **respiratory rate**, the **tidal volume** delivered, the **peak inspiratory flow rate**, and the **fraction of inspired oxygen (FiO$_2$)**. **Positive end-expiratory pressure (PEEP)** is sometimes added to improve oxygenation, partly by "recruiting" otherwise collapsed alveoli. However, high levels of PEEP can be deleterious, through decrease in CO and barotrauma (e.g., pneumothoraces).

Most modes of mechanical ventilation in adults are volume-limited, in which a preset volume of air is delivered with each inspiration, at which time inspiration is terminated. Other modes use a maximum pressure or flow rate. In **controlled mechanical ventilation**, minute ventilation is completely dependent on the rate and tidal volume of the ventilator, with no patient triggering; such a mode of ventilation is most appropriate for a patient with no respiratory effort, such as a severe drug overdose or those with neuromuscular paralysis and for patients who should expend minimum energy breathing (e.g., acute myocardial infarction [MI] or septic shock). In **assist-controlled** mode, a minimum rate and tidal volume are set, but the patient can trigger the ventilator over and above that minimum rate, receiving a set tidal volume each time. Such a modality is appropriate for a conscious patient. **Intermittent mandatory ventilation (IMV)** likewise entails a minimum ventilator-generated breath, but the patient can breathe spontaneously by triggering a demand valve between machine-generated breaths. **Synchronized IMV (SIMV)** is a modification of IMV, in which the ventilator synchronizes machine breaths with patient effort. In **pressure-support ventilation**, the ventilator assists the patient's inspiratory effort with a preset pressure, but the patient determines the rate, inspiratory time, and tidal volume. This is considered a comfortable form of ventilation for patients, but obviously entails a patient not in extremis. Pressure support is often added to IMV, with the pressure support allowing for overcoming the endotracheal and circuitry resistance encountered during spontaneous breaths.

MANAGEMENT

Successful management of ICU patients can be summed up by these steps:

1. ABCs—assess and manage airway, breathing, and circulation.
2. Diagnose and treat the underlying illness.
3. Prevent and recognize iatrogenic complications and treat them rapidly.

The importance of speed and precision cannot be overemphasized. Management of the ABCs often requires the use of large amount of fluids or blood products and a number of vasoactive agents, the use of which is unique to the intensive care setting. In choosing therapeutic procedures and phar-macologic treatments one has to be mindful of the interaction of these strate-gies with other treatments as well as the patient's own deranged physiology.

Since a large number of patients in the ICU are unable to communicate, decisions regarding treatment are often made after discussion with their family members or health care surrogates. This can sometimes raise inter-esting ethical issues which must be resolved with the patient's best interest in mind (see Chap. 65).

Challenges of serious illness that the patients and their loved ones face in the technologically threatening intensive care environment can be indeed daunting. It is the physician's duty to provide emotional support and help them navigate the treacherous path of critical illness. All measures to exact a cure with minimum morbidity should be aggressively pursued but when this goal is not achievable it is equally important to help patients and their loved ones face mortality with dignity.

ADVANCED CARDIAC

LIFE SUPPORT

Eric Alper

KEY POINTS

- ACLS is a series of specific algorithms that are performed in specific scenarios by skilled providers.
- The ABCDs of ACLS are "Airway, Breathing, Circulation, Defibrillation (or Differential Diagnosis)."
- Providers who deliver ACLS need to be able to recognize key arrhythmias in order to deliver the most appropriate therapy.

INTRODUCTION

Coronary artery disease remains the most common cause of death in the United States. Cardiac arrest is a common presentation for coronary artery disease and may occur for other reasons as well. Respiratory arrest may happen as a consequence of many common problems, including pneumonia, chronic lung disease, and pulmonary embolism.

These arrests may happen in or out of hospital. While in children respiratory failure is more common, in adults cardiac arrests are much more common. Advanced cardiac life support (ACLS) is a series of algorithms that help the provider to deliver care during these serious life-threatening events. While Basic Life Support can be administered anywhere, provision of ACLS is generally limited to medical environments where there is access to special equipment and devices.

PATHOPHYSIOLOGY

A variety of problems can lead to cardiac or respiratory arrest. Myocardial ischemia/infarction leading to an arrhythmia is the most common cause of cardiac arrest. The following are some of the common types of dysfunctions that can occur with abnormal myocardial perfusion:

- **Complete heart block (CHB):** Poor AV node perfusion (the right coronary artery supplies the SA and AV nodes). Patients typically have marked bradycardia.
- **Ventricular tachycardia (VT):** An ischemic focus or previously scarred focus beats on its own at a rapid rate. Patients typically are pulseless but may have a normal blood pressure.
- **Ventricular fibrillation (VF):** Rapid, highly disorganized electrical activity in the heart. Patients are always pulseless.
- **Torsades de pointes** ("twisting of points"), also known as polymorphic VT: A form of VT with characteristic appearance, usually related to a prolongation of the QT interval.
- **Asystole:** Complete failure of the electrical system of the heart.
- **Pulseless electrical activity (PEA):** Electrical activity seen on the monitor but without pulse or blood pressure; is seen in variety of conditions discussed under treatment.

Respiratory arrests typically occur with progressive respiratory failure. Some of the more common causes include pneumonia, chronic lung disease especially chronic obstructive pulmonary disease, pulmonary embolus, and asthma. The final common pathway leading to arrest is respiratory fatigue with progressive respiratory acidosis and hypoxia.

CLINICAL PRESENTATION

The presentation of these patients is variable. They may be sudden (e.g., due to a ventricular arrhythmia) or gradual (e.g., worsening asthma exacerbation or myocardial infarction). The history will vary significantly depending on the cause. In many cases, the patient is unconscious, so no history can be obtained.

Despite the requirement for urgent action, a rapid focused physical examination (accomplished in a matter of seconds) should be performed. The goal is to identify potential causes for the arrest and assess for extent of injury due to the arrest. After assuring that the airway has been opened, assess if the patient is breathing. If so, note the respiratory rate, pattern, and use of accessory muscles such as sternocleidomastoid contractions, intercostal muscle contractions, nasal flaring, or abdominal breathing. If the patient's respiratory rate is low, this may be an indication of central hypoventilation, frequently from opiates or benzodiazepines. Measure pulse oximetry to assess oxygenation. Auscultate the lungs to assess whether breath sounds are present bilaterally and consider performing percussion to assess if hypertympany is present on one side, which may indicate pneumothorax.

Next, check for a pulse at the radial, carotid, or femoral artery. In general, a radial pulse suggests a systolic blood pressure of at least 80 mmHg, a femoral pulse at least 70 mmHg, and a carotid pulse at least 60 mmHg. A Doppler device to measure blood pressure may be necessary if a pulse cannot be palpated. Assess jugular veins for distention (suggests either cardiogenic shock, pericardial tamponade, or tension pneumothorax). Auscultate the precordium for new murmurs or diminished heart sounds (may be a sign of pericardial effusion or cardiac tamponade). Feel the abdomen rapidly to assure that the patient doesn't have peritoneal signs. Examine the legs to evaluate for evidence of edema (fluid overload, heart failure) or asymmetric swelling (deep venous thrombosis). A brief neurologic examination, including examining pupils for reactivity, extremities for flaccidity, and reflexes for hyperreflexia may be helpful if trying to determine if the patient has suffered a major stroke or has already sustained severe neurologic damage due to prolonged cardiac arrest.

EVALUATION

Laboratory studies should be sent shortly after the onset of the arrest. An arterial blood gas analysis usually will reveal a respiratory acidosis (due to respiratory failure) and metabolic acidosis (due to hypoperfusion). A complete blood count will determine if severe anemia is present, perhaps from hemorrhage, while severe electrolyte abnormalities, especially hypo- or hyperkalemia, should be the focus of electrolyte analysis. CPK-MB (MB isoenzyme of creatinine phosphokinase) and troponin are sent in most adults to evaluate for myocardial infarction. Blood cultures should be drawn if sepsis is suspected. Type and cross blood and send coagulation studies if hemorrhage is suspected. A cardiac monitor is attached rapidly to determine underlying cardiac rhythm followed by a 12-lead ECG to further define rhythm and look for ischemia or infarction. A stat chest x-ray is usually indicated to evaluate for pneumothorax, pericardial effusion, pulmonary edema, and other common problems (particularly in patients who already received cardiopulmonary resuscitation [CPR] with chest compressions).

MANAGEMENT

The management of arrests should follow a series of specific guidelines established by the American Heart Association. When you encounter a patient that has arrested, the first thing to do is to **call for help**, whether this means notifying the nurse at the nursing station, pressing the Code button, or calling 911. As soon as one can, verify the patient's code status. If the patient has requested no life-sustaining measures, efforts should not proceed. Be aware of state laws regarding advanced directives, and be aware that patients may have specific requests with regard to such measures (e.g., no intubation).

Apply the **ABCDs—airway, breathing, circulation, defibrillation**. While presented below sequentially, in practice these efforts go on simultaneously by multiple members of the team and occur within seconds/minutes of one another. As the team arrives, the senior member usually takes the role of team leader. One person, frequently the respiratory therapist, is assigned to manage airway and breathe for the patient. One person is assigned to deliver chest compressions. One or more people work to establish peripheral and central access. One person measures blood pressure, attaches the monitor, and administers medications. One person records the events that take place. Depending on personnel, people may serve multiple roles.

- Airway: Assess whether the airway is open. If no air is moving, tilt the head back to try to open the airway. There may be a need for use of devices to secure the airway, such as use of a nasal trumpet or an oropharyngeal airway. If resuscitation is prolonged or has a respiratory origin, it is likely that the patient will require oral endotracheal intubation to secure an airway.
- Breathing: Once an airway is established and it is determined that the patient is not breathing adequately, ventilation is initiated usually beginning with a bag-valve-mask device, like an Ambu-bag connected to high flow oxygen. If the patient is intubated, proper tube placement is confirmed using a CO_2 detector and the bag-valve-mask is attached to the endotracheal tube. Oxygenation is monitored by a pulse oximeter.
- Circulation: The responding providers will rapidly assess for a pulse and measure blood pressure. If there is no pulse in the carotid or femoral and blood pressure is not measurable (including using a Doppler device), chest compressions are initiated at a rate of 100 per minute. IV access is established as rapidly as possible. (A central line may need to be placed and the femoral vein is used frequently in this setting due to ease of access.) A cardiac monitor is connected to the patient to determine the rhythm. There are a number of specific algorithms for the type of cardiac rhythms that one is likely to find in a cardiac arrest. Most providers carry a pocket-sized manual of ACLS that contains all the details of the algorithms. Key features of these algorithms will be highlighted for the most common arrest scenarios. Updates can be accessed at: www. americanheart.org.
- **Defibrillation**

VF or unstable VT: These are by far the most common causes of arrest and survival is directly correlated with the rapidity of defibrillation. Begin defibrillation using 200 J. If ineffective, repeat at 300 J and if needed again at 360 J. If the patient remains in VF/VT, a pattern of drug-CPR (30–60 seconds)-shock (360 J) is repeated until a stable rhythm is obtained or efforts are discontinued. First-line drugs are epinephrine 1 mg IV or vasopressin 40 units IV but amiodarone, lidocaine, magnesium (especially in *torsades de pointes*), and procainamide are also used. Because VF is the most common rhythm found during cardiac arrest and recovery is much more likely with early defibrillation, automated external defibrillators (AEDs) can now be found in many public areas for first responders.

Differential diagnosis: The following causes of arrest do not rely on defibrillation for resuscitation but rather require identification and treatment of the underlying cause of the arrest to maximize success:

- **Asystole** (no electrical activity detectable on the monitor and confirmed in more than one lead): Initiate transcutaneous pacing and assess if capture and pulses occur. Administer epinephrine 1 mg IV every 3–5 minutes and atropine 1 mg every 3–5 minutes. The differential includes hypoxia, hyper- or hypokalemia, preexisting acidosis, drug overdose, and hypothermia. Asystole tends to be a terminal rhythm.
- **PEA**: This is the most complex ACLS scenario and relies solely on treating the underlying cause. The differential includes hypovolemia, hypoxia, hydrogen (severe acidosis), hyper- or hypokalemia, hypothermia, tablets (drug overdoses), tamponade, tension pneumothorax, thrombosis of coronary artery (acute myocardial infarction), and thrombosis in pulmonary artery (pulmonary embolism).

Bradycardia and tachycardia can be medical emergencies but the important distinction is whether or not the patient is unstable. Signs and symptoms or an unstable arrhythmia include hypotension, shock, mental status changes, chest pain, and pulmonary edema. Only the treatment of unstable cases will be addressed in this chapter.

- **Bradycardia**: Perform a 12-lead ECG to diagnose the underlying etiology (e.g., sinus bradycardia, third-degree heart block, and infarction). Administer atropine 0.5–1 mg IV. If ineffective, initiate transcutaneous pacing. (Patients who are awake when this is initiated may require sedation, as transcutaneous pacing may be uncomfortable.) Dopamine, epinephrine, or isoproterenol IV infusions are sometimes used to preserve blood pressure and heart rate followed by transvenous pacing. In many cases, patients ultimately require a permanent pacemaker.
- **Tachycardia**: Perform a 12-lead ECG to determine whether it is a wide or narrow complex and if possible the actual rhythm (e.g., atrial fibrillation).

Narrow complex tachycardia is almost always supraventricular and treatment focuses on rate control. Wide complex tachycardia (in unstable patients) is assumed to be VT. This is treated with "synchronized cardioversion," or shock delivered at the same time as the QRS complex to avoid shocking on the T wave. Start with 100 J, followed by 200, 300, then 360 J if necessary. Consider adding antiarrhythmic medication as well, such as amiodarone or procainamide.

Finally, for any given cardiac arrest, it may be necessary to use multiple algorithms sequentially. For example, if the patient is found in VF, defibrillation may produce PEA, which degenerates into asystole. Resuscitation efforts should be discontinued if a perfusing rhythm has not been restored by 20 minutes. The exception is arrests accompanied by hypothermia (exposure, cold water drowning), in which case resuscitation efforts continue until a core body temperature of at least 90°F is achieved. Many patients will be successfully resuscitated and it is important to perform a prompt evaluation for what may have caused the arrest in order to initiate definitive therapy for the underlying problem. Unfortunately, not every patient who suffers an arrest will survive resuscitation. It is important to notify the next of kin as soon as possible. They may want to come to the hospital. Notify the attending physician and/or the primary care physician as well.

CHAPTER 6

INTERPRETATION OF THE ELECTROCARDIOGRAM

Alison L. Bailey

INTRODUCTION

Regardless of their specialty, all physicians must be familiar with basic electrocardiogram (ECG) interpretation. To prevail over the ECG, one simply needs a plan for each ECG encountered. In this chapter, a basic plan for reading ECGs will be detailed. A systematic method for reading each ECG is essential, otherwise one will become lost. For each ECG, determine the **rate, rhythm, axis, hypertrophy, ischemia/injury patterns,** and **other patterns**.

The standard format for obtaining an ECG is a 12-lead ECG, obtained by positioning the ECG electrodes on all four limbs and the chest as follows:

- V_1: Right 4th intercostal space
- V_2: Left 4th intercostal space
- V_3: Halfway between V_2 and V_4
- V_4: Left 5th intercostal space in midclavicular line
- V_5: Halfway between V_4 and V_6
- V_6: Left 5th intercostal space in midaxillary line

Each electrode or series of electrodes will reflect activity of different areas of the heart. The ECG tracing produced is actually a recording of the electrical activity inside myocytes as the heart contracts. At rest, each myocyte has a net internal negative charge. When it is affected by an electrical stimulus, it becomes positively charged, or depolarized. This causes contraction of the myocyte, and when groups of myocytes contract together, either atrial or ventricular contraction occurs. After this wave passes, the cells become repolarized and regain their negative intracellular charge.

The wave of depolarization, or positive charge, is seen as an upward deflection on the surface ECG recording as it moves toward a positive electrode.

The deflection represents either the **P wave,** if the atria are being depolarized and contracting, or the **QRS complex** if the ventricles are involved (Fig. 6-1). The repolarization of the atria is buried in the QRS complex, but the repolarization of the ventricles is depicted by the **T wave**. After the atria and ventricles are repolarized, the myocytes regain their intracellular negative charge and are ready for the next depolarization. (See Table 6-1.)

When looking at an ECG, remember that the X-axis is time and the Y-axis is voltage. Conventionally, ECGs are recorded at a speed of 25 mm/s and signal calibration of 1 mV/10 mm. Each large box represents 0.20 seconds and is comprised of five smaller boxes, each representing 0.04 seconds (Fig. 6-2).

Rate

- Normal heart rate is 50–100 beats per minute (bpm).
- Bradycardia is defined as <50 bpm.
- Tachycardia is defined as >100 bpm.

The most efficient way to estimate rate is by counting the distance between successive R waves. Locate an R wave that falls on a thick line. Begin counting at the next thick line after this complex; this is 300, the next is 150, and so on until a second R wave is located (Fig. 6-3). If the R wave is not

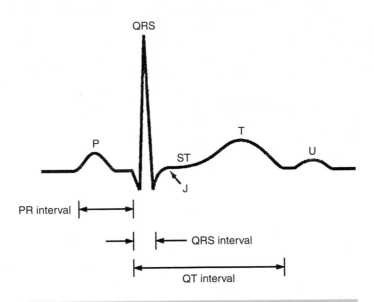

Figure 6-1 **Basic ECG waveforms and intervals.** (*Source:* Reproduced with permission from Kasper DL, Braunwald E, Fauci A, et al. *Harrison's Principles of Internal Medicine*, 16th ed. New York: McGraw-Hill, 2005, Figure 210-2.)

Table 6-1 **Major Waves, Complexes, and Segments**

Name	What Does It Correspond To?	Should Be
P wave	Atrial depolarization	<3 mm height, <2.5 mm (0.10 s) wide
PR interval	Time from depolarization of the atria to depolarization of the ventricles; measure from start of P wave to start of QRS	0.12–0.20 s
PR segment	Atrial systole	Isoelectric at rest
QRS complex	Ventricular depolarization; endocardium to epicardium	<0.10 s wide
Q wave	First downward deflection of the QRS complex	<1/3 the QRS complex and <0.04 s wide
R wave	First upward deflection of the QRS complex	Should increase from V_1 to V_6
S wave	Downward deflection following the R wave	
ST segment	Isoelectric segment between S wave and T wave	Flat without elevation, depression, or sloping
T wave	Ventricular repolarization	Broad, upright; not peaked
QT interval	Ventricular depolarization and repolarization or ventricular systole; measure from start of QRS to end of T wave	<1/2 R-R interval; must be corrected for rate. $QT_c = QT/\sqrt{R-R}$ (Bazett formula)
U wave	Possibly repolarization of Purkinje fibers	Not always present
R-R interval	Ventricular depolarization cycle; measure from one R wave to the next	

on thick line, one can extrapolate between the two numbers. This works because each thick line represents 1/300th of a minute (60 seconds/ 0.2 seconds). So, the first line is 1/300th or 300; the second line is 2/300ths or 150; the third line is 3/300ths or 100, and so on.

If the rate is <50 or is erratic, then one will need to use the 3-second marks on the ECG to obtain the rate (Fig. 6-4). Count the number of QRS complexes contained between the two 3-second marks and multiply by 10. If there are not any 3-second marks on the ECG, then 15 large boxes equal 3 seconds.

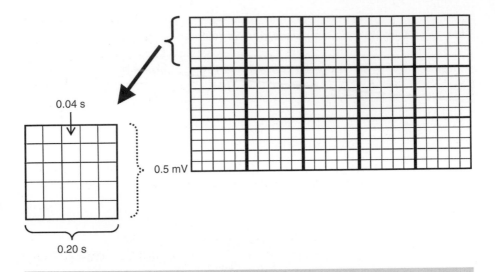

Figure 6-2 **Measurements on the ECG paper.**

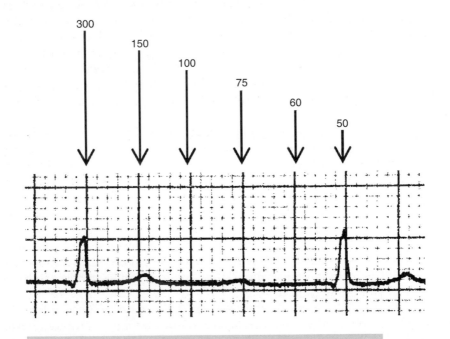

Figure 6-3 **Rate determination.**

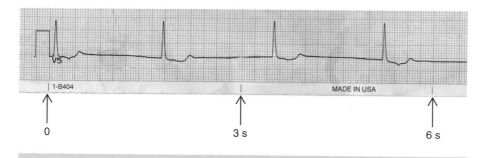

Figure 6-4 **Rate determination in bradycardia or with erratic rhythms.**

Rhythm

- Sinus rhythm is defined as having one P wave for each QRS complex and having upright P waves in lead II.
- Premature atrial contractions (PACs) have normal QRS duration and lack a compensatory pause, whereas premature ventricular contractions (PVCs) have a wide QRS and a compensatory pause.
- First-degree atrioventricular (AV) block is a prolonged PR interval.

To address abnormalities in cardiac rhythms, the normal conduction system of the heart must be understood. The heartbeat originates in the sinoatrial node (SA node), located in the right atrium. An electrical impulse is generated here which is relayed down the conducting tissue of the atria to the AV node causing atrial contraction. From the AV node, the impulse travels down the His bundle then to the right bundle branch and left bundle branch and finally to the Purkinje fibers. This process causes ventricular contraction.

The SA node has an inherent rate, usually 60–80 bpm, and is the dominant pacemaker of the heart when the conduction system is functioning properly. However, the heart has several backup plans should the SA node fail: the AV node can take over, and if the AV node fails, then the ventricle can take over as the dominant pacemaker. The inherent pacemaker rate becomes slower in the more distal conduction system. At the level of the AV node, or junction, it is about 40–60 bpm and at the level of the ventricle it is about 20–40 bpm.

Any discussion of rhythm must begin with sinus rhythm, in which each P wave is followed by a QRS complex and P waves are positive (upright) in lead II. There are some modifiers for sinus rhythm related to rate and regularity.

- Regular pattern (same R-R interval) and rate 50–100 bpm → normal sinus rhythm
- Rate <50 bpm → sinus bradycardia

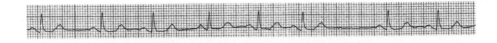

Figure 6-5 **Sinus arrhythmia.**

- Rate >100 bpm → sinus tachycardia
- Irregular R-R interval with >10% variation → sinus arrhythmia (Fig. 6-5)
  - Rate increases with inspiration and decreases with expiration

Any rhythm other than sinus is described as an arrhythmia (see Chap. 11). Evaluation of the underlying rhythm can be made more difficult by the presence of premature beats. These complexes occur because either the atria or the ventricles depolarize prematurely and are considered to be normal variants.

- **PAC:** Abnormal P wave occurring before the expected sinus beat, usually followed by a normal QRS complex, and lacking a compensatory pause before the next normal beat.
- **PVC:** A wide QRS complex beat not preceded by a P wave and followed by a compensatory pause (Fig. 6-6).

Heart blocks are interruptions of the normal electrical conduction system that prevent passage of a stimulus to produce depolarization. There are two main categories, AV blocks and bundle branch blocks. With an AV block, the normal electrical conduction between the atria and the ventricles is either delayed or completely prevented depending on the severity. This is assessed with the PR interval, and is measured from the start of the P wave to the start of the QRS complex. The normal range is 0.12–0.20 seconds.

- **First-degree AV block:** PR interval >0.20 seconds indicating a delay in conduction from the SA node to the AV node. It is not treated nor is it considered pathologic.

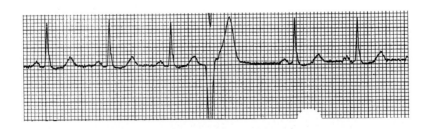

Figure 6-6 **PVC with compensatory pause.**

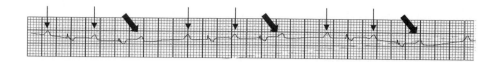

Figure 6-7 **Second-degree AV block (type I or Wenckebach). Note the increasing PR interval (small arrows) prior to the dropped QRS complex (large arrows).**

- **Second-degree AV block:** Some P waves that are intermittently nonconducted:
  - Type I (Wenckebach): Gradual increase of the PR interval from beat to beat until one of the P waves is not conducted (Fig. 6-7). This is generally a benign rhythm.
  - Type II (Mobitz): Constant PR interval from beat to beat until one of the P waves is not conducted. This is an unstable rhythm which can degenerate to third-degree AV block (Fig. 6-8).
- **Third-degree AV block:** Complete heart block with a lack of conduction from the atria to the ventricles, characterized by independent rates of the atria and ventricles (AV dissociation). Third-degree AV block requires close monitoring and a pacemaker (Fig. 6-9).

Bundle branch block is a form of heart block which occurs distal to the AV node during the depolarization of the ventricles. This is measured by the QRS interval, from the start of the Q wave to the end of the S wave, and should be <0.10 seconds. Normally, conduction occurs down the His bundle and then the right and left bundles simultaneously. This results in the right and left ventricles being depolarized at essentially the same time. When there is a delay in conduction down either of the bundle branches, a block occurs and is evident by a widening of the QRS complex on the ECG. This widening results from the blocked bundle depolarizing later and instead of one QRS complex (both ventricles depolarizing at the same time), there are now two QRS complexes superimposed on each other. QRS duration between 0.10 and 0.12 seconds is called an incomplete bundle branch block and a QRS duration >0.12 seconds is a complete bundle branch block.

- **Left bundle branch block (LBBB):** Late depolarization of the left ventricle. The blocked left ventricle depolarizes late so the terminal portion represents

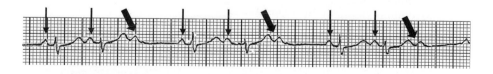

Figure 6-8 **Second-degree AV block (type II or Mobitz). Note the constant PR interval (small arrows) prior to the dropped QRS complex (large arrows).**

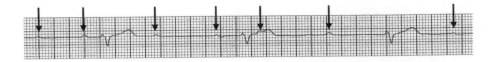

Figure 6-9 **Third-degree AV block. Note the P waves that are not conducted (small arrows) and the ventricular escape rhythm with a rate of 32.**

left ventricular depolarization. This is seen on the ECG as a wide QRS complex that is mostly negative in V_1 and V_2 and positive in V_5 and V_6 with a RSR(or "rabbit ear" morphology (Fig. 6-10).

- **Right bundle branch block (RBBB):** Late depolarization of the right ventricle. It is manifest as a wide QRS complex that is mostly positive and has a RSR morphology in V_1 and V_2 and a large S wave in V_5 and V_6 (Fig. 6-10).

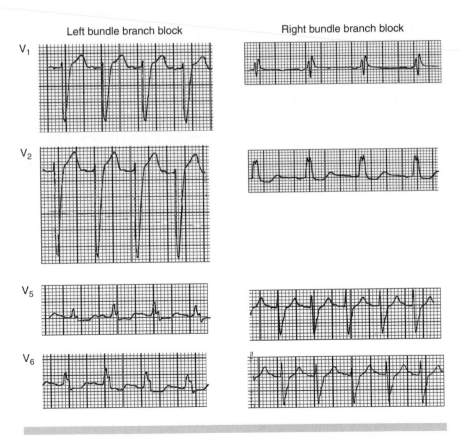

Figure 6-10 **Morphology of the QRS complex in LBBB and RBBB.**

Axis

- QRS positive in leads I and II → normal axis
- QRS positive in lead I but negative in lead II → left axis deviation (LAD)
- QRS negative in lead I but positive in lead II → right axis deviation (RAD)

Axis refers to the net direction of depolarization vectors spreading through the heart in the frontal plane, normally inferior and to the patient' left. Examining the QRS morphology in the limb leads can determine the axis of the heart. The limb leads can be superimposed on the heart to form four quadrants (Fig. 6-11). Each of the limb leads is represented by an arrow with the positive electrode at the arrow head. The wave of depolarization, or positive charge, is seen as an upward deflection as it moves toward a positive electrode on the ECG recording.

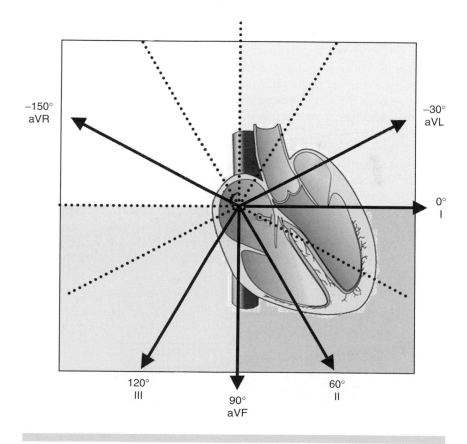

Figure 6-11 **Axis of the heart.**

The normal axis is between −30° and +90°. LAD is between −30° and −90°. RAD is between +90° and ±180°. Extreme axis deviation is between −90° and ±180°.

To determine axis, first examine the QRS complex in lead I. If it is mostly positive, then depolarization is headed predominantly toward the positive electrode of lead I. Next, look at lead II. If the QRS complex is mostly positive then it is going toward the positive electrode of lead II. QRS complexes positive in both leads I and II represent a normal axis because the axis must be between −30° and +90°. If the QRS is positive in lead I but negative in lead II, the axis is shifted to the left. If the QRS is negative in lead I but positive in lead II, the axis is shifted to the right. Last, if the QRS is negative in both leads I and II, an extreme axis is present.

Hypertrophy

- Left atrial enlargement (LAE) is present if the P wave is prolonged.
- Right atrial enlargement (RAE) is present if the P wave is too tall.
- Left ventricular hypertrophy (LVH) has increased QRS amplitude in the precordial leads.

Atrial activity (including hypertrophy) is best viewed in leads II and V_1. The atria have thinner walls than the ventricles and consequently tend to dilate rather than thicken. A normal P-wave duration is <0.12 seconds (three small boxes) and has an amplitude of <2.5 mm.

- **LAE:** Classically seen in mitral stenosis, mitral regurgitation, left ventricular dysfunction, and hypertensive heart disease. The P wave is prolonged with an "m" shape in lead II (p "mitrale") and a biphasic P wave in lead V_1 with a larger terminal than initial component (Fig. 6-12).
- **RAE:** Seen with an atrial septal defect, tricuspid stenosis, tricuspid regurgitation, pulmonary hypertension, chronic pulmonary disease, and acute pulmonary embolism. There is a tall (2.5 mm), peaked P wave in lead II (p "pulmonale") and a large or biphasic P wave in lead V_1 with a larger initial than terminal component (Fig. 6-13).

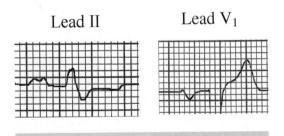

Lead II   Lead V_1

Figure 6-12 **Left atrial enlargement.**

Lead II   Lead V$_1$

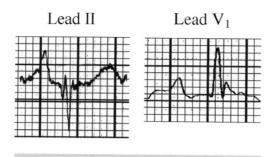

Figure 6-13 **Right atrial enlargement.**

Ventricular hypertrophy occurs when the muscular ventricles must contract against increased pressure. Unfortunately, the ECG is insensitive for detecting hypertrophy; however, it is specific (if the findings suggest hypertrophy, the heart is usually hypertrophied).

LVH: Commonly occurs with systemic hypertension, aortic stenosis, and in some hereditary cardiomyopathies. Numerous criteria are available to diagnose LVH but none are perfect.

- R wave in I plus S wave in III >25 mm
- R wave in aVL >11 mm (for men) or >9 mm (for women)
- Tallest S wave in V$_1$ or V$_2$ plus tallest R wave in V$_5$ or V$_6$ >35 mm
- R wave in aVL plus S wave in III >28 mm in men and 20 mm in women

Downsloping ST depression and T-wave inversion can be seen with LVH and are generally seen in leads I, aVL, and the precordial leads. This is referred to as a "strain" pattern (Fig. 6-14).

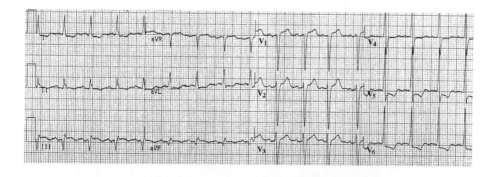

Figure 6-14 **Left ventricular hypertrophy. Note the downsloping ST depression and T-wave inversions seen laterally characteristic of a strain pattern.**

Right ventricular hypertrophy (RVH): Seen commonly with chronic lung disease and pulmonary hypertension and occurs transiently with an acute pulmonary embolism. RAD is usually present.

- Tall R wave in V_1 (R wave >S wave)
- Deep S waves in V_5 and V_6 (>7 mm)

A "strain" pattern can also be seen with RVH, consisting of downsloping ST depression and T-wave inversions in leads V_1–V_3 (Fig. 6-15).

Injury and Ischemia

- T-wave inversions and ST depression can signify either cardiac muscle ischemia or infarction.
- ST elevation classically occurs with infarction, but may occur with other conditions.
- The ECG leads with ST elevation localize the area of infarction.

T-wave inversion can be seen with myocardial ischemia but this finding is neither sensitive nor specific. The typical inversions seen with ischemia are deep and symmetric (Fig. 6-16). T-wave inversions tend to occur in the lateral leads but do not predict the anatomic distribution involved. ST depression is another marker of myocardial ischemia, typically seen with flow-limiting lesions in a coronary artery but not total occlusion. Similar to T-wave inversion, the location of ST depression does not predict the anatomic distribution involved (Fig. 6-17). T-wave inversion and ST depression are not specific for

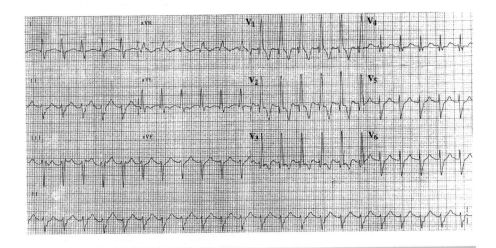

Figure 6-15 **Right ventricular hypertrophy.**

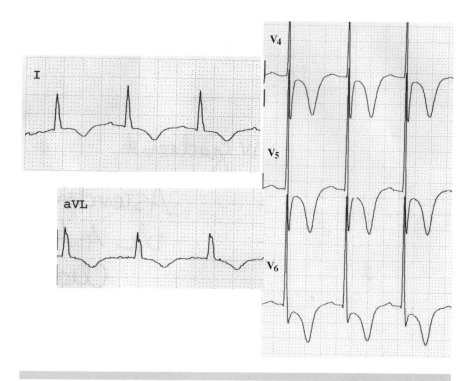

Figure 6-16 **Deep symmetric T-wave inversions seen in the lateral leads.**

ischemia and both may be present with a myocardial infarction or other disorders (hypokalemia).

ST elevation occurs as an acute injury pattern in the leads corresponding to the anatomic area where the injury is occurring. The most common cause of ST elevation is complete loss of blood supply to the myocardium from an occluded artery, but it may result from other conditions such as pericarditis, electrolyte abnormalities, LBBB, LVH, and often a normal finding in the anterior leads of healthy young men. The ST elevation seen with

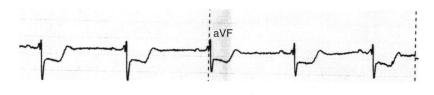

Figure 6-17 **Horizontal ST-segment depression in two contiguous leads.**

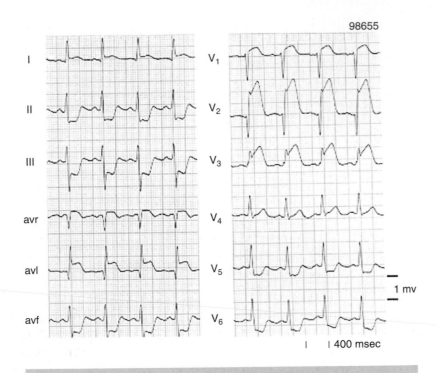

Figure 6-18 **Anterior myocardial infarction with ST elevation in leads V₂ and V₃.** (*Source:* Reproduced with permission from Kasper DL, Braunwald E, Fauci A, et al. *Harrison's Principles of Internal Medicine*, 16th ed. New York: McGraw-Hill, 2005, Online Figure 53-5.)

injury is typically described as being concave down and looking like a tombstone (Fig. 6-18).

- Leads II, III, and aVF → inferior wall of the left ventricle
- Leads I, aVL, V_5, and V_6 → lateral wall of the left ventricle
- Leads V_1–V_4 → anterior wall of the left ventricle
- Leads V_1–V_2 → anteroseptal portion of the heart

The posterior wall of the left ventricle can also be involved, but no lead is positioned over the posterior surface of the heart. A posterior infarction is seen as ST depression and tall R waves in V_1 and V_2.

In pericarditis, the ST elevation is generally diffuse. With the other causes, the ST elevation does not resolve nor does it fit clinically with an acute myocardial infarction; however, ischemia must be ruled out.

Q waves indicate myocardial infarction. To be significant, a Q wave should be >0.04 seconds wide or >1/3 the amplitude of the QRS complex. If

Q waves are seen with ST elevation then at least a portion of the myocardium has already been irreversibly injured.

Other Patterns

Potassium is the main intracellular cation and is responsible for maintaining the resting state of the cardiac myocyte, particularly from the intracellular influx of potassium during repolarization. Low potassium levels will actually delay repolarization. The typical signs of hypokalemia on the ECG include flattening or inversion of the T wave, prominent U waves, and ST-segment depression. By contrast, high potassium levels will increase the ratio of extracellular to intracellular potassium, resulting in an unstable membrane at rest which is prone to depolarization. The typical ECG manifestations of hyperkalemia include peaked T waves, widening of the QRS complex, and loss of P waves. The ECG changes can progress to the classic sine wave pattern lacking P waves, but consisting of large T waves and broad QRS complexes.

After depolarization of the myocyte, the slow influx of calcium maintains the action potential. Thus, high extracellular calcium levels will increase the influx of calcium and shorten the ventricular action potential, whereas low calcium levels will decrease calcium influx and prolong the action potential. Therefore, hypercalcemia will shorten the QT interval and hypocalcemia will prolong the QT interval.

Digitalis is an inhibitor of the Na-K cotransporter located on cellular surfaces. This will directly increase intracellular Na, but also indirectly increase intracellular Ca, because of consequent greater activity of a Na-Ca cotransporter. The main effects of digitalis are slowing of the SA node and prolonging the refractory period of the AV node. However, the influx of intracellular calcium also makes ventricular myocytes more excitable and predisposes to ventricular arrhythmias. Classic changes on the ECG when a patient is taking digitalis include a prolonged PR interval, a distinctive "scooped" ST depression, and flattening of the T wave. High digitalis levels may result in bradyarrhythmias (from sinus bradycardia and increased AV nodal block) or tachyarrhythmias (from increased ventricular excitability).

CARDIOVASCULAR

CHEST PAIN

D. Stephen Goggans

KEY POINTS

- Chest pain has a wide differential diagnosis which includes problems in multiple organ systems and which range from benign to life-threatening.
- A complete history, including associated symptoms and risk factors, is the key to narrowing the differential and choosing appropriate studies.
- In acute chest pain, diagnosis and management focus on ruling out the most life-threatening causes.

INTRODUCTION

Chest pain is a common reason for presentation to doctor's offices and emergency departments in the United States. For the patient with chest pain, the possibility of myocardial infarction is often the main concern. For the physician evaluating such pain, a much broader differential diagnosis must be considered. Sources of chest pain range from the completely benign to the catastrophic. The workup of a patient with chest pain requires being able to confidently exclude the most severe causes before diagnosing a more benign origin. Like most areas of medicine, a thorough history and physical examination are essential to making a correct diagnosis. In particular, understanding the historic features of, and risk factors for, the critical sources of chest pain will allow a judicious use of lab and imaging tests.

PATHOPHYSIOLOGY

Determining the etiology of chest pain is sometimes difficult, because the differential diagnosis is very broad, reflecting the complexity of the underlying pathophysiology. Somatic pain fibers innervate the musculoskeletal components of the chest wall and the parietal pleura. Pain originating from stimulation of these fibers (musculoskeletal pain; pulmonary embolism [PE] or infections involving the pleura) tends to produce well-localized, sharp pain. In contrast, visceral structures (which include the heart, blood vessels, pericardium, esophagus, visceral pleura, and the diaphragm) have overlapping innervation, reflecting common embryologic development. Therefore, an abdominal process irritating the diaphragm (cholecystitis, pancreatitis) may be perceived as chest pain. To further complicate matters, visceral pain is difficult to localize, resulting in vague pain sensations such as heaviness, pressure, aching, or burning, all of which can be from relatively benign causes or from catastrophic causes. In addition, different organs will have similar patterns for referred pain. For example, cardiac pain may be perceived in the left shoulder, but so might diaphragmatic disease. One should also remember that the lung parenchyma has no sensory innervation, so primary lung processes (pneumonia, PE) will not produce pain unless involving the pleura.

CLINICAL PRESENTATION

An important consideration in evaluating chest pain is that "pain" may not be the right word to use. In coronary artery disease, for example, the sensation many patients experience is uncomfortable and unpleasant, but they do not characterize it as "pain." Therefore, when asking about chest pain it is helpful to question broadly. "Do you have any pain or discomfort in your chest?" is more likely to identify all of the salient symptoms.

The history from a patient with chest pain includes the common historic elements (location, character, aggravating/alleviating factors, and associated symptoms), which are detailed in Table 7-1. In addition to these historic features, it is also very important to ascertain whether the patient is currently having the chest pain symptom, as that will affect the immediate evaluation (e.g., ECG should be obtained while the patient is symptomatic).

Understanding the **risk factors** for diseases which cause chest pain is essential for estimating the risk of a particular patient. Risk factors for coronary artery disease and PE are especially important to ascertain (see Chaps. 8 and 15). Risk factors for pneumothorax include a large number of chronic lung diseases such as chronic obstructive pulmonary disease (COPD), asthma, cystic fibrosis, and sarcoidosis. Tall, thin males in their teens or twenties may develop a primary pneumothorax. Risks for aortic dissection include coarctation of the aorta, Marfan syndrome, bicuspid aortic valve, and pregnancy.

The physical examination of a patient with chest pain can provide clues to the etiology though it is rare to diagnose the cause of chest pain by physical

Table 7-1 **Historic Features of Important Causes of Chest Pain**

	Location	Character Factor	Aggravating Factor	Alleviating Symptom	Associated
Cardiac	Retrosternal; radiates to left arm or jaw	Pressure, heaviness, squeezing, tightness	Exertion, activity	Rest, NTG	SOA, nausea, diaphoresis, dizziness
Aortic dissection	Center of chest; radiates to back, abdomen, or groin	Severe even at onset; tearing or ripping	None	None	Syncope or hemiplegia possible
PE	Variable	May be sharp, pleuritic	Deep breathing, cough	None	Hemoptysis. Symptoms of DVT
Pneumothorax	Unilateral	Variable severity; pleuritic	None	None	SOA, often primary symptom
Pericarditis	Substernal; may radiate to neck, back, arms, and epigastrium	Pleuritic	Lying down. Deep breathing, cough, and so forth	Sitting up, leaning forward	SOA, cough—especially in tamponade. Fever—depending on cause
Pneumonia	Unilateral	Pleuritic	Deep breathing, cough	None	SOA. Fever, purulent sputum
GERD	Epigastric, retrosternal	Burning or sharp	Large meals, lying down, particular foods, NSAIDs	Antacids	Belching, dyspepsia, bitter taste in throat
Anxiety panic attacks	Variable	Variable	Stressful situations	Spontaneous resolution	Feeling of impending doom, dizziness, SOA

Abbreviations: NTG, nitroglycerin; SOA, shortness of air; DVT, deep venous thrombosis; GERD, gastroesophageal reflux disease.

Table 7-2 **Specific Physical Examination Findings in Important Causes of Chest Pain**

Disease	Physical Examination Findings
ACS	Diaphoresis Shock or cardiac arrest in severe cases Signs of vascular disease—arterial bruits, diminished peripheral pulses
Aortic dissection	Most patients are hypertensive. May have asymmetric pulses or aortic insufficiency murmur
PE	Hypoxia, tachypnea Shock or cardiac arrest in massive PE Signs of right ventricular failure—RV heave Signs of DVT—asymmetric peripheral edema
Pneumothorax	Tachycardia, hypoxia Decreased breath sounds; tympanic to percussion; decreased tactile fremitus Hypotension and tracheal shift suggest tension pneumothorax
Pericarditis	Friction rub Diminished heart sounds if effusion Jugular vein distention (JVD), pulsus paradoxus if effusion progresses to tamponade
Pneumonia	Fever Hypoxia possible Focal crackles Decreased breath sounds and dullness to percussion with effusion or consolidation Tactile fremitus increased in consolidation, decreased in effusion
GERD	Epigastric tenderness
Anxiety	No specific physical findings
Chest wall pain	Tenderness to palpation (if the tenderness does not exactly reproduce all of the patient's symptoms, the evaluation must continue to look for other, nonmusculoskeletal etiologies)

examination alone. Many of these findings are listed in Table 7-2—next to the clinical context in which they are most frequently found. However, one of the most critical aspects of examining a patient with chest pain is the vital signs, specifically pulse and blood pressure, as these can be the first clues that the patient needs urgent treatment.

EVALUATION

There are many tests which may be useful in the evaluation of chest pain. None are absolutely universal; for example, if the history and physical examination strongly support costochondritis, no further testing may be needed. Otherwise, the tests ordered depend on which items remain in the differential after the history and examination. However, as a general rule **any patient having chest pain should at least have an ECG** and this includes patients who are recently symptomatic and have never had an ECG. The ECG may show signs of ischemia or infarction (ST-segment elevation or depression), signs of coronary heart disease or cardiomyopathy (old Q waves; left bundle branch block; left ventricular hypertrophy), or classic (although usually not present) signs of PE (signs of right heart strain such as right axis deviation or right atrial or ventricular hypertrophy; an S wave in lead I, Q in lead III, and inverted T wave in lead III). The ECG in acute pericarditis shows diffuse ST elevation throughout multiple leads, progressing to T-wave inversion late. A **chest x-ray** is indicated for many patients with chest pain, as it will demonstrate pneumonias, pneumothoraces, and sometimes aortic dissection (widened mediastinum). Further testing depends on suspicion for the underlying disease (e.g., cardiac enzymes for suspected cardiac pain; D-dimers, CT angiogram for PE; and transesophageal echocardiogram for aortic dissection), many of them discussed in detail in other chapters (e.g., Chaps. 8, 15) of the textbook.

MANAGEMENT

The main consideration in management is determining critical and sometimes life-threatening causes of chest pain from more benign causes. The critical causes include myocardial infarction/acute coronary syndrome (ACS), aortic dissection, PE, pericarditis, pneumothorax, and pneumonia (see specific chapters for details). If no critical cause is likely, either initially or after appropriate studies have been completed, further workup to identify a specific cause of the pain can occur at a routine pace.

Regarding a few specific conditions, for **aortic dissection**, blood pressure and heart rate reduction are the keys to the medical management. Intravenous beta-blockers are the preferred treatment but nitroprusside may also be required to reach the target systolic blood pressure of 100–120 mmHg. Proximal, ascending aortic lesions (Stanford type A) require emergent surgery, while distal lesions (Stanford type B) may be managed medically or surgically, depending on severity. Management of **pericarditis** depends on its etiology. Viral pericarditis, the most common acute variety, is treated with high-dose nonsteroidal anti-inflammatory drugs (NSAIDs) or corticosteroids. **Costochondritis** and other musculoskeletal chest pain can be treated with NSAIDs.

ACUTE CORONARY

SYNDROMES

Pat F. Bass

KEY POINTS

- ACS generally occur from rupture of an atherosclerotic plaque, with subsequent thrombus formation, leading to myocardial ischemia and sometimes infarction.
- Patients with chest pain or chest discomfort require risk stratification focusing on previous cardiac history, description of symptoms, physical examination, ECG findings, and biochemical markers of cardiac injury.
- All patients with possible ACS should promptly receive ASA, oxygen, nitrates, and beta-blockers.
- Clopidogrel, anticoagulation, GP IIb/IIIa inhibitors, ACE inhibitors, and statins may be added to hospitalized patients in specific conditions.
- Certain high-risk patients may benefit from an early invasive strategy.

INTRODUCTION

Coronary artery disease (CAD) is the leading cause of death in the United States and chest pain is a common reason for presentation to an emergency department. Patients require risk stratification to determine their likelihood of having an acute myocardial infarction (MI). Acute coronary syndrome (ACS) represents a spectrum of disease encompassing both unstable angina (UA) and non-ST-elevation MI (NSTEMI). UA and NSTEMI have similar pathophysiology except NSTEMI leads to biochemical evidence of myocardial damage, while UA does not. UA and NSTEMI are grouped together under the term ACS because the pathogenesis, clinical presentation, and treatment are similar.

PATHOPHYSIOLOGY

Angina occurs when myocardial oxygen demand exceeds myocardial oxygen supply. Stable angina results from fixed coronary arterial stenosis causing coronary perfusion compromise with exertion and relief with rest. In contrast, ACS generally occurs from plaque rupture, resulting in thrombus formation and subsequent myocardial ischemia, which if prolonged will lead to infarction. Although large plaques are more likely to rupture than small plaques, the greatest risk of infarction is actually from rupture of small plaques. Part of this paradox lies in the fact that persons with large obstructing plaques, or "significant" CAD, will develop collateral circulation around the areas of stenosis in response to repeated bouts of ischemia. Therefore, less myocardium is at risk if these plaques rupture because of these collateral vessels. In addition, small plaques are more common than large plaques. Finally and most importantly, significant plaque rupture is less a function of plaque size than of plaque composition. Plaques that tend to rupture and cause ACS/MI are characterized by a thin fibrous cap, large lipid core (which is extremely thrombogenic), and a high density of macrophages (which release matrix metalloproteinases that digest collagen further thinning the fibrous cap). The lipid core results from the death of lipid-laden macrophages, or foam cells, and the accumulation of lipids in the extracellular matrix. Plaques appear to go through repetitive cycles of localized rupture and fissuring, followed by inflammation and healing—advanced plaques have layers from healed plaque rupture which contribute to the instability of the plaque and propensity to rupture. Rupture may occur because of the nature of the plaque, but may also occur from other factors, such as shear forces, coronary arterial tone, and perfusion pressure. Many of these episodes of rupture and fissuring are clinically silent. However, with significant plaque rupture and tearing of the fibrous cap, the necrotic lipid core is exposed to blood in the arterial lumen, setting off an acute cascade of inflammatory and thrombogenic mediators, promoting platelet aggregation, adhesion, and ultimately thrombosis. Activation of the platelet-surface glycoprotein (GP) IIb/IIIa receptor is the final common pathway in this process. Thrombus formation either partially or completely obstructs the arterial lumen causing ischemia and potentially, infarction.

CLINICAL PRESENTATION

Patients with suspected ACS may present with a heterogeneous group of symptoms ranging from classic angina to vague feelings of fatigue and tiredness. One must decide whether the patient's symptoms represent acute ischemia, chronic ischemia, or some noncardiac process (see Chap. 7). Angina may be characterized as a poorly localized pain, pressure, or discomfort in the left arm or chest. Patients classically have associated dyspnea, nausea, or diaphoresis; however, some patients may have no symptoms at all or vague symptoms such as abdominal complaints, indigestion, jaw pain, and feelings of tiredness. Women, diabetics, and the elderly may have more atypical symptoms. Symptoms less suggestive of a cardiac origin include prolonged (many hours or days) or fleeting (few seconds) pain, reproducible chest wall pain or chest pain the patient is able to point to with one finger, and pain radiating to the lower extremities. Stable angina is generally incited by physical exertion or emotional stress and is relieved by rest. In contrast, ACS/UA is characterized by a change in one's anginal (or angina-equivalent) pattern, such as: (1) chest pain (or symptoms) at rest; (2) new onset of severe and compromising chest pain in the last 2 months; and (3) an accelerated anginal pattern (more frequent, longer duration, and/or occurring at a lower threshold).

Key aspects of the history include known CAD and risk factors for CAD. One should remember that diabetes, peripheral vascular disease, symptomatic carotid artery disease, and end-stage kidney disease are considered cardiac risk-equivalents, meaning these patients carry the same risk as someone with known CAD. Patients with higher risk are more likely to have poor outcomes and thus require more aggressive intervention. Cocaine use inquiry is important as it can cause coronary vasoconstriction and promote thrombus formation. New physical examination findings (e.g., S_3 or pulmonary edema) are ominous and connote an increased risk of death.

EVALUATION

For patients presenting with acute chest pain, evaluation occurs concomitant with the history and physical examination. An **ECG** is obtained promptly, and is an important determinant of subsequent management. **ST-segment elevation** suggests acute MI, with urgent need for reperfusion either through angioplasty or thrombolysis. **Q waves** suggest infarcted tissue, either recent or remote. **ST-segment depression and T-wave inversion** suggest myocardial ischemia, which if unabated can result in infarction (see Chap. 6). The presence of a new left bundle branch block also suggests ischemia and makes subsequent interpretation of ischemia of the ECG difficult. The affected area of the heart can be suggested by the location of changes on the ECG. Changes in leads V_1–V_6 suggest anterior wall involvement, classically from the left anterior descending artery or circumflex artery. Changes in leads II, III, and aVF suggest inferior wall involvement, classically from the right coronary artery. Posterior changes are rarer and more challenging to interpret, suggested by large R waves in V_1 and V_2 with ST-segment depression. Patients with inferior changes should also have a right-sided ECG performed, to look for right ventricle involvement. A right side ECG entails a mirror reversal of the chest leads, leaving the limb leads unchanged. ST changes in rV_3 or rV_4 suggest right ventricular involvement. **Echocardiography** can detect evidence of cardiac ischemia by demonstrating wall motion abnormalities, which can precede ECG changes.

Cardiac biomarkers should be obtained, usually **troponin-I** and **creatine kinase MB isoenzyme (CK-MB)**. These markers become detectable 4–6 hours after infarction has occurred and peak by 12–24 hours. Therefore, markers obtained shortly after the chest pain has begun will often not be detectable, necessitating repeat measurement, such as three sets obtained every 6–8 hours. Troponin-I is more specific for cardiac injury than CK-MB; however, levels remain elevated for 7–10 days, so troponin-I is less useful for ascertaining repeated episodes of myocardial ischemia or infarction.

MANAGEMENT

Initial management entails risk-stratifying patients to high-risk, intermediate-risk, or low-risk patients, based on history, physical examination, ECG, and cardiac marker findings (Table 8-1).

Once one is suspicious of or diagnoses ACS, anti-ischemic therapy must be initiated. The main treatment difference between ACS and the ST-elevation MI is that there is no indication for thrombolysis in ACS. Patients should be placed on bed rest and receive cardiac monitoring. Because of increased myocardial oxygen demand, **oxygen** should be administered in all patients.

Patients with chest pain should be given sublingual **nitroglycerin** (three times 5 minutes apart) and switched to IV nitroglycerin if pain persists. Nitrates are arterial vasodilators that increase oxygen delivery and decrease oxygen demand. **Morphine sulfate** is indicated when patients fail to respond to sublingual nitroglycerin. Morphine functions as an anxiolytic and decreases oxygen demand by decreasing heart rate. **Beta-blockers** decrease myocardial oxygen demand and workload by blocking catecholamine receptors on the cell membrane.

Three types of **antiplatelet therapy** have been used in ACS: (1) aspirin (ASA), (2) clopidogrel, and (3) GP IIb/IIIa antagonists. Patients should be instructed to chew a 325 mg **ASA tablet** as soon as possible after onset of chest pain. ASA prevents the formation of thromboxane A_2, a potent vasoconstrictor and platelet aggregator. Aspirin alone decreases mortality rates and further decreases mortality when used in combination with other agents. Addition of **clopidogrel** to ASA provides improved outcomes in patients with ACS, albeit with an increased risk of bleeding. Clopidogrel works by inhibiting platelet aggregation through the blockade of adenosine diphosphate-dependent platelet aggregation. The **GP IIb/IIIa receptor blockers** (tirofiban, eptifibatide, abciximab) inhibit the final common pathway for thrombus formation. High-risk patients and those proceeding with a percutaneous intervention should receive a GP IIb/IIIa infusion

Table 8-1 *Risk That Signs and Symptoms Represent ACS Related to Cardiac Disease*

	High Risk, Any of the Following:	Intermediate Risk, Absence of High-Likelihood Features and Any of the Following:	Low Risk, Absence of High- or Intermediate- Risk Features but may Have:
History	Previous history of CAD Chest or left arm pain similar to previous angina	Chest or left arm pain as main symptom Male Age >70 Diabetes mellitus	Probable ischemic symptoms in absence of other intermediate characteristics Recent cocaine use
Physical examination	Transient mitral regurgitation, hypotension, diaphoresis, pulmonary edema	Extra cardiac vascular disease	Chest discomfort reproducible on examination
ECG	New ST-segment or T-wave abnormalities	Fixed Q waves; old ST-segment/ T-wave abnormalities	Normal; some T-wave flattening
Cardiac markers	Elevated CK-MB or troponin	Normal	Normal

Source: Braunwald E, Mark DB, Jones RH, et al. Unstable angina: diagnosis and management. Rockville, MD: Agency for Health Care Policy and Research and the National Heart, Lung, and Blood Institute, U.S. Public Health Service, U.S. Department of Health and Human Services; 1994; AHCPR Publication No.94–0602.

for 48–72 hours; for lower-risk patients, the risk of bleeding offsets the benefits of these agents.

Anticoagulation should be added to antiplatelet therapy. Both unfractionated and **low molecular weight heparins (LMWH)** stabilize ruptured plaques by preventing progression of thrombus formation. In general, LMWH are preferred unless there is severe renal insufficiency or possible percutaneous intervention within 8 hours.

Angiotensin-converting enzyme (ACE) inhibitors have a demonstrated benefit in acute MI, especially MIs associated with decreased left ventricular function. The American Heart Association/American College of Cardiology (AHA/ACC) recommends ACE inhibitors in patients with symptoms of congestive heart failure (CHF), diabetics, and hypertension that persist despite treatment. However, one must closely monitor for hypotension and worsening myocardial ischemia. **"Statins"** are indicated in all patients prior to hospital discharge. In addition to their lipid-lowering benefits, these agents are felt to be helpful in ACS from their anti-inflammatory properties, improving the stability of plaques.

Early invasive versus conservative therapy: Certain patients with ACS may benefit from early angiography/revascularization after initial stabilization with the previously discussed medications. While there are a number of different risk classifications, the TIMI (thrombolysis in myocardial infarction) score is one of the most commonly used and is presented below. The score is based on the following risk factors:

- Age >65
- Three risk factors for CAD
- Previous coronary stenosis >50%
- ST-segment depression or elevation
- ASA use in the last 7 days
- Elevated serum markers of myocardial injury
- Two or more anginal episodes in 24 hours

Patients with three or more risk factors may benefit from an early invasive approach.

Patients with ST-segment elevation and MI who do not have access to angioplasty can be treated with **thrombolytic therapy**. Thrombolytics do not demonstrate benefit in NSTEMI or UA.

For the most up-to-date recommendations, the reader is referred to the ACC/AHA guideline update for the management of patients with UA and NSTEMI available at: http://www.acc.org/clinical/guideline.

CONGESTIVE HEART FAILURE

Charles H. Griffith

KEY POINTS

- CHF is a progressive disorder, and effective treatment entails not only symptom control, but early recognition and preventive strategies.
- Current pharmacologic therapy of CHF recognizes the pivotal role of an activated neurohumoral system as deleterious to the failing heart.
- Therapies which target the neurohumoral system will improve survival: ACE inhibitors, beta-blockers, ARBs, aldosterone antagonists, and hydralazine/nitrates.
- The echocardiogram is critical in determining causes of CHF, with a normal EF strongly suggesting causes referable to diastolic dysfunction, as opposed to systolic dysfunction.

INTRODUCTION

Congestive heart failure (CHF) is a constellation of signs and symptoms resulting from dysfunction of the heart or factors affecting the heart, culminating in pulmonary congestion, fluid overload, and poor end-organ perfusion. Nearly 5 million people in the United States have heart failure today, and the prevalence is increasing as our aged population increases. CHF is the most common reason for hospitalization in older adults, and represents a substantial portion of subsequent readmissions. Further, symptomatic heart failure confers a worse prognosis than most metastatic cancers, with a 1-year mortality of 30–50% in advanced disease (i.e., those individuals most often being admitted).

PATHOPHYSIOLOGY

Congestive heart failure is often classified as primarily **systolic dysfunction** (classic "pump" failure, or the inability of the left ventricle to contract normally and expel sufficient blood) characterized by a decreased ejection fraction (EF), usually <40% or **diastolic dysfunction** (inability of the left ventricle to relax and/or fill normally), characterized by a preserved EF, usually >50%. Most patients have elements of both systolic and diastolic dysfunction, although a third or more of patients have primarily diastolic dysfunction. Diastolic dysfunction results from two different abnormalities: slowed ventricular relaxation (which primarily affects early diastole) and increased myocardial stiffness (which primarily affects late diastole). These both result in the inability to fill the left ventricle at normal left atrial pressures causing backflow into the lungs and the symptoms of CHF. Last, **high-output heart failure** can occur when a normally functioning heart decompensates while trying to keep up with extreme metabolic requirements.

The progressive nature of CHF arises from a complex interplay of structural, functional, and biologic alterations (Fig. 9-1). Structurally, ventricular size and shape are altered by the process of left ventricular remodeling, often provoked by ischemia, infarction, hypertension (HTN), cardiomyopathy, or valvular disease. **Left ventricular remodeling** involves hypertrophy, loss of myocytes, and increased interstitial fibrosis, with subsequent dilation and change of the shape of the left ventricle into something more spherical, which in turn adversely affects pump function. With increased left ventricular dilation into a more globular shape, the geometric relation between the papillary muscles and the mitral leaflets changes, with subsequent increase in the severity of mitral regurgitation. This results in increasing left ventricular filling pressures and volume overload, further remodeling of the heart, further symptoms, spiraling into end-stage symptoms and disease. An ominous sign is when cardiac output is so reduced to cause decreased end-organ perfusion, manifested by hypotension and progressive renal dysfunction. This hemodynamic model was the predominant model for the pathogenesis of CHF until recently, when more attention has been focused on the role of **neurohumoral system activation**, and its deleterious effects on the failing heart. The neurohumoral system includes the complex interplay of the renin-angiotensin-aldosterone system, the sympathetic nervous system (norepinephrine), as well as other local and circulating biologically active substances, such as brain natriuretic peptide (produced by the ventricular myocardium in response to stretch), vasodilators (nitric oxide, prostaglandins, bradykinin), cytokines, and matrix metalloproteinases. As will be discussed below, deactivation of the neurohumoral system is a key focus of much current CHF therapy.

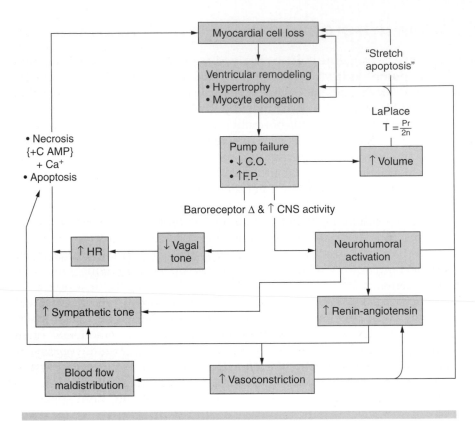

Figure 9-1 **Pathophysiology of heart failure.** (*Source:* Reproduced with permission from Tierney LM, McPhee SJ, Papadakis MA, et al. *Current Medical Diagnosis & Treatment*, Online Edition (45th ed.). New York: McGraw-Hill, 2006, Cardiology Section.)

CLINICAL PRESENTATION

Patients presenting with CHF generally have symptoms referable to pulmonary venous congestion, such as dyspnea at rest or with exertion, fatigue, and chronic cough. Pulmonary venous congestion is classically worse at night, from redistribution of peripheral edema into the central circulation, resulting in characteristic nightly symptoms: orthopnea (having to sleep more upright or with more pillows), paroxysmal nocturnal dyspnea (waking breathless, classically running to the window for air), and nocturia (from greater perfusion of the renal vasculature). Symptoms referable to right heart failure include peripheral edema, right upper quadrant pain (from passive congestion of the liver), and anorexia/nausea (from edema of the gut or impaired gastrointestinal perfusion).

The physical examination of patients with CHF can be quite variable. Many hospitalized patients will appear short of breath, with difficulty finishing sentences and perhaps even diaphoretic with cold extremities from high sympathetic tone. The blood pressure may be elevated, especially with diastolic heart failure, but in end-stage CHF, cardiac output is so poor that the patient is hypotensive (see Chap. 12). Patients are usually tachycardic and tachypneic, and have an elevated weight from fluid retention. The classic signs of venous congestion may be noted with wet crackles or wheezing ("cardiac asthma") in the lungs, elevation of the jugular venous pressure, right upper quadrant tenderness and hepatomegaly from passive congestion, ascites, and peripheral edema. Certain examination procedures may make venous HTN more obvious, such as sustained pressure on the liver which causes an increase in jugular venous pressure by >1 cm (positive hepatojugular reflux). The cardiac examination may reveal a displaced and sustained left ventricular impulse, indicating left ventricular hypertrophy (LVH) or murmurs from various valvular diseases, such as mitral regurgitation and stenosis, and aortic regurgitation and stenosis. Realize that murmurs of mitral regurgitation and tricuspid regurgitation are often functional murmurs caused from the heart failure (and not causing the heart failure). As mentioned above, left ventricular dilatation stretches the mitral valve annulus resulting in functional regurgitation. Likewise, tricuspid regurgitation is most likely the result of pulmonary venous HTN. Special attention should be made to auscultate at the apex for a gallop as an S_3 is indicative of ventricular dilatation and an S_4 gallop indicates an atrium contracting against a stiff noncompliant left ventricle.

The severity of heart failure has traditionally been defined by degree of symptoms, using the New York Heart Association (NYHA) functional classification. However, with the recognition that heart failure is a progressive disorder that begins long before symptoms develop, and the subsequent need to ideally intervene in these preclinical stages, the American College of Cardiology (ACC) and the American Heart Association (AHA) have suggested a four-stage classification of heart failure (Table 9-1). This new classification underscores the fact that certain risk factors and structural abnormalities are necessary for the development of heart failure, emphasizes the progressive nature of CHF, and highlights the critical importance of prevention in treatment strategy.

Chest x-ray classically shows cardiomegaly (the heart size is greater than half the thoracic diameter on a posterior-anterior [PA] film) and pulmonary venous congestion, especially noted in the upper lobe veins ("cephalization"; Fig. 9-2). Frank pulmonary edema will appear as confluent opacities in the central lung fields resembling butterfly wings, often with pleural effusions and Kerley B lines (1–2 cm horizontal lines in the lower lung fields near the costophrenic angles, thought to be from thickened interlobular septa due to edema). The **ECG** may show LVH, evidence of old infarctions, or

Table 9-1 **Classification and Staging of Heart Failure**

ACC/AHA Stage	NYHA Functional Class	Patient Condition
A: High risk of developing heart failure, but without structural heart disease		HTN Atherosclerotic disease Diabetes Obesity Metabolic syndrome
B: Structural heart disease but no signs or symptoms of CHF	I: No symptoms with ordinary physical activity	Previous myocardial infarction (MI) Left ventricular remodeling (LVH, low EF) Asymptomatic valve disease
C: Structural heart disease and current or past symptoms of CHF	II: Symptoms on ordinary exertion III: Symptoms with minimal exertion	Known structural heart disease AND Shortness of breath, fatigue, or reduced exercise tolerance
D: End-stage symptoms of heart failure refractory to standard treatments	IV: Symptoms at rest	Marked symptoms despite maximal medical therapy or requiring specialized interventions

underlying secondary or precipitating arrhythmias, especially atrial fibrillation. The **serum B-type (brain) natriuretic peptide (BNP)** is generally elevated, although false positive elevations do occur. A very low BNP (<50–100 pg/mL) is useful in making CHF very **unlikely** in a patient presenting with dyspnea.

EVALUATION

The initial clinical evaluation of the patient with symptomatic heart failure should focus on determining the underlying cause of the CHF (Table 9-2) and the cause of the current exacerbation (Table 9-3). Determining the cause

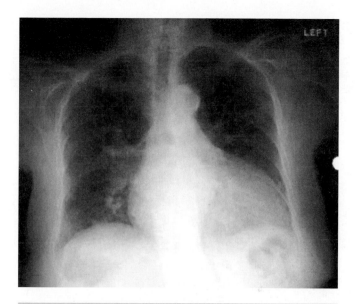

Figure 9-2 **Chest x-ray of heart failure with cardiomegaly and pulmonary venous congestion. (Courtesy of H. Goldberg.)** (*Source:* Reproduced with permission from Tierney LM, McPhee SJ, Papadakis MA, et al. *Current Medical Diagnosis & Treatment*, Online Edition (45th ed.). New York: McGraw-Hill, 2006, Cardiology Section.)

of an acute exacerbation of heart failure is important to try to prevent future exacerbations and admissions.

The most useful test to aid in diagnosis is an echocardiogram. The echocardiogram will of course assess valves, identifying any unrecognized valvular disease as a cause of CHF. Importantly, the echocardiogram provides the EF, which can help differentiate systolic from diastolic (normal EF) dysfunction. In addition, the echocardiogram can provide information on the presence of LVH (suggesting long-standing HTN or hypertrophic cardiomyopathy), as well as noting regional wall motion abnormalities suggesting prior infarction. If high output heart failure is a consideration, measuring the serum hematocrit and thyroid function tests is important. Low serum sodium and an increased creatinine are poor prognostic findings, both suggesting end-stage CHF with poor end-organ perfusion. Further diagnostic tests could include cardiac catheterization, especially if ischemic cardiomyopathy is suspected.

Table 9-2 **Causes of Heart Failure**

Systolic dysfunction	Ischemic cardiomyopathy, such as patients with CAD, especially post-MI, the most common cause in the United States
	Dilated (nonischemic) cardiomyopathy results from alcohol, postpartum, postviral (myocarditis), anthracycline-induced (postchemotherapy with doxorubicin), or idiopathic
Diastolic dysfunction	Hypertrophic cardiomyopathy, most commonly from long-standing HTN
	Restrictive cardiomyopathy from infiltrative processes (amyloid, hemochromatosis, sarcoid), postradiation or post-open heart surgery myocardial fibrosis
Valvular heart disease	Volume overload: mitral regurgitation, aortic insufficiency
	Pressure overload: aortic and mitral stenosis
High-output heart failure	Sepsis
	Severe anemia (usually hematocrit <20%)
	Thyrotoxicosis (may be subtle in the elderly)
	Paget's disease of bone (blood flow requirements through disorganized bone)
	Massive arteriovenous malformations
	Beriberi (thiamine deficiency)

Table 9-3 **Precipitators of Acute Heart Failure**

Cardiovascular	*Patient-Related*	*Medication*	*Other Stressor*
Acute MI	Nonadherence to	Nonsteroidal	Infections
Myocardial ischemia	medications	anti-inflammatory	Blood loss
Uncontrolled HTN	Excessive salt	drugs (NSAIDs)	Pulmonary
Cardiac arrhythmias	Excessive fluid	Thiazolidinediones	embolism
(especially atrial	Excessive	Corticosteroids	
fibrillation)	alcohol	Negative inotropes	
Valvular disease	Physical stress		
	Emotional stress		

MANAGEMENT

Therapy for patients with chronic heart failure consists of progressive step therapy depending on the patient's ACC/AHA stage. Therapy for stage A heart failure consists of aggressive risk factor modification and reduction, such as optimal control of HTN, smoking cessation, and modification of other cardiovascular risk factors. Medical therapy is usually with angiotensin-converting enzyme inhibitors (ACEIs) or angiotensin-receptor blockers (ARBs) as these may prevent the development of heart failure. In keeping with the current pathophysiologic paradigm, for patients with stage B and C heart failure, the goal of therapy is to deactivate the neurohumoral system, and indeed, medications that accomplish this goal are the ones which have been demonstrated to improve survival. Patients with stage D heart failure are by definition refractory to standard medical therapy, but may benefit from left ventricular assist devices and cardiac transplantation, if indicated.

ACEIs are the cornerstone of therapy for chronic CHF, and should generally be prescribed for all patients. Contraindications to ACEIs include worsening renal failure (especially provoked in those with bilateral renal artery stenosis) and severe hyperkalemia. Chronic cough is a well-recognized side effect, but one should make sure the cough is not from poorly controlled CHF before stopping an ACEI for cough. ACEIs of proven survival benefit in clinical trials include captopril, enalapril, ramipril, and trandolapril.

In the older paradigm focusing on cardiac hemodynamics, **beta-adrenergic receptor blockers** were considered a contraindication in patients with CHF. However, beta-blockers deactivate the neurohumoral system by counteracting the harmful effects of the sympathetic nervous system activated during heart failure, and indeed, reverse cardiac remodeling, and improve survival. It is generally recommended not to start beta-blockers during the acute throes of an exacerbation, but begin these medicines once the patient is more stabilized. Recent Cochrane System Database analyses suggest that contrary to long held belief, beta-blockers generally do not worsen symptoms in most patients with asthma or chronic obstructive pulmonary disease (COPD), and should be used in patients with CHF (and coronary artery disease [CAD]) even with these coexisting conditions. Cardioselective beta-blockers which have demonstrated survival benefits include long-acting metoprolol (succinate, not the short-acting tartrate) and bisoprolol. Carvedilol is a nonselective beta-blocker with alpha-blockade and antioxidant properties, and has been proven efficacious in many clinical trials.

Several **ARBs** have demonstrated survival benefit in clinical trials, including candesartan, losartan, and valsartan. In general, because more extensive data exist for ACE inhibitors and ARBs are usually more expensive, current guidelines suggest ARBs as a second-line alternative to an ACE for those who cannot tolerate an ACE, usually because of cough (ARBs are similar to ACEs in the potential for provoking renal insufficiency and hyperkalemia). Studies adding an ARB to ACE therapy with or without beta-blockers have yielded mixed results; such therapy is usually reserved for those with difficult-to-control CHF.

Two **aldosterone antagonists**, spironolactone and eplerenone, have demonstrated a survival benefit for patients with moderate to severe CHF. Eplerenone selectively blocks mineralocorticoid receptors, and therefore does not have the gynecomastia and sexual dysfunction side effects sometimes seen with spironolactone (which also nonselectively blocks androgen and progesterone receptors); however, eplerenone is much more expensive. Both agents can worsen renal insufficiency and hyperkalemia. A common mistake prescribing these drugs is treating them as diuretics, as in ascites. Over-diuresis will activate the neurohumoral system, and higher doses will result in greater incidence of hyperkalemia. Relatively small doses of these medicines (i.e., 25 mg of spironolactone) is all that is needed to deactivate the neurohumoral system, as opposed to diuretic level doses (100–200 mg commonly prescribed in ascites from liver failure).

A large study from the 1980s demonstrated a survival benefit from the combination of **hydralazine/isosorbide dinitrate**, but they had generally been relegated to use when ACE inhibitors were not tolerated (i.e., advanced renal insufficiency), given that survival benefit was greater with ACE inhibitors, and the troubling side effects of hydralazine (tachyphylaxis, which is often detrimental in heart disease, and drug-induced lupus). With the emergence of the neurohumoral model which includes the role of nitric oxide in CHF, and given the lower bioavailability of nitric oxide in patients of African heritage, a recent study of African American patients demonstrated a survival benefit of adding hydralazine and nitrates to standard CHF therapy. Whether this benefit will apply to other groups of patients is unknown at this time.

Although they do not confer a mortality benefit, several other agents are important for symptom control, quality of life, prevention of admissions, and therapy of exacerbations. **Digoxin** is no longer first-line therapy for systolic dysfunction, but is useful in reducing the rate of hospitalization and improving the clinical status of patients, especially those with very low EFs. **Diuretics** such as the loop diuretics furosemide and bumetanide have not been shown to improve survival, and indeed, would be predicted as such given that diuresis activates the neurohumoral system. Nevertheless, for symptom control, most patients with moderate to severe CHF need daily diuretics.

Patients with ischemic myocardium may greatly improve their systolic function with **coronary revascularization**. Finally, the implantation of certain devices has been shown to improve survival in certain patients with CHF. One of the major causes of death in patients with CHF is ventricular arrhythmias, so **automatic implantable cardiac devices (AICD)** to prevent sudden death may benefit certain patients. Candidates for AICD include those with ischemic cardiomyopathy, an EF <30%, and NYHA class I–III (not IV), although the financial implications of such prophylactic insertions are huge. Patients with cardiac dyssynchrony (a QRS duration on ECG longer than 0.12 ms) may be candidates for **cardiac resynchronization therapy**, a special pacemaker which triggers both ventricles to pump in unison. Patients with persistent symptoms despite maximal medical therapy who receive cardiac resynchronization therapy have an improved EF, functional class, and quality of life.

Patients presenting with symptomatic heart failure require intravenous diuretics, most improving dramatically within 24 hours with IV furosemide (with careful monitoring of urine output, renal function, and potassium). Nitroglycerin is also effective in treating an exacerbation of heart failure and may be a useful adjunct to diuretics. Low-dose nitrates induce venodilation which reduces pulmonary congestion, whereas higher doses cause arterial dilation of the coronary arteries. Nitrates are particularly effective if patients have concomitant myocardial ischemia. The recombinant human natriuretic peptide (hBNP) nesiritide has demonstrated more rapid improvement in symptoms and hemodynamics during exacerbation, but has not demonstrated shorter hospitalizations or morbidity/mortality benefits (indeed, it may be deleterious, with worsening of renal insufficiency and increased mortality), and is generally reserved for refractory patients.

HYPERTENSIVE
URGENCY/EMERGENCY

Christopher A. Feddock

KEY POINTS

- Hypertensive urgency occurs when a patient has a severely elevated blood pressure.
- Hypertensive emergency occurs when a patient has end-organ damage.
- Hypertensive emergencies require immediate medical therapy with a goal of a 10–15% reduction in blood pressure.
- Aggressive treatment of hypertension after an ischemic stroke results in worse clinical outcomes.

INTRODUCTION

Hypertensive urgency is defined as a severely elevated blood pressure without any signs of end-organ damage. Sources vary on the values which represent "severely elevated," but one common definition uses the stage 2 hypertension as defined by The Seventh Report of the Joint National Committee on Prevention, Detection, Evaluation, and Treatment of High Blood Pressure (JNC VII), a systolic blood pressure (SBP) ≥160 mmHg or diastolic blood pressure (DBP) ≥100 mmHg. **Hypertensive emergency**, on the other hand, is defined not by the elevation of blood pressure but by the **presence of end-organ damage** (Table 10-1).

PATHOPHYSIOLOGY

The initial physiologic response to an elevation in blood pressure is vasoconstriction of arteries and arterioles. This **autoregulation** prevents the transmission of the higher pressure to more distal vessels and maintains a

Table 10-1 **Hypertensive Emergencies and Appropriate Antihypertensive Medications**[*]

Hypertensive Emergency	Frequency (%)	Antihypertensive
Left ventricular failure with pulmonary edema	37	Nitroglycerin + Lasix
Cerebral infarction	25	Labetalol
Hypertensive encephalopathy	15	Multiple
Myocardial infarction/unstable angina	12	Nitroglycerin + beta-blocker
Intracranial or subarachnoid hemorrhage	5	Labetalol
Severe preeclampsia or eclampsia	5	Hydralazine or labetalol
Acute aortic dissection	2	Labetalol + nitroprusside
Acute renal failure		Multiple[†]
Microangiopathic hemolytic anemia		Multiple[†]

[*]Note that acute renal failure and hemolytic anemia typically occur in combination with other diagnoses.

[†]Such as labetalol, hydralazine, beta-blocker, calcium channel blocker, clonidine, and fenoldopam.

normal level of perfusion. In most individuals, normal cerebral blood flow can be maintained across a wide spectrum of blood pressure, typically mean arterial pressures between 60 and 120 mmHg (Fig. 10-1). However, once arteries and arterioles maximally constrict, rising pressure is transmitted to distal vessels. This increased hydrostatic pressure within the capillaries damages the endothelium, leading to fibrinoid necrosis. The disruption of the vascular endothelium coupled with the high hydrostatic pressure causes the leakage of plasma into the perivascular space (edema). The level of pressure which causes endothelial damage and edema is highly variable, because chronic hypertension results in vessel adaptations and a "rightward shift" in cerebral autoregulation (Fig. 10-1). Pathologically, arterioles become thickened allowing them to maintain normal cerebral blood flow with higher pressures. Thus, patients with poorly controlled chronic hypertension may only develop symptoms when their DBP exceeds 130 mmHg, whereas a normotensive individual with a sudden acute elevation of DBP to 100 mmHg may develop complications. This rightward shift in autoregulation also makes patients with chronic hypertension more susceptible to hypoperfusion as blood pressure decreases. The vascular hypertrophy results in vessels which cannot achieve

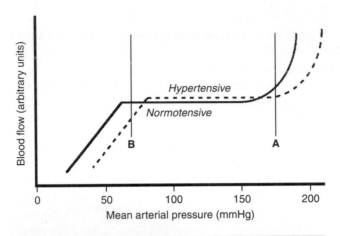

Figure 10-1 **Cerebral blood flow autoregulation in hypertensive and normotensive individuals. Chronic hypertension results in a rightward shift of autoregulation
such that elevated mean arterial pressures may no
longer result in cerebral edema (point A). However, this
shift with chronic hypertension also results in a
decreased ability to maintain cerebral blood flow with
lower mean arterial pressures (point B).** (*Source:* Fuster V,
et al. *Hurst's the Heart,* 11th ed. New York: McGraw-Hill,
2001.

the same degree of vasodilatation to maintain perfusion. This issue is critically important in the management of hypertensive emergency.

CLINICAL PRESENTATION

If they are symptomatic, patients with severely elevated blood pressure most
commonly have neurologic signs from ischemic cerebral infarction, intracerebral or subarachnoid hemorrhage, or hypertensive encephalopathy.
Hemorrhagic and ischemic strokes are discussed elsewhere (see Chap. 58), so
this chapter will concentrate on hypertensive encephalopathy. **Hypertensive
encephalopathy** typically presents with generalized findings as opposed to
the focal findings associated with ischemic or hemorrhagic strokes. Initially,
patients usually complain of headache, nausea, and vomiting. As edema
progresses, patients become restless and confused then develop a coma and
seizures if blood pressure remains uncontrolled. On examination, the fun-
doscopic examination is essential because it usually shows **papilledema,**
retinal hemorrhages, and retinal exudates.

The single most common diagnosis causing hypertensive emergency is **acute heart failure** with pulmonary edema (see Chap. 9). Other cardiac presentations include unstable angina or myocardial infarction (see Chap. 8) and **aortic dissection**. Patients with aortic dissection need to be differentiated from acute coronary syndromes. These patients typically describe a centrally located chest pain radiating to the intrascapular area of the back and described as "ripping" or "tearing." The pain is sudden in onset and usually worst at its onset (as opposed to ischemic pain which has a more crescendo development). Physical examination findings vary on the location of the dissection and can include: pericardial tamponade (from a proximal dissection), focal neurologic signs (from disrupted flow through the carotid arteries), or a pulse deficit (from disrupted flow through either subclavian artery).

The diagnosis of **preeclampsia** is based on having elevated blood pressure and gross proteinuria during the third trimester of pregnancy. Although most women with preeclampsia also have edema, it is not a diagnostic criterion because of its high prevalence during pregnancy. Severe preeclampsia is characterized by end-organ damage, such as oliguria, encephalopathy (altered consciousness, headache, blurred vision), and pulmonary edema, or HELLP (hemolysis, elevated liver enzymes, low platelets) syndrome. Eclampsia is defined as preeclampsia with the addition of generalized seizures.

EVALUATION

The initial evaluation of patients with elevated blood pressures should concentrate on identifying any end-organ damage and determining the history of hypertension and its treatment. All patients should be asked about prior diagnosis of hypertension, their usual blood pressure range, and their antihypertensive regimen and compliance. Noting recreational drug use is important, particularly use of cocaine, amphetamines, and phencyclidine. Symptoms of secondary hypertension should also be elicited. A laboratory evaluation must be performed in order to definitively identify individuals with hypertensive emergencies. A **complete blood count and peripheral blood smear** will detect microangiopathic hemolytic anemia (schistocytes and red cell fragmentation). **Electrolytes** and **renal function** may give clues to secondary causes of hypertension and acute renal failure. A **urinalysis** with attention to the presence of proteinuria and hematuria may be the only initial signs of hypertensive nephropathy. An **electrocardiogram** may detect signs of ischemia or infarction. A **chest x-ray** may reveal cardiomegaly with pulmonary edema (heart failure) or enlarged mediastinum (aortic dissection). Cardiac enzymes should be obtained in any patient with chest pain. A head computed tomographic scan should be obtained if the patient has an abnormal neurologic examination.

MANAGEMENT

Hypertensive urgency can be treated using oral medications over the next 24–48 hours. More aggressive blood pressure control is necessary if the clinician suspects that a hypertensive emergency will develop imminently. Treatment of a hypertensive emergency requires immediate intravenous medication and close monitoring of blood pressure. Although an optimal timing of lowering blood pressure is unknown, most suggest lowering the mean arterial pressure by 10–15% within 2 hours and an ultimate goal blood pressure of **160/100 mmHg** within 6 hours of presentation. More aggressive reductions in blood pressure must be avoided because it can precipitate cerebral, renal, or cardiac ischemia. The choice of antihypertensive agent often depends on the clinical situation (Table 10-1).

In patients with thromboembolic **cerbrovascular accidents** (CVAs), persistent hypertension does not worsen clinical outcomes. When an area of the brain becomes ischemic, perfusion of the surrounding area is maintained by collateral vessels, which become maximally dilated after the stroke. Lowering blood pressure in these flow-dependent areas only diminishes perfusion and causes further ischemia. Current guidelines advise against treating high blood pressure for 10 days following a stroke unless the DBP exceed 120 mmHg and/or the SBP exceeds 220 mmHg. **Labetalol** is considered the drug of choice in acute stroke. After a **hemorrhagic stroke**, the risk of hypoperfusion also exists with low blood pressure; however, elevated blood pressure can perpetuate bleeding and worsen outcomes. Therefore, patients with hemorrhagic strokes have a goal SBP between 140 and 160 mmHg.

Two drug-related causes of severe hypertension deserve special mention. Patients with chronic use of sympathetic blockers, such as **clonidine**, develop an upregulation of sympathetic receptors during treatment. An abrupt discontinuation of such agents can result in a sudden increase in blood pressure. The most appropriate action is to readminister the drug which has been discontinued. Increased adrenergic activity also occurs as a result of increased release of catecholamines. Examples of this include pheochromocytoma or the use of sympathomimetic drugs such as amphetamines, phencyclidine, or cocaine. The drug of choice in these conditions is a direct-acting alpha-blocker, such as phentolamine. Administration of beta-blockers is contraindicated, because this also blocks beta-receptor vasodilatation resulting in unopposed alpha-receptor vasoconstriction and worsening of hypertension.

ARRHYTHMIAS

Carabeth W. Russell

KEY POINTS

- Arrhythmias can be classified into tachyarrhythmias and bradyarrhythmias.
- Goals of AF treatment are to obtain rate control, consider rhythm control, and provide anticoagulation to prevent stroke.
- Atrial flutter has a classic sawtooth ECG pattern and treatment is similar to AF.
- Sinus tachycardia will resolve with treatment of the underlying etiology.
- WPW syndrome is caused by conduction through an accessory pathway and may lead to sudden death; the treatment of choice is radiofrequency ablation of the accessory pathway.

INTRODUCTION

Cardiac arrhythmias are commonly encountered on internal medicine inpatient services and in the ambulatory setting. They range from benign findings on examination or ECG to life-threatening disturbances such as ventricular tachycardia (VT) or ventricular fibrillation. Arrhythmias can be classified as tachyarrhythmias and bradyarrhythmias, each requiring different treatment strategies.

TACHYARRHYTHMIAS

Tachyarrhythmias are defined as heart rates >100 beats per minute (bpm) and can be further subdivided into **narrow complex** and **wide complex** depending on the duration of the QRS complex.

Narrow-Complex Tachycardia

Atrial fibrillation (AF) is the most common arrhythmia requiring treatment. The prevalence is estimated as 0.4% of the population and increases with age. It is classified into three main categories:

- **Paroxysmal**—episodes of AF that last <7 days and are self-terminating (do not require electrical or pharmacologic intervention).
- **Persistent**—AF that fails to self-terminate and requires electrical or pharmacologic cardioversion.
- **Permanent**—AF that consistently lasts more than 1 year.

AF can cause hypotension, myocardial ischemia, syncope, pulmonary edema, or tachycardia-induced cardiomyopathy with rapid ventricular rates. It also increases the risk of embolic stroke.

Pathophysiology

Atrial fibrillation is characterized as a chaotic, irregular atrial rhythm with varying conduction to the ventricle. The atrial rate is 400–600/minute, but most impulses are blocked by the AV node. The ventricular response can be rapid, rates usually ranging from 80 to 180 bpm. There are two generally accepted principles:

- A **trigger** (i.e., ectopic beat) must occur to initiate the arrhythmia.
- A **substrate** (i.e., vulnerable atrium) must exist to perpetuate the arrhythmia.

Ectopic beats can originate from several areas including the atrial free wall, interatrial septum, crista terminalis, ostium of the coronary sinus, and the pulmonary veins. After initiation and prolonged duration of AF, electrical and contractile remodeling occurs in the atrium. This includes shortening of atrial refractoriness and histologic/ultrastructural changes such as an increase in atrial fibrotic tissue. These changes make the atrium more vulnerable to further perpetuation of AF which can explain the reason paroxysmal AF can progress to chronic AF. Several studies have implicated the role of vagal and autonomic influences on the initiation of AF from focal triggers. Table 11-1 lists common causes of AF.

Table 11-1 **Causes of AF**

Hypertension	CAD
Cardiomyopathy/CHF	Valvular disease (i.e., mitral stenosis or regurgitation)
Postcardiac surgery	Congenital heart disease
Myocarditis/pericarditis	Pulmonary embolism/COPD exacerbation
Infection (i.e., pneumonia)	Hyperthyroidism
ETOH intake/withdrawal	Idiopathic AF (lone)

Clinical Presentation

Patients with AF can range from asymptomatic to severely symptomatic. Symptoms may include palpitations, chest pain, dyspnea, dizziness, or fatigue. Physical examination findings include an irregularly irregular pulse, varying intensity of the first heart sound, irregularly irregular jugular venous pulsations (JVP) with absence of an A wave, and a **pulse deficit**, which is a difference between the apical rate and the pulse due to varying stroke volumes from differing periods of diastolic filling causing not all ventricular beats to produce a palpable peripheral pulse. The difference is enhanced when the ventricular rate is rapid. One may also see signs of heart failure (lower extremity edema, increased JVP, and inspiratory wet crackles at the bases).

Evaluation

Atrial fibrillation is confirmed by **ECG**, which classically shows **absence of P waves** and an **irregular rhythm** (Fig. 11-1A). Initial evaluation of AF requires a thorough investigation into possible causes, such as ETOH (ethanol) use/abuse. In addition, an **echocardiogram** should be performed to evaluate for structural heart disease and **thyroid function tests** should be obtained to assess for hyperthyroidism.

Management

There are two main goals in the treatment of AF: **treatment of the arrhythmia** and **prevention of thromboembolism/stroke**. Treatment should be divided into acute and chronic management based on patient presentation and stability.

ACUTE MANAGEMENT

On initial presentation, if there are signs of **hemodynamic instability** (severe hypotension, pulmonary edema, myocardial ischemia or infarction), the patient must be hospitalized and undergo **immediate electrical cardioversion**. The initial shock should be 100–200 J in synchrony with the R wave, with 360 J in subsequent attempts. IV load with antiarrhythmics, such as ibutilide and procainamide, can increase the success rate. Patients with **rapid ventricular rates** and less hemodynamic instability should also be hospitalized to obtain **rate control**. Acute decrease in ventricular rate can be accomplished with IV formulations of beta-blockers (i.e., **metoprolol** and **esmolol**), calcium channel blockers (i.e., **diltiazem** and **verapamil**), **digoxin**, or **amiodarone**. Anticoagulation is not required prior to electrical cardioversion in a patient with hemodynamic instability, as the risk of persistent arrhythmia outweighs the risk of thromboembolism.

CHRONIC MANAGEMENT

Rate control: Several studies have evaluated whether converting and maintaining a patient in sinus rhythm is preferable to allowing the patient to stay

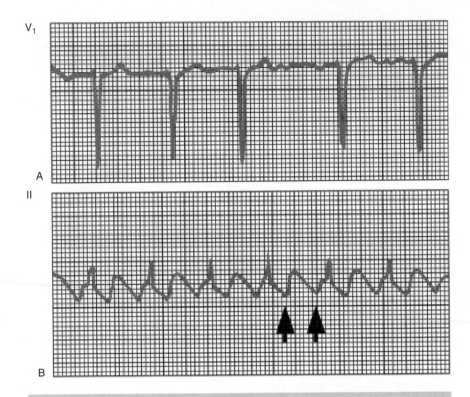

Figure 11-1 **AF and atrial flutter. (A) Lead V₁ demonstrating an irregular ventricular rhythm associated with poorly defined irregular atrial activity consistent with AF. (B) Lead II demonstrates atrial flutter, identified by the regular "sawtooth-like" activity (arrows) at an atrial rate of 300 bpm with 2:1 ventricular response.** (*Source:* Reproduced with permission from Kasper DL, Braunwald E, Fauci AS, et al. *Harrison's Principles of Internal Medicine*, 16th ed. New York: McGraw-Hill, 2005, Figure 214-5.)

in AF with ventricular rate control. The overall consensus is that rhythm and rate control are equal in preventing morbidity/mortality, and therefore simple rate control is preferred in most patients due to increased risk of side effects with antiarrhythmic agents. Rate control can be accomplished with several different medications alone or in combination. **Calcium channel blockers** (verapamil, diltiazem) and **beta-blockers** (metoprolol, atenolol), are the primary agents used for rate control in AF. Historically, digoxin has been used for rate control. However, it is only effective for rate control at rest and not exertion. Amiodarone can also control rate. Each of these agents has a similar action of slowing down conduction through the AV node to decrease ventricular response.

Rhythm control may be preferred in patients who are highly symptomatic while in AF. Rhythm control can be accomplished by pharmacologic or nonpharmacologic means (i.e., electrical cardioversion). Several antiarrhythmics have been used for pharmacologic conversion (i.e., sotalol, amiodarone, dofetilide, propafenone, and flecainide). The majority of these drugs have a risk of proarrhythmia (mostly in patients with structural heart disease) and risk/benefit analysis must occur. **Amiodarone** has the least proarrhythmic effects, but has serious side effects such as **thyroid disease (hypothyroidism and hyperthyroidism) and pulmonary fibrosis**. Recently, there has been great interest in eradicating AF through surgical means (i.e., Maze and Corridor procedures), or catheter radiofrequency ablation. A last option to treat AF when other therapies have failed is to ablate the AV node causing a complete block and implanting a permanent pacemaker.

Anticoagulation

Atrial fibrillation causes uncoordinated atrial activity that promotes stasis of blood in the atrium and thrombus formation. If the patient is converted to sinus rhythm, atrial activity becomes organized and the thrombus may be dislodged and travel through the circulation, causing embolization. AF, whether chronic or intermittent, increases the risk of thromboembolism. The most serious adverse event related to AF is **stroke** from cerebral emboli. Most patients with AF are treated with **warfarin** to prevent thromboembolism, with a target international normalized ratio (INR) of **2.0–3.0**. However, patients <60 years old without structural heart disease (i.e., lone AF) have a very low risk of stroke, and **aspirin (ASA)** may suffice for primary prevention of stroke. In addition, other low-risk patients can be identified by calculating a CHADS2 score (consists of 1 point for congestive heart failure (CHF), hypertension, age >75, diabetes, and 2 points for prior stroke or transient ischemic attack [TIA]). A CHADS2 score of 0–1 suggests low stroke risk, and ASA prophylaxis may be sufficient.

Anticoagulation ought to be performed prior to cardioversion if AF has been present for **more than 48 hours or is of unknown duration** due to risk of thromboembolism. Anticoagulation is started 3–4 weeks before cardioversion and maintained for 4 weeks after the procedure. An alternative approach is to perform transesophageal echocardiography (TEE) to evaluate for atrial thrombus prior to cardioversion. If no atrial thrombus is demonstrated, cardioversion without precardioversion anticoagulation is generally safe in terms of stroke risk. However, even if the TEE shows no atrial thrombus, anticoagulation must be maintained for 4 weeks after conversion to sinus rhythm due to slow recovery of normal atrial contractions and continued risk of thromboembolism.

Atrial flutter is characterized by a classic sawtooth pattern on ECG (Fig. 11-1B). The atrial rate is usually 250–350 bpm and the ventricular rate is a fraction of the atrial rate (i.e., 2:1, 3:1, and 4:1), and therefore atrial flutter can present as a regular or irregular rhythm (if the ventricular conduction is variable, i.e., variable 3:1 and 4:1). Etiologies of atrial flutter include coronary artery disease (CAD), rheumatic heart disease, chronic obstructive pulmonary disease (COPD), CHF, or atrial septal defect. Management is similar to AF: rate or rhythm control and anticoagulation is necessary. Atrial flutter responds well to ibutilide for rhythm control and has a high success rate of electrical cardioversion to sinus rhythm.

Sinus tachycardia is defined as sinus rhythm with rates >100 bpm. Causes include fever, anxiety, hypoxia, dehydration, hypotension, pulmonary embolism, sepsis, hyperthyroidism, and stimulant use. Sinus tachycardia usually resolves with treatment of the underlying cause.

Wolf-Parkinson White syndrome (WPW) is commonly seen in young patients without structural heart disease. WPW is caused by conduction through an accessory pathway that causes preexcitation of the ventricle with heart rates up to 150–200 bpm, with a risk of deterioration into ventricular fibrillation. WPW can present as a narrow or wide-complex tachycardia. Characteristic ECG findings include **wide QRS complex (>0.12 seconds) with a delta wave (initial slurring of the R wave)**. PR interval shortening is usually present (Fig. 11-2). The usual treatment of supraventricular tachycardias (i.e., digoxin, calcium channel blockers, and beta-blockers) should be avoided due to risk of accelerating conduction through the accessory pathway with decreased AV node conduction. Lidocaine can be used for emergent treatment. Definitive treatment is **radiofrequency ablation of the accessory pathway**.

Multifocal-atrial tachycardia is commonly seen in patients with severe COPD. The arrhythmia is caused by increased automaticity throughout the atrium resulting in chaotic atrial contraction. This chaotic activity results in multiple different looking P waves, varying PR intervals, and an irregularly irregular tachycardia. Treatment of the underlying condition (COPD or CHF) is the mainstay of therapy.

Other narrow-complex tachyarrhythmias include AV nodal re-entrant tachycardia and AV re-entrant tachycardia.

Wide-Complex Tachyarrhythmias

Tachyarrhythmias associated with a wide QRS complex can be either supraventricular (i.e., atrial or nodal) or ventricular in origin. Ventricular arrhythmias range from benign premature ventricular contractions (PVCs) to life-threatening arrhythmias such as ventricular fibrillation.

PVCs are caused by ectopic ventricular impulses and are usually benign. Etiologies of PVCs include hypoxia, stimulant use, myocardial ischemia, and electrolyte abnormalities (i.e., hypokalemia). Resolution of PVCs will likely occur with treatment of the underlying cause. Otherwise no treatment is necessary unless the patient is symptomatic and then the treatment of choice is beta-blockers.

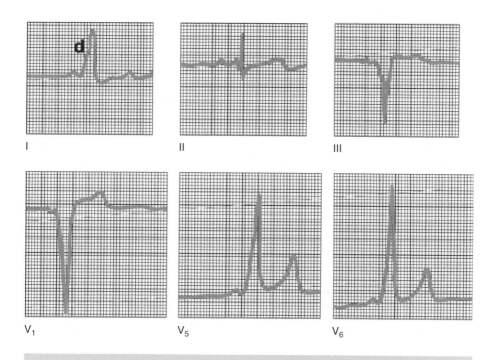

Figure 11-2 **ECG in WPW syndrome. There is a short PR interval (0.11 s), a wide QRS complex (0.12 s), and slurring on the upstroke of the QRS produced by early ventricular activation over the bypass tract (delta wave, d in lead I). The negative delta waves in V₁ are diagnostic of a right-sided bypass tract. Note the Q wave (negative delta wave) in lead III, mimicking myocardial infarction.** (*Source:* Reproduced with permission from Kasper DL, Braunwald E, Fauci AS, et al. *Harrison's Principles of Internal Medicine*, 16th ed. New York: McGraw-Hill, 2005, Figure 214-10.)

VT is defined as greater than or equal to three consecutive PVCs (Fig. 11-3), and is classified as sustained VT when it lasts more than 30 consecutive beats. VT is associated with structural heart disease including CAD, dilated cardiomyopathy, acute myocardial infarction, hypertrophic cardiomyopathy, and myocarditis and stimulant use. The hallmark of VT is **AV dissociation**. When this occurs, AV synchrony is lost and causes severe impairment of cardiac output. This leads to hypotension and cardiac collapse. Sustained VT can lead to ventricular fibrillation and sudden death if not treated. The treatment for nonsustained VT in an asymptomatic person is similar to treatment of PVCs (treat the underlying cause, otherwise, no acute treatment necessary). However, if the patient has structural heart disease, the patient should undergo electrophysiologic evaluation to evaluate the risk for inducible-sustained VT, in which case, an implantable cardioverter-defibrillator (AICD) is

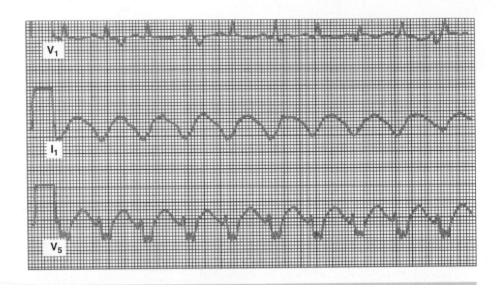

Figure 11-3 **VT with AV dissociation. P waves are dissociated from the under-lying wide-complex rhythm (best seen on lead V₁).** (*Source:* Reproduced with permission from Kasper DL, Braunwald E, Fauci AS, et al. *Harrison's Principles of Internal Medicine*, 16th ed. New York: McGraw-Hill, 2005, Figure 214-11.)

necessary. Acute treatment of sustained VT and ventricular fibrillation are discussed in Chap. 4.

Bradyarrhythmias are defined as heart rates below 50 bpm. They can occur due to slowing of conduction through the AV node or when normal sinus impulses cannot be conducted effectively due to a block. These arrhythmias are usually of concern only when symptomatic, such as fatigue, dyspnea, chest pain, dizziness, and syncope.

Sinus bradycardia is defined as normal rhythm with a heart rate <50 bpm. Bradycardia can be a normal finding, especially in athletes. Symptomatic bradycardia can occur from age-related changes in the sinus node and cardiac conduction system ("sick sinus syndrome") or medications (i.e., beta-blockers) that cause excessive slowing of conduction through the AV node. For life-threatening bradycardia, the immediate treatment of choice is **atropine**. **Permanent pacemaker implantation** may be necessary.

Atrioventricular blocks are described in Chap. 6. Mobitz type II second-degree heart block and third-degree heart block often require transcutaneous pacing in the acute setting.

SHOCK

Dan Henry

KEY POINTS

- Shock is a physiologic state characterized by a systemic reduction in tissue perfusion, resulting in decreased tissue oxygen delivery.
- Hypovolemic, cardiogenic, and septic are the most common causes of shock.
- Early recognition and aggressive treatment of shock is important to prevent end-organ damage.
- Mortality is high, especially in cardiogenic and septic shock.

INTRODUCTION

Shock is a clinical syndrome characterized by inadequate tissue perfusion. Based on the predominant physiologic derangement, four types of shock states are recognized:

- **Hypovolemic shock** (from inadequate circulating volume)
- **Cardiogenic shock** (from inadequate cardiac pump function)
- **Distributive shock** (from massive peripheral vasodilatation)
- **Obstructive shock** (from extracardiac obstruction to blood flow)

Regardless of the cause of shock, inadequate tissue perfusion results in decreased tissue oxygen delivery and an imbalance between tissue oxygen supply and oxygen demand, resulting in lactic acidosis. Although the effects of inadequate tissue perfusion are initially reversible, prolonged oxygen deprivation leads to cellular dysfunction, which can produce inflammatory mediators that further compromise perfusion through functional and structural changes within the microvasculature. Organs frequently affected include the kidney (prerenal azotemia, which can progress to acute renal failure), lung (adult respiratory distress syndrome, which is usually seen with septic shock or pancreatitis), liver (ischemic hepatitis), and brain (altered mental status). Aggressive treatment of shock is important to reduce the severity of end-organ damage.

PATHOPHYSIOLOGY

Global tissue perfusion depends on cardiac output (CO) and systemic vascular resistance (SVR). CO is the product of heart rate and stroke volume. Stroke volume depends on preload, myocardial contractility, and afterload. SVR is dependent on vessel length, blood viscosity, and importantly for the pathophysiology of shock, the inverse of the vessel diameter. Therefore, **shock is due to either decreased CO with inability of SVR to compensate or decreased SVR with CO not able to increase adequately to compensate**. Less common are patients who have decreases in both CO and SVR. Table 12-1 summarizes the differences in shock type depending on preload (the pulmonary capillary wedge pressure [PCWP] is a marker for preload); cardiac index (CI) (the CO divided by the patient's body surface area in meters squared, to adjust for patient size); SVR; and for obstructive shock, pulmonary artery pressures (PAP).

CLINICAL PRESENTATION

Early in the development of shock, there may only be a decrease in blood pressure relative to patient's baseline blood pressure. Tachycardia is often a subtle early sign of impending shock, but despite the subtlety, may reflect a serious underlying condition. For example, a patient with a gastrointestinal bleed may not be tachycardic until he or she has lost 20% of the blood volume. Mental status changes are often seen ranging from agitation to obtundation and even coma. Specific types of shock are discussed as follows:

- **Hypovolemic**: The diagnosis of nonhemorrhagic hypovolemic shock is usually readily apparent from the history of gastrointestinal losses (vomiting and/or diarrhea), fluid losses (increased urine output due to diabetes, diuretics), or insensible losses (burn patients). On examination, patients may exhibit dry mucous membranes and poor skin turgor. Most patients will show evidence of prerenal azotemia with blood urea nitrogen (BUN)/creatinine (Cr) ratio >20. Hemorrhagic shock is often apparent due to history of hematochezia, hematemesis, or melena, although sometimes blood loss may be occult (into the retroperitoneum, the thigh, or the chest). In addition, in patients with acute gastrointestinal hemorrhage, the initial hematocrit may not be low if enough time has not elapsed for equilibration.

Table 12-1 Shock Characteristics and Management

Type of Shock	Example	Hemodynamic Parameter				Management
		CI (2–4 L/min/m²)	PAP 9–18 (mmHg)	PCWP (6–12 mmHg)	SVR (700–1600 dynes·s/cm⁵)	
Hypovolemic	Diarrhea Vomiting Hemorrhage	N or ↓	N	↓	↑	Volume with crystalloids or colloids; blood products as indicated
Cardiogenic	Acute MI Endocarditis with acute regurgitation	↓↓	N or ↑	↑	↑↑	Diuretics Inotropes IABP
Distributive	Sepsis/SIRS Anaphylaxis	N to ↓ ↑ after fluids	N	N or ↓	↓↓	Volume replacement Vasopressors Rx underlying condition
Obstructive	Hypoadrenal Massive PE Cardiac tamponade	N ↓	N ↑	N or ↓ N or ↑	→ N	Hydrocortisone Thrombolysis Pericardiocentesis

Abbreviations: N, normal; CM, cardiomyopathy; IABP, intra-aortic balloon pump; SIRS, systemic inflammatory response syndrome.

- **Cardiogenic**: Myocardial causes of shock are caused by failure of the heart to be an effective pump. Most patients have had a myocardial infarction (MI) and will present with symptoms of chest pressure or pain, dyspnea, diaphoresis, nausea or vomiting. Patients may have an ECG showing ST elevation and possibly Q waves. Chest x-ray (CXR) will often have evidence of pulmonary congestion. Bradyarrhythmias (severe bradycardia, second- or third-degree heart block) can also cause shock if the ventricular rate is very low. Rupture of papillary muscles or chordae tendineae can cause acute mitral regurgitation and a shock-like picture.
- **Distributive**: Two classic causes of distributive shock are **sepsis** (see Chap. 49) and **adrenal insufficiency**. Adrenal insufficiency is important to consider because it is often not rapidly identified. In patients with **Addison's disease**, the lack of cortisol decreases the activity of cate-cholamines and angiotensin (AII), which decreases their ability to increase SVR in the setting of volume depletion. Also, cortisol normally decreases activity of tumor necrosis factor alpha (TNF-α), a potent vasodilator, so increased activity of TNF-α also contributes to a decrease in SVR. Lack of aldosterone further contributes to hypovolemia due to sodium depletion. Usually, shock is precipitated by an acute stressful event such as infection or surgery. Prior symptoms may include fatigue and abdominal pain. There may be a previous history of thyroid disease or pernicious anemia suggesting polyglandular autoimmune disease. Increased skin pigmentation may be noted due to an increased adreno-corticotropic hormone (ACTH) level (which stimulates melanocytes). Patients with Addison's disease will often have hyponatremia, hyper-kalemia, metabolic acidosis, and eosinophilia (due to decreased cortisol levels). If Addison's disease is suspected, an ACTH stimulation test is indicated—measure ACTH, cortisol and aldosterone levels at baseline, and measure cortisol and aldosterone again 30 minutes after ACTH administration. If Addison's disease is present baseline levels of corti-sol and aldosterone will be low with high ACTH levels, and cortisol and aldosterone levels will not increase after ACTH administration. Patients may also present with an **isolated glucocorticoid deficiency**, most commonly from chronic glucocorticoids suppressing endogenous cortisol production. These patients still make mineralocorticoids through the renin-angiotensin system. When the patient is stressed due to surgery or infection there may be an inadequate cortisol production. They will be hypotensive secondary to a decrease in SVR related to isolated glucocor-ticoid deficiency. Patients with isolated glucocorticoid deficiency may have hyponatremia, but should not be hyperkalemic since the renin-angiotensin-aldosterone system is intact.
- **Obstructive**: **Pulmonary embolism (PE)** is an uncommon cause of shock, but may cause obstructive shock if it is massive or there is underlying left or right ventricular dysfunction. Patients often have an underlying reason

for PE (postoperative, deep venous thrombosis, malignancy; see Chap. 15). **Pericardial tamponade** is most common after heart surgery or in patients with malignancy (especially lung and breast). Patients with pericardial tamponade will have a narrow pulse pressure with pulsus paradoxus (an exaggeration of the normal 10 mmHg drop in systolic blood pressure which occurs in inspiration), tachycardia, decreased heart sounds, increased jugular venous distention (JVD), and peripheral edema. With pericardial tamponade the CXR will show an enlarged cardiac silhouette; an echocardiogram will show evidence of pericardial fluid, and sometimes collapse of the right atrium and ventricle during diastole due to increased pressure in the pericardium.

MANAGEMENT

Management of shock entails initial stabilization (Airway, Breathing, Circulation) and treatment of the underlying condition (e.g., antibiotics for septic shock; cardiac catheterization and angioplasty for acute MI). Therapy is summarized in Table 12-1.

PULMONARY

CHRONIC OBSTRUCTIVE PULMONARY DISEASE

Lisa Bellini

KEY POINTS

- COPD is a disease state characterized by airflow limitation that is not fully reversible.
- The severity of COPD is defined by degree of symptoms, often using the Global Initiative for Chronic Obstructive Lung Disease.
- Smoking is the leading cause of COPD.
- Smoking cessation is the single most effective—and cost-effective—intervention to reduce the risk of developing COPD and stop its progression.
- The diagnosis of COPD is based on a history of exposure to environmental risk factors and the presence of airflow limitation that is not fully reversible, with or without the presence of symptoms.
- Spirometry is the gold standard for the evaluation and ongoing assessment of COPD.
- None of the existing medications for COPD has been shown to modify the long-term decline in lung function that is the hallmark of this disease.
- Oxygen is the only therapy shown to improve survival in COPD if it is used a minimum of 15 hours a day.

INTRODUCTION

Chronic obstructive pulmonary disease (COPD) is a disease state characterized by airflow limitation that is not fully reversible. The airflow limitation is usually both progressive and associated with an abnormal inflammatory response of the lungs to noxious particles or gases.

The severity of COPD has often been defined by degree of symptoms, using the Global Initiative for Chronic Obstructive Lung Disease. The GOLD suggests the following stages:

Stage	Characteristics
0: At risk	Normal spirometry Chronic symptoms (cough, sputum)
I: Mild	FEV_1/FVC <70%; FEV_1 ≥80% predicted With or without chronic symptoms (cough, sputum)
II: Moderate	FEV_1/FVC <70%; FEV_1 50–79% predicted With or without chronic symptoms (cough, sputum, dyspnea)
III: Severe	FEV_1/FVC <70%; FEV_1 30–49% predicted With or without chronic symptoms (cough, sputum, dyspnea)
IV: Very severe	FEV_1/FVC <70%; FEV_1 <30% predicted or FEV_1 <50% predicted plus chronic respiratory failure

COPD is the fourth leading cause of death in the United States (behind heart disease, cancer, and cerebrovascular disease). The number of hospitalizations for COPD in 2000 was estimated to be 726,000. Medical expenditures in 2002 were estimated to be $18.0 billion. The economic impact of COPD will continue to increase as the world's population continues to age, smoking becomes more prevalent, and health care becomes more expensive.

PATHOPHYSIOLOGY

Both individual (host) and environmental factors are responsible for the development of COPD. Host factors include genetic abnormalities such as **α1-antitrypsin deficiency**, airway hyperresponsiveness, and improper lung growth during gestation. Environmental factors include **tobacco smoke**, occupational dusts and chemicals, respiratory infections, as well as socioeconomic status. Cigarette smoking is the primary cause of COPD. All of these factors promote inflammation at the level of the small airways and in the pulmonary parenchyma. The inflammation in COPD is mediated by CD8 T cells, neutrophils, and macrophages. This is in contrast to the inflammation seen in asthma that is mediated by CD4 T cells and eosinophils. This ongoing inflammation promotes the following sequence of physiologic changes characteristic of the disease: mucus hypersecretion, ciliary dysfunction, airflow limitation, pulmonary hyperinflation, gas exchange abnormalities, pulmonary hypertension, and cor pulmonale. Chronic cough and sputum production are caused by mucus hypersecretion and ciliary dysfunction and can be present for many years before other symptoms or physiologic abnormalities develop.

The relative proportion of inflammation between the small airways and the alveolar parenchyma is responsible for the clinical manifestations of

Table 13-1 **Characteristics of Irreversible and Reversible Airflow Limitation**

Irreversible	Reversible
Loss of elastic recoil due to alveolar destruction	Accumulation of inflammatory cells and mucous
Airway fibrosis and subsequent narrowing	Airway smooth muscle contraction
Loss of alveolar support to maintain small airway patency	Hyperinflation with exercise

chronic bronchitis and emphysema. This concept emphasizes that both chronic bronchitis and emphysema exist on the continuum of obstructive lung diseases and most patients will have symptoms of both. Airflow limitation can be either irreversible or reversible (Table 13-1).

CLINICAL PRESENTATION

The diagnosis of COPD is based on a history of exposure to environmental risk factors and the presence of airflow limitation that is not fully reversible, with or without the presence of symptoms. Patients who have chronic cough and sputum production with a history of exposure to environmental risk factors should be tested with spirometry for airflow limitation, even if they do not have dyspnea.

On general examination, patients may have shortness of breath with difficulty finishing sentences. Patients with advanced disease may use the accessory muscles in the neck as well as their intercostal muscles to facilitate breathing, and may appear cyanotic if they are hypoxic. Tachycardia and tachypnea may be present. On lung examination, hyperinflation of the airways and air trapping may lead to reduced diaphragmatic excursion and less audible breath sounds. Coarse crackles (interrupted sounds heard on inspiration) may be heard in those with significant mucous production. Wheezing (continuous sounds heard on expiration) suggests airflow limitation. On cardiac examination, the left ventricular impulse can be displaced medially due to an increase in right-sided pressure. A right ventricular heave may be present due to right heart overload from pulmonary hypertension. The pulmonic component of S_2 may be increased in intensity due to pulmonary hypertension. A right-sided S_3 gallop (a ventricular filling sound) may be heard. The most typical murmur is that of tricuspid regurgitation from right ventricular pressure overload. Patients with cor pulmonale will have elevated jugular venous pressure and peripheral edema.

EVALUATION

A **PA and lateral chest radiograph** is a necessary part of any initial evaluation. In early disease, that is, GOLD stages 1 and 2, it may be normal. As the disease progresses and hyperinflation and air trapping become more severe, several findings become apparent: flattening of the hemidiaphragms, increased number of ribs visible on the anterior-posterior (AP) film (normal is 8–9), and increased size of the retrosternal airspace on the lateral film. **Spirometry** is gold standard for the initial evaluation and ongoing assessment of COPD. The main measurements obtained are: the **forced vital capacity (FVC)**, which is the volume of air that can be exhaled going from maximal inhalation to maximal exhalation; the **forced expiratory volume in 1 second (FEV_1),** which is the volume of air exhaled in the first second of exhalation, starting at maximal inhalation; and the **FEV_1/FVC ratio**. The American Thoracic Society defines the presence of **obstruction as an FEV_1/FVC ratio of <70%**. The severity of airflow obstruction is graded by the FEV_1 percentage.

Oxyhemoglobin saturation should be measured both at rest and with ambulation. The latter is to rule out exercise-induced hypoxemia caused by impaired diffusion of oxygen across the alveolar capillary bed.

An **arterial blood gas** should be obtained to look for hypercarbia in individuals with an FEV_1 <40%, signs of right heart failure, or respiratory failure.

Laboratory studies that might be useful include a **hemoglobin** to help assess oxygen-carrying capacity and a **bicarbonate** level to determine whether metabolic compensation is present for a chronic respiratory acidosis. An **ECG** might reveal decreased voltage from severe air trapping, right axis deviation, or right ventricular hypertrophy. An ECG is also important to look for signs of coronary artery disease, as smoking is a major risk factor for both. **Echocardiograms** are not ordered routinely unless there is concern for pulmonary hypertension and right heart failure.

MANAGEMENT

Chronic Stable COPD

The overall approach to managing stable COPD should be characterized by a stepwise increase in treatment, depending on disease severity. Disease severity is determined by the severity of symptoms and airflow limitation, as well as the frequency and severity of exacerbations, complications, respiratory failure, comorbidities, and the general health status of the patient. The management strategy is based on an individualized assessment of disease severity and response to various therapies. None of the existing medications for COPD has been shown to modify the long-term decline in lung function that is the hallmark of this disease. Therefore, pharmacotherapy for COPD is used to decrease symptoms and/or complications. The following summarizes key features in the management of stable COPD.

1. **Smoking cessation** is the single most effective—and cost-effective—intervention to reduce the risk of developing COPD and stop its progression.
2. **Inhaled bronchodilators** are the mainstay of management in COPD. There are three classes: **β2-agonists** (e.g., albuterol), **anticholinergics** such as ipratropium or tiotropium bromide, and the **methylxanthines** (e.g., theophyllines). The choice between these or combination therapy depends on availability and individual response in terms of symptom relief and side effects. Generally, the longer-acting anticholinergic medications are the initial choice for maintenance therapy, given their lower side effect profile and prolonged duration of effect, with shorter-acting agents such as albuterol used on an as-needed basis. None of these drugs will improve survival but they will provide relief of symptoms and improve exercise capacity.
3. **Glucocorticoids** can be administered orally or via inhalation. The oral administration is typically reserved for the management of acute exacerbations. Inhaled glucocorticoids are appropriate for symptomatic COPD patients with an FEV_1 <50% predicted (GOLD stage 3 or 4). Although inhaled glucocorticoids do not modify the long-term decline of FEV_1, regular administration does result in reduced frequency of exacerbations. The combination of an inhaled glucocorticoid with a long-acting β2-agonist is very effective in GOLD stages 3 and 4.
4. **Oxygen** therapy has been the **only therapy shown to improve survival in COPD** if used a minimum of 15 hours a day. Patients must qualify for oxygen therapy by meeting the following criteria:
   - An SaO_2 below 88% or PaO_2 below 55 mmHg
   - An SaO_2 of 89% or PaO_2 between 55 and 60 mmHg in the presence of pulmonary hypertension, peripheral edema suggesting congestive heart failure, or polycythemia (hematocrit >55%)

   The goal of oxygen therapy is to maintain an SaO_2 >90%, roughly equivalent to a PO_2 of 60 mmHg. Most oxygen therapy is delivered by nasal cannula. When patients require oxygen at levels >6 L, they often will need the placement of a transtracheal oxygen catheter. Such catheters are inserted through the neck into the trachea and will reduce the concentration of oxygen necessary by eliminating the dead space ventilation of the upper airway and oral cavity.
5. **Diuretics** are helpful in managing the fluid retention associated with pulmonary hypertension and right heart failure.
6. **Nutrition** support is important in patients with advanced disease. As COPD progresses, the work of breathing becomes very high thus increasing caloric needs. Patients with severe disease will become dyspneic after eating due to abdominal distention and a resultant change in pulmonary mechanics. Such patients should be advised to eat multiple small meals per day and consume foods lower in carbohydrates that are less likely to promote hypercarbia.

7. **Pulmonary rehabilitation** is a structured exercise and education program designed to improve quality of life by reducing symptoms and
   increasing physical activity to allow independence in activities of daily
   living. Patients typically undergo a baseline assessment of exercise
   capacity and then begin a 12-week program of pulmonary conditioning
   that focuses on upper and lower extremity strength as well as breathing
   techniques. Most patients will attend two to three times per week. There
   is an added advantage of reducing social isolation often associated with
   COPD. All stages of disease benefit from pulmonary rehabilitation by
   improving exercise tolerance and symptoms of dyspnea and fatigue.
   Once the initial program is completed, patients need to enter a maintenance phase or the benefit derived from improved conditioning will
   slowly dissolve.
8. **Surgical options** include bullectomy, lung volume reduction surgery
   (LVRS), and lung transplant. In patients with large bullae, a bullectomy
   (surgical removal of the bulla) is effective in reducing dyspnea and
   improving lung function. LVRS is a surgical procedure in which parts of
   the lung are resected to reduce hyperinflation and thus help to restore
   normal pulmonary mechanics. LVRS does not improve mortality but
   improves exercise capacity in patients with predominant upper lobe
   emphysema and a poor functional status. This procedure is not recommended for most patients with COPD due to its high cost and limited
   benefit. In appropriately selected patients with very advanced COPD,
   lung transplantation has been shown to improve quality of life and functional capacity.
9. **Influenza vaccines** can reduce serious illness and death in COPD
   patients by about 50%. Annual influenza vaccines should be administered each fall to patients in all stages of disease. **Pneumococcal vaccine**
   is recommended in all patients with COPD.
10. **Advanced directives** should be discussed with all COPD patients. COPD is
    a chronic, progressive disease with exacerbations that can be life threaten-
    ing. Hospice programs are appropriate when life expectancy is <6 months.

Acute Exacerbations of COPD

The risk of death from a COPD exacerbation is related to the presence of
underlying comorbidities, respiratory acidosis, and the need for invasive
mechanical ventilation. The following key features should be addressed in
patients with an acute COPD exacerbation.

Oxygen therapy is the mainstay of treatment for COPD exacerbations.
Oxygen should be administered at the minimum level required to achieve a
PaO_2 >60 mmHg or SaO_2 >90%. Oxygen therapy can cause CO_2 retention
due to relief of hypoxic vasoconstriction in the pulmonary vascular bed and
thus increased perfusion of nonventilated alveolar units. However, oxygen
therapy should not be withheld for fear of worsening respiratory academia,

as profound hypoxemia is more an immediate threat to life than hypercarbia. Nevertheless, arterial blood gas monitoring should be performed in any patient with a history of hypercarbia approximately 30 minutes after institution of oxygen therapy to ensure satisfactory oxygenation without CO_2 retention or acidosis. Venturi masks should be used in patients with baseline hypercarbia as they are a more controlled oxygen delivery system than are nasal prongs.

Short-acting **bronchodilators** are important in improving the symptoms of dyspnea caused by bronchoconstriction and mucous production. The most commonly used are short-acting, inhaled β2-agonists.

Oral or IV **glucocorticoids** are recommended in the treatment of COPD exacerbations. The dose of oral steroids should be between 30 and 40 mg a day for 10–14 days. Higher doses lead to more frequent complications of steroid therapy. Adrenal insufficiency does not occur with this duration of steroid use so tapering is not necessary. Many physicians will taper the steroids because a taper is better tolerated by patients than abrupt cessation of therapy.

Antibiotics are only indicated when patients with worsening dyspnea and cough also have increased sputum volume and purulence. Antibiotic choice should reflect local patterns of antibiotic sensitivity among *Streptococcus pneumoniae*, *Haemophilus influenzae*, and *Moraxella catarrhalis*.

Ventilatory support can occur in the form of noninvasive positive pressure ventilation (NIPPV) or invasive mechanical ventilation requiring intubation. NIPPV is appropriate when the following is present:

- Moderate to severe dyspnea with use of accessory muscles and paradoxical abdominal motion
- Moderate to severe acidosis (pH <7.35) and hypercapnia (PaCO$_2$ >45 mmHg)
- Respiratory rate >25 breaths per minute

NIPPV is usually successful in such patients and will lead to decreased morbidity and mortality related to intubation.

Invasive mechanical ventilation is the standard treatment for patients with impending acute respiratory failure and those with life-threatening acid-base status abnormalities and/or altered mental status.

RESPIRATORY FAILURE

David M. Hiestand

KEY POINTS

- Respiratory failure is a syndrome resulting from the inability of the lungs to perform one or both of their gas exchange functions: uptake of oxygen or removal of carbon dioxide.
- Respiratory failure is a medical emergency, requiring prompt identification of gas exchange abnormality and institution of therapy to correct it.
- Treatment of respiratory failure may include supplemental oxygen and/or noninvasive ventilation.
- Severe respiratory failure requires intubation and mechanical ventilation.

INTRODUCTION

Respiratory failure is generally defined as failure of the respiratory system to perform one or both of its gas exchange functions: **uptake of oxygen** or **removal of carbon dioxide**. In **hypoxemic respiratory failure**, the predominant abnormality is impaired oxygen uptake from the lung, and it is typically defined as an arterial PO_2 of ≤ 60 mmHg. In **hypercapnic respiratory failure**, the predominant abnormality is impaired carbon dioxide removal, and it is typically defined as arterial PCO_2 of ≥ 50 mmHg. Of course, these two conditions may coexist in severely ill individuals. Respiratory failure may be further classified into acute or chronic. Acute respiratory failure typically occurs in otherwise healthy individuals with acute neurologic, respiratory, cardiovascular, or metabolic illness. Chronic respiratory failure more frequently occurs in individuals with chronic neurologic, muscular, respiratory, or cardiovascular disease.

Respiratory failure should be regarded as a syndrome, not a disease process. Therefore, describing the morbidity and mortality of respiratory failure requires the context of the underlying disease. For example, acute respiratory distress syndrome (ARDS) is a condition resulting in noncardiogenic pulmonary edema with noncompliant lungs. It can result from primary or secondary lung injury, and carries a mortality rate up to 50% (see Chap. 19). Chronic obstructive pulmonary disease (COPD) exacerbations with respiratory failure have a mortality approaching 30% (see Chap. 13). In general, all disease processes are associated with greater morbidity and mortality when occurring with respiratory failure and conversely, respiratory failure occurring with other organ dysfunction (e.g., renal, hepatic, and cardiovascular) is associated with excess morbidity and mortality. Thus, the syndrome of respiratory failure requires prompt attention to etiology and associated organ failure, as well as institution of supportive care.

PATHOPHYSIOLOGY

Hypoxia is defined on a cellular level as insufficient oxygen delivery to tissues to meet metabolic needs. **Oxygen delivery** is the product of cardiac output (CO) and arterial oxygen content (CaO_2):

$$DO_2 = CO \times CaO_2$$

As the equation below illustrates, arterial oxygen content is mostly a function of hemoglobin concentration (Hgb) and saturation with oxygen. Dissolved O_2 in the blood contributes slightly:

$$CaO_2 = (1.34 \times Hgb \times SaO_2) + (0.0031 \times PaO_2)$$

Therefore, oxygen delivery can be represented as:

$$DO_2 = CO \times [(1.34 \times Hgb \times SaO_2) + (0.0031 \times PaCO_2)]$$

From this equation we can see that tissue hypoxia can result from four categories of disorders:

1. **Hypoxemic hypoxia**—arterial oxygen saturation is insufficient to maintain tissue oxygen delivery.
2. **Anemic hypoxia**—gas exchange is satisfactory, but there is insufficient hemoglobin for effective oxygen transport.
3. **Circulatory hypoxia**—arterial oxygen content is adequate, but the circulatory pump or blood vessel dysfunction interferes with oxygen delivery.
4. **Histotoxic hypoxia**—oxygen delivery is adequate, but metabolic pathways are poisoned, and oxygen cannot be utilized (such as in cyanide poisoning).

From a practical standpoint, however, tissue oxygen delivery cannot be rapidly determined and blood oxygen is used as a surrogate assessment for tissue oxygenation. **Hypoxemia** is defined as low oxygen content in the blood, and occurs when there is inadequate transfer of oxygen from the environment to the alveolus or from the alveolus to the pulmonary circulation. Arterial oxygen content can be measured directly and alveolar oxygen content can be determined from the alveolar air equation:

$$P_AO_2 = P_IO_2 - P_aCO_2/R$$

where P_AO_2 is alveolar partial pressure of oxygen; P_IO_2 is partial pressure of oxygen in inspired air; $P_IO_2 = F_IO_2 \times (P_B - P_{water})$; P_aCO_2 is arterial partial pressure of CO_2; and R is respiratory quotient (usually 0.8 depending on dietary intake).

The calculated alveolar oxygen content should be compared to the measured arterial oxygen content, the P_AO_2, which represents the **alveolar-arterial (A-a) gradient**. The A-a gradient serves as a rough indicator of the lung's capacity to transfer gas. The normal A-a gradient is generally considered to be about 12, but it does increase with age (normal ~0.29 × age). Hypoxemia can be classified into conditions in which the gradient is normal or elevated.

When a patient has **hypoxemia with a normal A-a gradient**, either hypoventilation or reduced inspired oxygen (as in high altitude) is responsible. More commonly, patients will have **hypoxemia with a widened A-a gradient** secondary to either ventilation-perfusion (V/Q) mismatch or a right to left shunt.

Ventilation-perfusion mismatch occurs when lung units are *poorly* ventilated in relation to perfusion. Common causes of V/Q mismatch include airway obstruction, atelectasis, consolidation, or edema. The important point regarding V/Q mismatch is that these lung units are *partially* ventilated. Increasing oxygen supply (via supplemental F_IO_2) is an effective means to overcome hypoxemia, because the oxygen content in the poorly ventilated units can be raised enough to fully saturate hemoglobin at the alveolar-capillary membrane. By contrast, right-to-left shunts have an absolute bypass of lung units as venous blood shunts directly into the arterial circulation, so hypoxemia will not improve with supplemental oxygen. This occurs in various conditions such as intracardiac shunts (right-to-left congenital heart disease) and intrapulmonary shunts (A-V fistulae). Common anatomic disturbances leading to hypoxemic respiratory failure include:

- Air spaces/alveoli—cardiogenic pulmonary edema, ARDS, pulmonary hemorrhage, pneumonia
- Interstitium—pulmonary fibrosis, extrinsic allergic alveolitis
- Heart/pulmonary vasculature— pulmonary embolism (PE), intracardiac or intrapulmonary shunt, pulmonary hypertension, congestive heart failure (CHF)

- Airways—asthma, COPD, mucous plugging
- Pleura—pneumothorax, pleural effusion

Hypercapnia is defined as elevated blood CO_2 and results from insufficient excretion of CO_2, often leading to the development of respiratory acidosis. It can result from one of three possible scenarios: **increased CO_2 production, increased dead space ventilation, or decreased tidal ventilation**. Individuals with normal lungs generally develop hypercapnia from inadequate minute ventilation, because compensatory mechanisms can adapt to the other changes. However, individuals with impaired lung function have inadequate compensatory mechanisms and hypercapnia can develop as a result of one or more of these scenarios. Increased dead space ventilation requires physiologically significant increase in the amount of dead space in the lung. Individuals with normal lungs have structures that do not participate in gas exchange (upper airway); however, individuals with ventilation-perfusion inequality have an increase in physiologic dead space. Ventilation-perfusion inequality represents a state in which either ventilation of alveoli is preserved but perfusion of those alveoli is limited, or ventilation is impaired but perfusion is preserved. Either will result in an increase in dead space ventilation and lead to hypercapnia. Although increased CO_2 production occurs in hypermetabolic states such as exercise, fever, and sepsis, it rarely is clinically significant. Most patients are able to increase their effective alveolar ventilation to handle the increased CO_2 production. Thus, hypercapnic failure is generally divided into two basic forms:

1. Decreased minute ventilation (pure hypoventilation) which can result from:
   a. Impaired central drive to breath
   b. Neuromuscular weakness
2. Ventilation-perfusion mismatch

Several mechanisms can lead to hypercapnic respiratory failure (Table 14-1).

CLINICAL PRESENTATION

The clinical presentation of acute respiratory failure can vary slightly depending on the gas exchange abnormalities. In hypoxemic respiratory failure, the classical clinical symptom is **dyspnea**. Confusion, restlessness, anxiety, and delirium are also associated with hypoxemia, though these features may not be helpful in the acutely ill individual. In hypercapnic respiratory failure, dyspnea may also occur, although a **decreased level of consciousness** may be the sole clinical symptom.

The onset of symptoms generally relates to the underlying disorder. In general, when symptom onset is rapid, the underlying disorder is more life

Table 14-1 **Mechanisms of Hypercapnic Respiratory Failure**

Defect	Mechanism and Clinical Example
Ventilatory drive	Pharmacologic—drug overdose (opioids, sedatives, alcohol), general anesthesia
	Acquired—CVA, neoplasm, carotid body resection
	Combination—obesity hypoventilation syndrome
Neural transmission to ventilatory muscles	Cervical spinal cord injury—trauma, tumor, vascular accident
	Demyelinating peripheral neuropathy—Guillain-Barre syndrome
	Anterior horn cell disease—poliomyelitis, ALS
	Phrenic nerve lesion—trauma, cardiac surgery, neoplasm, idiopathic
Ventilatory muscles	Pharmacologic—neuromuscular blocking agents
	Muscle disorder—muscular dystrophy, polymyositis, dermatomyositis
	Disorders of neuromuscular junction—myasthenia gravis, botulism, tetanus, tick paralysis
	Metabolic disturbances—hypophosphatemia, hypokalemia, hypomagnesemia, myxedema
Chest wall	Decreased mobility—kyphoscoliosis, tight casts or bandages, severe obesity, circumferential burns
Pleural disorders	Extrapulmonary restriction—pneumothorax, pleural effusion, pleural thickening, or malignancy
Airway obstruction	Upper airway—epiglottitis, foreign body, tumor, vocal cord paralysis
	Lower airway—COPD, acute severe asthma
Increased dead space ventilation	Very high V/Q—COPD
	Very low V/Q and right-to-left shunt—severe ARDS
	Generalized pulmonary hypoperfusion—shock, pulmonary hyperinflation (intrinsic or exogenous PEEP)
	Localized pulmonary hypoperfusion—PE, air embolism, fat embolism
Increased CO_2 production (with an inability to increase overall ventilation)	Hypermetabolism—fever, sepsis, burns, severe trauma
	Increased muscle activity—shivering, tetany, seizures, malignant hyperthermia
	Excessive caloric intake (especially carbohydrate intake)
Exogenous CO_2	Increased inspired PCO_2—laboratory or industrial accident

Abbreviations: CVA, cerebrovascular accident; ALS, amyotrophic lateral sclerosis; PEEP, positive end-expiratory pressure.

threatening. Typical scenarios include sudden, massive PE, myocardial infarction with acute pulmonary edema, or pneumothorax. More gradual onset of symptoms (on the order of hours) is associated with most other etiologies of pulmonary edema, exacerbations of obstructive airways disease, and pneumonia. The onset of respiratory failure in the context of central nervous system (CNS) depression is related to the onset of the event: acute CNS infarctions and rapid-acting drugs may occur swiftly, whereas slow-onset drugs and space-occupying CNS lesions may occur gradually.

An appropriate physical examination should include brief assessments of general appearance, neurologic, respiratory, and cardiac systems, as well as oxygen saturation via pulse oximetry.

Physical findings related to respiratory failure include cyanosis (occurs when the concentration of deoxygenated hemoglobin is >5 g/100 mL), tachycardia, tachypnea, hypertension, tremor, and dysrhythmias. The specificity of these physical examination findings, however, is rather low. A key assessment is the patient's level of alertness; if the patient is confused or somnolent, this could portend an impending need for mechanical ventilation.

EVALUATION

The evaluation of the patient with acute respiratory failure includes a rapid assessment of severity, determination of etiology, and identification of the most effective means of therapy.

The rapid history and physical findings will provide guidance to further diagnostic tests. Under most circumstances an arterial blood gas (ABG) should be obtained. From the ABG, one can determine the respiratory function abnormality (e.g., respiratory acidosis) and ascertain the A-a gradient. Additional tests should include a 12-lead ECG and chest x-ray.

MANAGEMENT

The management of acute respiratory failure depends on the primary respiratory disturbance. For disorders limited to hypoxemic failure, institution of supplemental oxygen may be sufficient to provide tissues oxygen while treatment of the underlying abnormality (e.g., CHF and COPD) is begun. Oxygen can be administered through several mechanisms. **Nasal cannula**, at 1–5 L/min of flow can reliably deliver supplemental oxygen to raise arterial PO_2 to 60 mmHg in many instances. A very crude estimate of F_IO_2 is 0.04 × flow (in L/min) + 0.2; however, this estimate is not valid at higher flow rates (above ~5 L/min). Limitations to this delivery system include the drying effect to nasal mucosa, inability to deliver high F_IO_2, and variation with respiratory variables (mouth breathing, respiratory rate, tidal volume).

Other oxygen delivery devices include simple face mask, "Venti" masks, face tents, and nonrebreather masks. **Simple face masks** deliver low flow oxygen with open expiratory vents to minimize CO_2 accumulation. These masks can deliver higher flow than nasal cannula, but can be uncomfortable; interfere with eating, speaking, and expectorating; and can allow CO_2 rebreathing. The **"Venti" mask** is a simple air-entrainment mask that delivers high flow through a sized jet orifice in conjunction with an air entrainment port to deliver a specified F_IO_2. These masks are useful because they deliver a specified F_IO_2 which is beneficial for patients with hypercapnic COPD. **Nonrebreather masks** incorporate a one-way valve allowing exhalation and a reservoir bag for inhalation. This device is capable of higher F_IO_2 delivery (60–80% at flow rates of 8–15 L/min), but the exact F_IO_2 cannot be determined accurately.

In more severe hypoxemic failure or in early hypercapnic failure, institution of noninvasive ventilation may be warranted. **Bilevel positive airway pressure** can be instituted in patients with more severe forms of pulmonary edema and COPD. This therapy should be limited to those patients in which consciousness is preserved, and to those patients in whom rapid improvement of the underlying etiology is anticipated. Noninvasive ventilation should not be considered for individuals with pneumonia, ARDS, or other conditions associated with a slow rate of clinical improvement. Inspiratory pressure should be initiated at a level that allows for adequate ventilation (typically 12–20 cmH$_2$O), and expiratory pressure initiated at a level that provides improved oxygenation (typically 6–14 cmH$_2$O). Patients should show improvement within 1–2 hours, which can be assessed by improvements in pH, respiratory rate, and PCO$_2$. For patients in whom improvement is not observed, or in whom the level of alertness declines, intubation and mechanical ventilation is warranted.

For patients with more severe respiratory impairment, rapid **intubation** and **mechanical ventilation** are indicated. This should be considered for individuals who cannot achieve oxygen saturations >88% despite supplemental oxygen with or without noninvasive ventilation. Intubation is also indicated in individuals who have developed respiratory acidosis from hypercapnic failure. Intubation should also be considered for individuals with increased respiratory effort combined with other metabolic or hemodynamic derangements such as acute myocardial infarction or septic shock. In these situations, decreasing the work of breathing is likely beneficial in improving overall outcome. The final indication for intubation is depressed mental status with loss of ability to protect the airway. In this situation, intubation will protect the lower respiratory tract from massive contamination with gastrointestinal (GI) or oropharyngeal contents. It will not prevent (and may worsen) aspiration of all oral and gastric secretions.

DEEP VENOUS THROMBOSIS AND PULMONARY EMBOLISM

Thomas D. Painter

KEY POINTS

- DVT and PE represent major causes of morbidity and mortality.
- The clinical diagnosis of both conditions is difficult, so physicians should use prediction models to direct their workup.
- Prophylaxis should be considered in all inpatients with risk factors.
- Both heparin and LMWH are effective initial therapies.
- Thrombolytic therapy is reserved for patients with life-threatening conditions.
- Vena cava interruption devices should be restricted to a few specific situations.

INTRODUCTION

Deep venous thrombosis (DVT) and pulmonary embolism (PE) are major causes of morbidity and mortality. Venous thrombosis is a very common event—approximately 5 million persons are affected each year. Many of these occur in hospitalized patients, making prevention an important issue for any inpatient. In addition, a single DVT can lead to postphlebitic syndrome, a significant cause of morbidity for those affected. Autopsy studies have consistently shown pulmonary emboli to be a major cause of inpatient mortality, frequently not diagnosed premortem.

PATHOPHYSIOLOGY

The classic risk factors (Virchow's triad) for the development of DVT include **venous stasis**, **hypercoagulability**, and **vascular injury**. Certainly, all three do not need to be present for thrombosis to occur, but some combination of those factors are usually identified. Frequently, patients are closely evaluated for hypercoagulable states, which are either inherited or acquired. Two of the most common inherited thrombophilias are factor V Leiden and prothrombin gene mutation. Factor V Leiden is a single point mutation which prevents activated factor V from being broken down by activated protein C. Prothrombin gene mutation G20210A results in an increase in prothrombin production. Although factor V Leiden and prothrombin gene mutation are quite common (5% and 2–4% of the population, respectively), most individuals with these conditions never have a thrombosis. Other inherited conditions to consider would be protein C deficiency, antithrombin III deficiency, protein S deficiency, and elevated levels of factor VIII. Two of the most common acquired hypercoagulable states occur in women who take oral contraceptives and patients with malignancy, especially adenocarcinoma (Trousseau's syndrome). Even when one of the hypercoagulable conditions is present, other factors are usually necessary for the development of a thrombosis. Other common acquired thrombophilias include pregnancy, antiphospholipid antibodies, and hyperhomocysteinemia.

The most common risk factor is venous stasis due to immobilization. As hospitalized patients are sedentary, both surgical and medical inpatients are at risk for thrombosis development. Sedentary individuals or those taking long trips are also at risk. Vascular injury is particularly important for trauma or surgery patients, particularly for those undergoing joint replacement.

PE should be considered a **complication** of DVT. Almost all clinically significant pulmonary emboli occur in patients with thrombosis in the veins of the leg. In at least one half of such patients, the leg vein thrombosis is asymptomatic. Thrombi present in the distal calf are rarely complicated by emboli. However, once thrombi extend to the proximal veins of the thigh (popliteal and femoral arteries), PE is likely. In fact, 50% of patients with proximal leg DVTs have evidence of PE on imaging studies, even though most do not have pulmonary symptoms. Arm vein thrombi very seldom lead to clinically apparent emboli.

Once a venous thrombus dislodges from the vascular wall, it invariably becomes trapped in the pulmonary vasculature, as it represents the smallest vessels to be encountered. The blockage will immediately result in an increase in pulmonary vascular resistance and right-to-left shunting of blood around the blockage. Next, irritant receptors are activated which cause hyperventilation. Also, bronchoconstriction occurs in the area of lung supplied by vessels distal to the embolus. Finally, over the next several hours, surfactant is lost in the affected area of lung resulting in atelectasis and edema. All of these contribute to the development of hypoxemia.

If the PE is large, the resulting hypoxemia and increased pulmonary vasculature resistance can cause right heart failure, a major cause of death in patients with a PE. Large obstructions will increase right heart wall tension and chamber pressures. The right ventricle is poorly adapted to increase its workload, so ischemia commonly develops resulting in a decreased cardiac output.

CLINICAL PRESENTATION

Patients with DVT will frequently complain of pain in the calf and possibly in the thigh with swelling of the soft tissues in the area involved. Examination of these patients may reveal tenderness in the musculature, erythema, and edema of the extremity which tends to be most severe in the most dependent portion of the extremity. Diagnostic maneuvers such as Homan's sign (rapid flexion of the foot leading to pain in the muscle of the calf) are nonspecific and not useful in determining whether or not a patient has a venous thrombosis. Unfortunately, the classic signs of pain, swelling, tenderness, and erythema are common with other causes for soft tissue pain. When the overall clinical presentation is evaluated, less than half of patients who are believed to have DVT ultimately are shown to have this syndrome. Alternatively, many patients with pulmonary emboli have no leg signs or symptoms at all but on diagnostic testing are found to have clots involving the deep veins of the lower extremities.

Rarely, patients with iliofemoral thrombosis may present with syndrome of phlegmasia cerulea dolens. There is swelling of the entire extremity and pain in the musculature of the thigh and the calf. These patients will have massive edema and their skin tends to be cool to the touch and violaceous. If the edema is severe, arterial flow can be restricted causing a pale leg with diminished or absent pulses (phlegmasia alba dolens).

The classic triad of PE includes chest pain (usually pleuritic), dyspnea, and hemoptysis. Unfortunately, a distinct minority of patients with pulmonary emboli have all three of these symptoms. The two most consistent symptoms are dyspnea (present in 75%) and pleuritic chest pain (present in 66%), whereas hemoptysis is unlikely.

On physical examination, the most consistent signs of PE are tachypnea and tachycardia. Fever has also been described, but is usually low grade and occurs several hours after the event. The lung examination is usually nonspecific—crackles are the most common finding. On cardiac examination, signs of right ventricular strain may be found if the PE was massive. A right ventricular heave may be palpated, the second heart sound may be accentuated, or the neck veins may be distended.

In PE, chest x-ray findings may be that of a normal chest x-ray (most common), atelectasis, or an infiltrate. If the patient has a wedge-shaped pleural-based density (Hampton's hump), the diagnosis of PE is likely. This finding is, unfortunately, very rare in patients with pulmonary emboli. Similarly, patients with marked ECG findings including the S1/Q3/T3 complex (S wave in lead I, Q wave in lead III, and T-wave inversion in lead III) and acute right ventricular strain are likely to have a PE but the ECG findings are seldom that specific. The most common abnormality on ECGs in patients with pulmonary emboli is tachycardia. Hypoxia is common but not a universal finding in patients with PE. Hypoxia may also be present in a variety of other conditions.

EVALUATION

The gold standard test for the demonstration of venous thrombosis is the venogram. Unfortunately, this test is expensive, invasive, and not universally available; therefore, noninvasive testing is usually performed. The compressive **ultrasound** can demonstrate the presence of clots in the proximal veins of the leg with a high level of sensitivity and specificity. The veins of the calf are more difficult to assess via this technique. However, the fact that calf vein thrombi seldom lead to pulmonary emboli unless there is extension of the clot leaves compressive ultrasound as the test of choice in the diagnostic approach to patients with possible venous thrombosis. Another option being used with greater frequency is computed tomography (CT) scanning of the legs, typically in conjunction with CT of the chest to evaluate for a pulmonary embolus. CT scanning is comparable to ultrasound in detecting DVT, but exclusively evaluates the proximal leg veins (not the calf veins).

The most thoroughly studied test for the diagnosis of PE is the nuclear **ventilation-perfusion (V/Q) scan**. More recently, **spiral CT scanning** has become more commonly utilized in patients with suspected PE. This test appears to be at least as good as the nuclear scan, is more readily available, and quicker to perform. The definitive test for PE is the **pulmonary angiogram**. Unfortunately, it is associated with significant morbidity and mortality and like the venogram, is not universally available.

Given the limitations of history, physical, and routine diagnostic tests, a definitive approach to the diagnosis of DVT or PE is difficult. What has improved diagnostic accuracy has been the development of clinical prediction rules which can accurately identify individuals at high risk for thromboembolism (Table 15-1). How aggressive the diagnosis of thromboembolism is approached is determined by the probability. For example, the Prospective Investigation Of Pulmonary Embolism Diagnosis (PIOPED) study has shown that in a patient with a low clinical suspicion history of PE and a low

Table 15-1 **Wells Clinical Prediction Model for Pulmonary Embolus**

Variable	Points
Clinical signs and symptoms of DVT	3.0
An alternative diagnosis is less likely than PE	3.0
Heart rate >100 beats/min	1.5
Immobilization or surgery in the previous 4 weeks	1.5
Previous DVT or PE	1.5
Hemoptysis	1.0
Malignancy (on treatment, treated in the last 6 months, or palliative)	1.0

Score	Clinical Assessment Probability
<2 points	Low probability
2–6 points	Intermediate probability
>6 points	High probability

Source: Adapted from Wells PS, Anderson DR, Rodger M, et al. Excluding pulmonary embolism at the bedside without diagnostic imaging: management of patients with suspected pulmonary embolism presenting to the emergency department by using a simple clinical model and D-dimer. *Ann Intern Med* 2001;135:98–107.

probability V/Q scan the chance the patient has had a PE is extremely small. In patients with a very strong clinical suspicion and a high probability scan the likelihood of PE is very high. However, other combinations of clinical suspicion and ventilation-perfusion outcome are less diagnostic.

A general approach to the elusive diagnosis of PE is described in Fig. 15-1. The **D-dimer**, a measurement of fibrin degradation products, has been studied extensively for evaluation of thromboembolic disease and new assays (enzyme-linked immunosorbent assay [ELISA]) have demonstrated respectable utility in certain clinical situations. For example, in the setting of a low to intermediate clinical suspicion (see Table 15-1), the D-dimer has sufficient sensitivity to exclude thromboembolic disease, and when combined with negative compression ultrasound, the negative predictive value is about 99%. However, in individuals with a high probability, a normal D-dimer has not been shown to rule out a PE. Further, elevated levels are not specific to thromboembolism and can be seen in a variety of conditions beyond clot formation. A V/Q scan and a spiral CT scan (PE protocol) are generally considered to be equivalent studies, but a negative result on either is not always sufficient to rule out a PE. Ultimately, only a pulmonary angiogram can definitively rule in or rule out a PE.

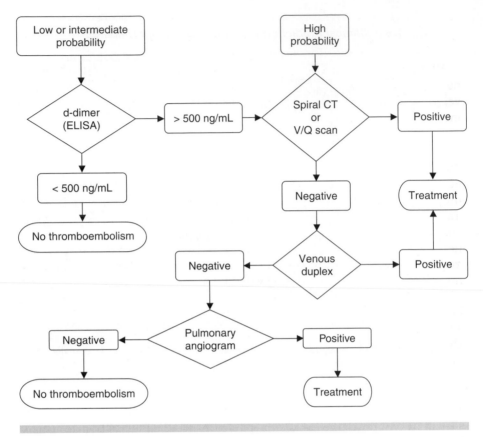

Figure 15-1 **Workup for a suspected PE.**

MANAGEMENT

Prevention

Given that most hospitalized patients have at least one risk factor for thromboembolism, prophylaxis should be considered in all inpatients. In studies, 10–40% of medical patients will develop a DVT during their hospitalization, most of whom will be asymptomatic. Recommendations suggest that the following patients should receive anticoagulation during their hospitalization:

1. Patients with congestive heart failure
2. Patients with severe respiratory disease
3. Patients who will be confined to bed and have one of the following risk factors:
   a. Active cancer
   b. Previous thromboembolism

c. Acute neurologic disease
d. Inflammatory bowel disease

Recommended anticoagulants include **low-dose unfractionated heparin** (heparin 5000 units sq q 8-12 h) or prophylactic doses of **low molecular weight heparin** (LMWH). If contraindications to heparin therapy exist, then pneumatic compression stockings should be used.

Initial Therapy

The treatment for venous thrombosis and PE utilize the same therapeutic modalities. The majority of patients are treated with anticoagulant therapy. Intravenous **heparin** is administered according to a weight-based nomogram. This dosage schedule allows the patient to reliably achieve a therapeutic anticoagulant level within 24 hours of beginning administration and therefore lowers the likelihood of embolization while on therapy. Traditionally, the desired effect is an increase in the partial thromboplastin time (PTT) to 1.5–2.5 the control value. However, considerable variability exists because of the various reagents used to perform the test. Ideally, the therapeutic PTT should be correlated to heparin levels (0.2–0.4 U/mL) or antifactor Xa activity (0.3–0.7 U/mL) to ensure adequate anticoagulation. Alternatively, **LMWH** has been shown to be as efficacious as heparin with a lower risk of bleeding. LMWH is made up of part of the heparin which has less effect on thrombin and therefore does not affect the PTT, making the monitoring of this value unnecessary. There is less protein binding and less endothelial binding which makes the response more predictable. The dosage is based on the patient's weight. LMWH is not lipid soluble and therefore dosing in morbidly obese patients is problematic. LMWH is also eliminated by the kidney, so it should not be used in patients with renal failure. The most significant advantage of LMWH is a considerable cost saving if it can be administered as an outpatient. Although LMWH is more expensive than IV heparin, the fact that it can be administered as an outpatient and thereby eliminating hospital cost has a dramatic impact on the overall cost of the therapy. LMWH has been safely utilized as outpatient therapy in patients with PE as long as the patient is hemodynamically stable and not hypoxic at presentation. Regardless of which heparin is selected, initial treatment should continue for at least 5 days.

Thrombolytic therapy has not reduced mortality or morbidity and is usually reserved for patients who are hemodynamically unstable with hypotension or refractory hypoxia.

Long-Term Therapy

Warfarin should be started the same day as heparin therapy. Loading doses of warfarin are not necessary to achieve the desired anticoagulant effect. The dosage of warfarin is monitored via the prothrombin time (PT) and the international normalized ratio (INR). The therapeutic goal for patients being treated for venous thromboembolic disease is an INR of 2–3. The patient needs to be maintained on heparin therapy for 24 hours after the INR time reaches the recommend therapeutic range. This is necessary because the effect of warfarin on the clotting cascade is not complete until 24 hours after the INR originally reaches its goal of level. The length of total anticoagulant therapy remains somewhat controversial. For patients with their first episode of uncomplicated DVT or PE secondary to a transient and reversible risk factor (i.e., immobilization), warfarin therapy is recommended for at least 3 months. If the patient has a first episode of DVT or PE which is idiopathic (no known risk factors), therapy is recommended for 6–12 months and lifetime anticoagulation should be considered. Any patient with a second episode of DVT or PE or a hypercoagulable state, warfarin therapy is recommended for life.

Devices such as the **Greenfield filter** and the bird's nest filter have been developed which can be inserted intravenously and be implanted in the vena cava. These devices provide short-term protection (as short as 2 weeks) against embolization in patients with venous thrombosis. The devices can become occluded which increases the likelihood of symptomatic postphlebitic syndrome. **Postphlebitic syndrome** is the development of venous insufficiency after a DVT. If at all possible, patient who have a vena cava interruption device inserted should be maintained on anticoagulant therapy. The accepted indications for insertion of one of these devices are:

1. Recurrent embolization on therapeutic anticoagulation
2. Absolute contraindications to anticoagulant therapy
3. Septic thromboembolism
4. Near fatal PE
5. Recurrent pulmonary emboli

EVALUATION
OF DYSPNEA

R. Scott Morehead

KEY POINTS

- Dyspnea is a symptom of multiple causes and varied pathophysiologic mechanisms.
- In acute onset dyspnea, evaluation begins with the ABCs: airway, breathing, and circulation.
- Normal (or nearly normal) blood gasses should not be the sole mechanism to exclude serious underlying pathology.
- Patients with dyspnea and a clear chest x-ray: consider airways disease (both small airways and central airways), pulmonary vascular disease, subtle interstitial lung disease, and diastolic heart failure (especially if dyspnea is chronic).
- Most important tests for patients with dyspnea out of proportion to chest x-ray findings: spirometry, echocardiography, and chest CT scanning (by appropriate protocol).

INTRODUCTION

Dyspnea is produced by pathologic processes of several organs, including the lungs, heart, upper airway, and neuromuscular system, and can occasionally be a manifestation of psychiatric, gastrointestinal, and hematologic disease. Despite its inherent poor specificity, new or worsening dyspnea must be viewed with utmost gravity.

121

PATHOPHYSIOLOGY

Shortness of breath (dyspnea) is often the patient's shorthand for one or more distinct sensations such as chest tightness, inability to get a deep breath, increased effort of breathing, difficulty with exhalation, shallow breathing, heavy breathing, and others. For example, investigators have determined that although patients with asthma and congestive heart failure (CHF) both report dyspnea, their subjective experience is demonstrably different. Dyspnea may be produced by the following mechanisms:

- Poorly functioning respiratory muscles (e.g., phrenic nerve disorders, amyotrophic lateral sclerosis, Guillain-Barre syndrome, myasthenia gravis, and polymyositis)
- Increased stiffness of the lungs and/or chest wall (i.e., pulmonary fibrosis and pulmonary edema)
- Increased resistance of the airways (e.g., asthma, emphysema)
- Stimulation of irritant receptors in the lung (e.g., interstitial edema from CHF)
- Inadequate cardiac output (e.g., CHF, primary pulmonary hypertension)
- Hypercarbia (increased arterial PCO_2)
- Hypoxemia (decreased arterial PO_2)

The brainstem respiratory center produces contraction of the diaphragm through neural output traversing the spinal cord and phrenic nerves, resulting in displacement of the chest wall, airflow into the lungs, alveolar gas exchange, and finally exhalation (together recognized as breathing). The respiratory center also produces a concurrent neural discharge to the cerebrum which is not consciously perceived in usual circumstances. Dyspnea is produced when the neural output of the respiratory center (the perceived "effort") does not conform to the expected outcome in terms of chest wall expansion and airflow. Contrary to popular opinion, hypoxemia is only a mild stimulus for the production of dyspnea. Alterations in blood gases, and their effect on chemoreceptors, due to altered respiratory physiology are just one part of this schema.

The following example demonstrates this principle: an asthmatic patient presents to the emergency department with wheezing and respiratory distress. Initial pulse oximetry reveals an oxygen saturation of 92% on room air. Inhaled β-agonists are administered, and the patient has improved airflow and subjective decrease in dyspnea. However, the oxygen saturation is observed to have decreased to 88%. What has transpired? Answer: β-agonists not only dilate airways resulting in improved airflow, they may also dilate pulmonary vessels, producing transient hypoxemia due to perturbed ventilation-perfusion relationships. But note that the patient feels better despite the lower PO_2!

One application of this concept is that blood gasses should not be the sole means of assessing the "reality" or significance of a patient's dyspnea; serious pathology may be missed or underestimated if this fallacy is practiced.

CLINICAL PRESENTATION

Dyspnea not surprisingly accompanies essentially all serious cardiorespiratory disease, and as such, is a common complaint. Dyspnea rarely remains an etiologic mystery for long, and generally speaking, the responsible disease will come to dominate the mind of the treating physician. Severity is assessed using the New York Heart Association classification (see Chap. 9), which places this symptom in the context of physical activity. Be aware that patients with slowly progressive disease may self-limit their activities to avoid the experience of dyspnea, and as such, their objective physiologic impairment may be far more severe than expected from history alone.

The medical literature is remarkably sparse concerning the subject of dyspnea of unknown cause. Case series, notably from pulmonary referral clinics, describe pulmonary disorders (i.e., asthma, emphysema, and interstitial lung disease) as the most common culprits followed by heart failure and pulmonary vascular disorders (i.e., pulmonary embolism [PE], pulmonary hypertension). Other responsible diseases include a grab bag of upper airway disorders (including postnasal drip), psychiatric conditions, neuromuscular disease, cardiac arrhythmia, thyroid dysfunction, deconditioning, and gastroesophageal reflux. Using this as guidance, the following is a suggested list of conditions to consider. Obviously, the patient's demography will modify the likelihood of each disorder.

Pulmonary Parenchymal Disorders

The most important diagnosis to consider is **asthma**, and the history to seek is: (1) temporal variability in dyspnea severity (i.e., time of day, nocturnal, and seasonal), (2) associated cough and wheeze, (3) relation to possible inhaled irritants/allergens and/or exercise. **Emphysema** should be considered in the elderly smoker; however, neither old age nor smoking is required for its development (i.e., α-1-antitrypsin deficiency). Environmental exposure history (i.e., silica, coal dust, asbestos) should prompt consideration of **interstitial lung disease**, as should a known history of collagen vascular disease. Most cases of emphysema and interstitial disease produce insidious onset of dyspnea with progression measured in months to years. Useful physical examination findings to seek include finger clubbing and abnormal auscultation. In particular, fine inspiratory crackles (Velcro-like) strongly suggest interstitial lung disease. The presence of wheezes, while suggesting pathologic involvement of the airways, does not equate to the diagnosis of asthma.

Heart Failure

The patient with heart failure may complain of air hunger, a feeling of suffocation, and rapid breathing, often with prominent easy fatigability. Up to half the patients with clinical heart failure retain fairly normal left ventricular systolic function; when compared to patients with impaired systolic function, these patients are disproportionately female and elderly, often with markers of the metabolic syndrome (i.e., diabetes and obesity). Examination findings consistent with cardiac failure should be sought (jugular vein distention [JVD], S₃ gallop, edema), but these are often lacking in patients with diastolic heart failure in part due to concomitant obesity (see Chap. 9).

Pulmonary Vascular Disease

For purposes of this discussion two entities should be considered, PE and primary pulmonary hypertension. While inflammation of the pulmonary vasculature (i.e., pulmonary vasculitis) produces dyspnea, the radiographic abnormalities tend to become the focus of the case presentation. **Pulmonary hypertension** occurs due to decreased aggregate vascular surface area with resultant increase in right ventricular afterload and limitation to cardiac output. If this increased vascular resistance occurs slowly and progressively, as in primary pulmonary hypertension, the patient's main complaint is exertional dyspnea. By contrast, if the increased resistance occurs rapidly, as in the case of a large **PE**, impressive symptoms such as central chest pain (simulating acute myocardial infarction [MI]), syncope, and sudden death may occur (see Chap. 15). In either situation, the patient's limitation/symptoms are out of proportion to the chest x-ray abnormalities and without evidence of left heart disease. Specific findings, including right-sided third heart sound, neck vein distention, loud second heart sound, and pulmonary insufficiency murmur, are often noted in long-standing pulmonary hypertension, but are completely unreliable in the assessment of a patient with suspected acute PE.

Upper Airway Disorders

Particularly in acute dyspnea, obstruction of the upper airway or trachea is important to consider. Obstruction can occur from the aspiration of food or a foreign body, or from angioedema. A history of allergy and other physical examination signs of anaphylaxis or angioedema (i.e., hives, facial edema) are important to elicit. **Paradoxical vocal cord dysfunction (PVCD),** a conversion disorder manifesting as a respiratory disease (a.k.a. pseudoasthma), more commonly presents as chronic dyspnea. Predominantly a disorder in women, there are associations with work in the health care field and experience with true asthma (either personal or family). PVCD may closely mimic asthma, and often these patients suffer horrendous complications of chronic steroid use. Consider this disorder in the appropriate setting, and especially when the patient with "difficult asthma" exhibits any of the following:

physician-seeking behavior, a demanding nature, wheezing predominantly over the larynx, and rapid cure by tracheal intubation. That said, be careful in quickly ascribing a patient's symptoms to PVCD; many patients have concomitant true asthma and PVCD.

EVALUATION

Dyspnea of uncertain etiology is by definition a diagnostic challenge. Evaluation should be guided by the patient's acuity of illness—priority is given to conditions of a life-threatening nature; as such, it is poor form for the patient to expire in the pulmonary function lab due to massive PE. What follows is a general plan for patients with dyspnea of uncertain etiology (prior history and examination is assumed):

Acute Dyspnea

The important concerns are the ABCs:

1. Ensure the patient's upper airway and trachea are not obstructed. Diagnoses such as laryngeal edema, foreign body, and epiglottitis should be excluded by direct visualization, assessment for stridor, and the ability to phonate.
2. Assess for acute cardiac disease with clinical examination and ECG. Remember that conditions other than acute MI (i.e., tamponade, acute valve rupture, and isolated right ventricular infarct) may present without diagnostic ECG findings, but the examination should be telling in these cases (see Chap. 7).
3. Obtain a chest x-ray; many diseases become immediately obvious after this step.

If the diagnosis is unclear after these steps, there are three tests to consider: imaging study to evaluate for PE, spirometry with flow-volume loop to assess asthma, emphysema, and tracheal obstruction, and echocardiography to assess cardiac function. Serum brain natriuretic peptide (BNP) testing has been applied to the evaluation of acute dyspnea. While high BNP levels help identify cardiac dysfunction, it is important to understand that right ventricular stretch (as may occur from PE) may produce an elevated BNP, and that chronic heart disease (with associated high BNP) does not preclude additional pathology.

Chronic Dyspnea

Practically speaking, chronic dyspnea has been present for more than a week and does not require acute intervention. Conditions producing chronic dyspnea may present acutely during an exacerbation, however, careful history and examination should disclose a disorder of longer duration. As for acute dyspnea, heart and lung disease are the most important conditions, whereas disorders such as laryngeal edema, MI, and PE are unlikely. The primacy of the history and examination is difficult to overstate in this evaluation.

If the chest x-ray suggests previously unrecognized heart or lung disease, testing for the presumptive diagnosis should be done (i.e., chest computed tomography [CT] scan and/or pulmonary function testing for lung disease), and evaluation of these patients will not be further discussed.

If the chest x-ray is normal (or nearly normal), diagnoses to be considered are asthma (and other obstructive diseases), upper airway disease, pulmonary hypertension, radiographically unapparent interstitial lung disease, and cardiac disease unassociated with an enlarged heart (i.e., diastolic heart failure). Spirometry provides numerical values for forced vital capacity (FVC) and forced expiratory volume in 1 second (FEV_1), with profiles including normal or abnormal, the latter grouped as either obstructive or restrictive. Visual inspection of the flow-volume loop may add valuable information beyond the numerical data (see Chap. 18 in the *First Exposure to Internal Medicine: Ambulatory Medicine*).

If normal spirometry and flow-volume loop are returned, airways disease is unlikely with the important exception of exercise-induced asthma; however, these patients should not complain of dyspnea with usual daily activities.

The next most useful tests are **echocardiography** and **chest CT scanning**. Echocardiography is the best screening test for pulmonary hypertension, and if the estimated pulmonary systolic pressure is ≥35–40 mmHg (elevated), CT pulmonary angiography (PE protocol CT) should be performed to exclude central thromboemboli. Chest CT scanning (high-resolution protocol) is also the best test to evaluate suspected but unapparent (by x-ray) interstitial lung disease.

If after the performance of spirometry, echocardiography, and chest CT scanning by both PE and high-resolution protocols no clear explanation for the patient's dyspnea is obtained, specialty referral should be contemplated. Often an integrated cardiopulmonary exercise test will be helpful in these cases.

PNEUMONIA

Simrit Bhullar
James R. McCormick
Malkanthie I. McCormick

KEY POINTS

- Pneumonia should be strongly considered in patients who present with an acute onset of fever, cough, dyspnea +/− chest discomfort, tachypnea, and bronchial breath sounds. The CXR will help confirm the diagnosis, but infiltrates may not be impressive early in the disease.
- CAP may be safely treated on an outpatient basis in patients who are otherwise healthy with stable vital signs and without respiratory distress; common first-line antibiotics are a macrolide or doxycycline.
- HAP and HCAP often involve multidrug-resistant organisms, such as *Pseudomonas, Acinetobacter,* and MRSA.

INTRODUCTION

In 1898, Sir William Osler characterized pneumonia as ". . . the friend of the aged. Taken off by it in an acute, short, often painless illness, the old escape those 'cold gradations of decay' that make the last state of all so distressing." While our treatment strategies for pneumonia have improved considerably since Osler's time, the mortality of pneumonia among the elderly is still a significant problem. Mortality rates approach 15% in hospitalized patients, and are much higher in certain populations (e.g., nursing home residents, patients with significant comorbidities). Pneumonia and influenza are noted to be the seventh leading cause of death in the United States. Approximately 4 million adult patients are diagnosed with community-acquired pneumonias (CAP) every year resulting in over $12 billion in annual health care costs.

PATHOPHYSIOLOGY

Pneumonia is the result of an infectious pathogen overwhelming a host's defense system. These infectious pathogens may be introduced to the host through microaspiration of material from a previously colonized oropharynx (pneumococcus, *Haemophilus influenzae*, *Staphylococcus aureus*, and *Pseudomonas*), inhalation (*Mycobacterium tuberculosis*, histoplasmosis, *Legionella*, *Pneumocystis jiroveci*, *Aspergillus*, and viruses), direct spread (some

Table 17-1 **Common Etiologies of Pneumonia**

Patient Population	Consider the Following Organisms
Healthy adult	Pneumococcus, *M. pneumoniae*, Chlamydia, viral
Smoker and/or COPD	Pneumococcus, *H. influenzae*, *Moraxella catarrhalis*
Alcoholic or nursing home resident	Pneumococcus, *H. influenzae*, *Klebsiella*, aspiration, *S. aureus*, TB
Neutropenia	Pneumococcus, gram negatives (*Escherichia coli*, *Klebsiella pneumoniae*, *Pseudomonas*, *H. influenzae*, *Enterobacter* species), *S. aureus*, fungi (*Candida*, *Aspergillus*)
Alcohol or IV drug abuse	Aspiration pneumonia, noncompliance with prior therapy
Altered mental status, seizures	Aspiration pneumonia—oral and anaerobic bacteria
Recent exposure to animals/birds	*Chlamydophila psitacci*, *Francisella tularensis*, *Coxiella burnetti*, or Hantavirus
Exposure to animal placentas	*C. burnetii*
HIV infection	Pneumococcus, *H. influenzae*, *P. jiroveci*, TB, aerobic gram-negative rods (*E. coli*, *Klebsiella*), MAC (Mycobacterium-avium complex), fungi (*Cryptococcus*, Histo, *Aspergillus*), cytomegalovirus (CMV), toxoplasmosis
Chronic disease history	Gram-negative bacilli or *S. aureus*
Travel to the Southwest or Ohio–Mississippi River Valley	*Coccidioides immitis* or *Histoplasma capsulatum*
Midwest or Southwestern Travel	Blastomycoses
Postviral (i.e., influenza).	Pneumococcus, *S. aureus*

viruses), hematogenous dissemination (i.e., bacterial endocarditis), and direct inoculation (from tracheal intubation).

Patients with an inadequate immune response (i.e., from underlying comorbidities such as diabetes, HIV, chronic obstructive pulmonary disease [COPD], and advanced age) or anatomic abnormalities (such as bronchiectasis or airway obstruction) are particularly susceptible to these pathogens. Even patients with relatively normal host defense systems may be afflicted with pneumonia if exposed to a particularly large inoculum of microorganisms or a particularly virulent strain.

The most common cause by far of CAP in all patient populations is *Streptococcus pneumoniae*. However, other pathogens should be suspected in different situations, as in Table 17-1.

CLINICAL PRESENTATION

Patients with a "typical" pneumonia syndrome (traditionally caused by *S. pneumoniae*) classically present with sudden onset of fever, cough productive of purulent sputum, dyspnea, pleuritic chest pain, signs of pulmonary consolidation, and a lobar infiltrate on chest x-ray (CXR). Patients with an "atypical" pattern (i.e., caused by *Mycoplasma pneumoniae*, *Chlamydophila pneumoniae*, also *S. pneumoniae*, and less commonly *Legionella*) classically present with a more gradual onset of symptoms, dry cough, more extrapulmonary symptoms (headache, myalgias, sore throat, gastrointestinal [GI] disturbances, and, especially in the elderly, confusion), less toxic appearing on physical examination with perhaps a few crackles, with a patchy or diffuse infiltrate on CXR. However, considerable overlap occurs between these patterns. In addition, patients with intact immune systems will generally present with the more typical symptoms such as productive cough, fever, and shortness of breath, while elderly or immunocompromised patients may present more atypically and subtly. In addition to characterizing the acute symptoms, the history should focus on any comorbid illnesses (i.e., diabetes, HIV), recent hospitalizations, recent contacts, travel, tuberculosis (TB) exposures, and diseases that may mimic pneumonia (i.e., congestive heart failure [CHF], pulmonary embolism [PE]; see Chap. 16). The physical examination should focus on the patient's general appearance (i.e., in severe distress or not), vital signs (fever, tachycardia, tachypnea), and the lung examination, as well as remembering to check the patient for any signs of disorders which may mimic pneumonia (i.e., jugular vein distention [JVD], pedal edema, S_3, new murmurs, and unilateral lower extremity swelling). The lung examination will generally show dry crackles. Dullness to percussion can represent areas of consolidation or pleural effusion. In areas of consolidation, one may note changes in tactile fremitus, increased whispered pectoriloquy (one can hear whispered words more clearly through consolidated tissue than fluid), and egophony ("e" to "a" changes).

EVALUATION

Lab studies include a **complete blood count (CBC) with differential** (the WBC count is usually elevated with a left shift, but may also be normal: a low WBC count is an ominous sign, as it may reflect an immune system that is overwhelmed) and an **arterial blood gas (ABG)** or some measure of oxygenation (i.e., pulse oximetry) if the patient is dyspneic. The ABG is not always performed, but may be helpful in determining whether or not to admit a patient (PO_2 <60 mmHg on room air is considered a standard criteria for hospital admission). Consider more focused serologic testing when clinically appropriate, such as an HIV test in patients with risk factors, a cold-agglutinin test or *M. pneumoniae* immunoglobulin M titer; or a *Legionella* test (urine antigen). **Blood cultures** should be performed, as especially patients with pneumococcal pneumonia may be bacteremic.

The role of sputum **Gram stain and sputum cultures** in patients with CAP is controversial. When deep respiratory cultures can be obtained (i.e., through an endotracheal tube, or a protected brush), the findings on these studies can be accurate and useful. However, such sputum retrieval is not practical for most uncomplicated CAP, and sputum obtained from a cough, passing through, and being contaminated by one's usual mouth flora, is less useful. Indeed, the poor positive and negative predictive values of sputum Gram stain and cultures have been documented in many studies. Nevertheless, expert panels suggest that sputum Gram stain be attempted in all patients with CAP, and sputum culture obtained for all those hospitalized, ideally before the administration of antibiotics. The value of the test will be enhanced if the specimen is truly sputum, not saliva; evidence of an "adequate" sputum sample is if the Gram stain has >25 WBCs and <10 squamous epithelial cells per high powered field. Classic Gram stain appearances include: pneumococcus (lancet-shaped gram-positive diplococci; see Fig. 17-1); *H. influenzae* (pleomorphic small coccobacillary gram-negative organisms); and *K. pneumoniae* (encapsulated gram-negative bacilli). Remember that the Gram stain may be negative in pneumonias caused by *Legionella*, viral, or some atypical pneumonias.

A **CXR** usually confirms the diagnosis, although it may be falsely negative within the first 24 hours or in patients with severe neutropenia. Contrary to popular belief, there is no evidence to suggest that dehydrated patients may have less of an infiltrate; any "blossoming" of an infiltrate over 24 hours most likely reflects the natural course of the inflammatory process, not a consequence of IV hydration. CXR patterns may be useful, with a lobar pneumonia classic for pneumococcus, and interstitial pneumonia suggesting *Mycoplasma* (or *Pneumocystis* in immunosuppressed patients), although no pattern is pathognomic of the specific cause. Apical infiltrates suggest TB (see Chap. 15 in the *First Exposure to Internal Medicine: Ambulatory Medicine*). Other findings may be pleural effusions, cavitations, or air-fluid levels (suggest

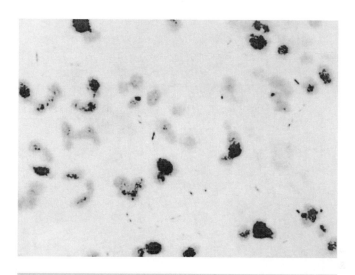

Figure 17-1 **Gram-stained sputum from a patient with pneumococcal pneumonia shows polymorphonuclear cells with no epithelial cells, indicating the origin of the sample in inflammatory exudate without contamination. Slightly pleomorphic gram-positive coccobacilli appear, generally in pairs. Displacement of stained proteinaceous background material outlines a capsule surrounding some of the organisms. When obtained from a patient with pneumonia, a sample like this one is highly specific in identifying the pneumococcus as the etiologic agent.** (*Source:* Reproduced with permission from Kasper DL, Braunwald E, Fauci AS, et al. *Harrison's Principles of Internal Medicine*, 16th ed. New York: McGraw-Hill, 2005, Figure 119-2.)

an abscess, as in aspiration pneumonia). Infiltrates will persist on CXR for up to 4–6 weeks, so unless there is clinical deterioration, there is no need for "following" serial x-rays in a patient (see Fig. 17-2).

Bronchoscopy may be important if the patient is not responding to appropriate antibiotic therapy within the first 48–72 hours, in immunocompromised patients or in patients with recurrent pneumonias in the same areas (the pneumonia may represent postbronchial obstruction from a cancer, for instance). For some severely ill patients, early bronchoscopy may be especially important. For example, in a patient with AIDS and a severe pneumonia, *P. jiroveci* sometimes warrants both antibiotics and systemic steroids. However, the patient could have other causes of pneumonia that steroids could worsen (TB, fungal), and therefore precise diagnosis may need to be made, and can sometimes be done from specimens obtained at bronchoscopy.

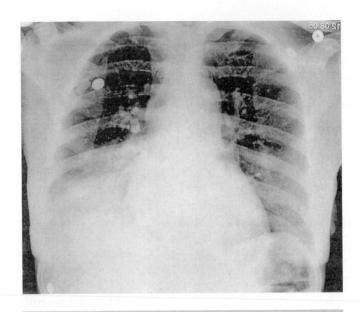

Figure 17-2 **Radiographic appearance of a right lower lobe pneumonia.** (*Source:* Reproduced with permission from Stone KC, Humphries RL. *Current Emergency Diagnosis & Treatment*, 5th ed. New York: McGraw-Hill, 2004, Figure 11-6.)

MANAGEMENT

Decision to admit: While most cases of CAP may be safely treated in an outpatient setting, recognizing CAP patients who are in need of hospitalization is a critical part of obtaining appropriate treatment for these patients. Several decision support tools have been developed to help identify patients at risk for death from pneumonia, and who therefore should be hospitalized. One commonly used tool was derived from the Pneumonia Patient Outcomes Research Team (PORT). In this schema, "points" are assigned for various risk factors, such as age (1 point for each year of life, minus 10 points for women, who tend to be hardier), risk factors (nursing home is 10 points), comorbidities (CHF, cancer, stroke, renal or liver disease), and various physical examination and laboratory findings. Persons with more than 90 "points" have 8–9% 30-day mortality, and therefore should be admitted. In general, older patients with the above comorbid conditions should be admitted. The decision to admit patients meeting criteria for physical examination or laboratory risk is generally straightforward, as these represent critically ill patients (i.e., hypoxic, hypotensive, and/or acidotic). One important question to ask as one considers therapy and admission is: "why is this not tuberculosis?" Certainly patients with fever, night sweats, weight loss, and apical infiltrates would be thought to have TB, but in less clear-cut situations, if one cannot give good reasons why the pneumonia is not TB, one should do further diagnostic testing, and if the patient is admitted, the patient should be in respiratory isolation until TB is ruled out.

Antibiotic choice needs to take into account the most likely organisms (always pneumococcus, but other organisms in other situations), but not choosing an antibiotic so broad as to select out resistant organisms, in that patient and in the public at large (see Chap. 50). In general, if you suspect a patient of having CAP, **do not delay** prompt treatment, starting appropriate empiric antibiotics therapy within 4–6 hours.

For otherwise **healthy patients** with no recent antibiotic use (within 90 days), appropriate initial therapy could include a **macrolide (azithromycin)** or **doxycycline**. For **older patients with comorbidities** (COPD, diabetes and/or renal failure), many experts recommend **both a macrolide and high-dose amoxicillin (or amoxicillin-clavulanate)**; some authorities recommend this combination even in young patients if they have had recent antibiotics, given the risk of drug-resistant pneumococcus. An alternative to a macrolide in these higher-risk patients would be a **respiratory fluoroquinolone** (gatifloxacin, levofloxacin, moxifloxacin).

For **inpatients** with no risk factors for pseudomonal infection (i.e., those without structural lung disease such as bronchiectasis/cystic fibrosis, or not recently hospitalized, especially in an ICU), options could include an advanced **macrolide** (azithromycin), generally with the addition of a **beta-lactam** (ceftriaxone, cefotaxime, ampicillin-sulbactam); alternatively one could use a respiratory fluoroquinolone, although many authorities try to reserve these for more serious infections, to prevent antibiotic resistance. Patients at risk for pseudomonas will be discussed in hospital-acquired pneumonia (HAP), below.

Any patient who does not respond appropriately to the initial treatment should be carefully reevaluated for other potential causes (i.e., endobronchial obstruction causing a postobstructive pneumonia, or extrapulmonary sites of infection such as an empyema or pericarditis). This evaluation may include CT scans, bronchoscopy, and/or consultation with a pulmonary or infectious disease specialist. Other indications for referral include a rapidly progressive pneumonia (infiltrates increasing by more than 50% within 48 hours), unusual pathogens, or relapse after initial response to therapy. Never forget that pneumonia is a serious, potentially fatal disease, and complications often occur, including pleural effusion, empyema, septic shock, and respiratory failure (see Chaps. 14, 18, and 49). Other supportive therapy includes supplemental oxygen as needed (to maintain O_2 saturation >90%), tight blood sugar control (see Chap. 39), proper nutrition, antipyretics, and analgesia. Before discharge, patients should be counseled on **smoking cessation**.

In addition, in those not immunized, **influenza and pneumococcal vaccinations** should be given before discharge from the hospital or at the 6-week follow-up examination. Patient should be advised that postinfectious cough may last for up to 8 weeks, although it should improve with time. Also, tell patients that it may take several months for them to return to their normal vigor.

HAP is defined as pneumonia that occurs 48 hours or more after admission which was not incubating at the time of admission. Patients with **early-onset HAP** (within 4 days of admission) with no risk factors for multidrug-resistant organisms (not in an ICU; no recent antibiotic use or hospitalizations) can be treated with similar antibiotics as CAP, such as a **beta-lactam antibiotic (i.e., ceftriaxone, ampicillin-sulbactam) or a respiratory fluoroquinolone. However, patients with ventilator-associated pneumonia, late-onset HAP, or those with recent antibiotic use or hospitalization are at risk for infection with multidrug-resistant organisms, such as methicillin-resistant** *Staphylococcus aureus* **(MRSA), resistant** *Pseudomonas, Acinetobacter*, **and other gram-negative organisms (e.g.,** *Enterobacter, Klebsiella*), **and are managed differently.** Every effort should be made to obtain deep respiratory quantitative cultures, ideally before antibiotics are administered. Antibiotics possibilities include **antipseudomonal carbapenems** (imipenem or meropenem), **fluoroquinolones** (levofloxacin, ciprofloxacin), or **beta-lactam inhibitors** (piperacillin-tazobactam), or an **aminoglycoside** (see Chap. 50). **MRSA** may require **vancomycin**, or considering the poor lung tissue penetration of vancomycin, **linezolid**. To prevent the pressure for resistance, antibiotics in general for HAP should not be given for more than 7–8 days. Recent guidelines make special mention of **health care-associated pneumonia (HCAP)**, who are presumed at risk for multidrug-resistant organisms, and should be treated like late-onset HAP. Those at risk for HCAP include those hospitalized for >2 days within 90 days of the infection; those residing in a nursing home or long-term care facility; those who have received IV antibiotics, wound care, or chemotherapy within 30 days of the infection; and those who attend a hospital or hemodialysis clinic.

Aspiration pneumonitis is frequently encountered in hospitalized and nursing home patients, with acute lung injury occurring from aspiration of regurgitated gastric contents. Acute symptoms can be dramatic, with wheezing, cough, dyspnea, accompanied by hypoxemia and CXR findings. In response to this chemical insult, some of these patients even progress to severe acute respiratory distress syndrome and death. However, the gastric contents aspirated are sterile, and antibiotics should NOT be administered in this situation, as they would only serve to select out resistant organisms. In contrast, **aspiration pneumonia** develops after the inhalation of large amounts of colonized oropharyngeal mouth flora. Risk factors include those with depressed consciousness (drug or alcohol intoxication or overdose; general anesthesia; seizures), those being intubated or extubated, those with neurologic disorders which depress gag reflex or swallowing (strokes), and those with nasogastric or enteral feeding tubes. If the patient has poor dentition, anaerobes are a big concern (although interestingly, patients with no teeth don't usually have periodontal disease). Antibiotic choice in this situation could include **clindamycin** or amoxicillin-clavulanate. Complications include the development of lung abscess, empyema, and necrotizing pneumonia.

The CDC (Centers for Disease Control), IDSA (Infectious Disease Society of America), and ATS (American Thoracic Society) are organizations which release guidelines regarding the appropriate treatment of pneumonias. These guidelines are revised frequently, so please review their recommendations periodically to make sure they haven't changed. The Web sites for these organizations are: www.cdc.gov, www.idsociety.org, and www.thoracic.org.

PLEURAL EFFUSION

Paula Bailey

KEY POINTS

- Diagnostic thoracentesis and subsequent pleural fluid analysis can help one distinguish transudative causes of pleural effusions from exudative causes.
- Transudative pleural effusions occur from CHF, ascites, nephrotic syndrome, and hypothyroidism, among other causes.
- Exudative causes include infection, malignancy, PE, pancreatitis, and connective tissue disease.
- Empyema warrants chest tube placement for drainage.

INTRODUCTION

The pleural space is the space that exists between the visceral pleura, which covers the entire surface of the lung except at the hilum, and the parietal pleura, which covers the inner surface of the chest wall, the diaphragm, and the mediastinum. This space is normally occupied by a very small amount of fluid (5–15 mL). This fluid is formed in the normal healthy individual at a rate of approximately 0.1 mL/kg/h. Movement of fluid in and out of the pleural space is dependent on hydrostatic and osmotic forces. When there is an abnormal increase in this fluid, the resulting condition is a pleural effusion. Pleural effusion is fairly common and is not a diagnosis in and of itself but rather a result of an underlying condition.

PATHOPHYSIOLOGY

Pathophysiology can best be discussed when broken down by type of effusion. There are two basic types of pleural effusion, **transudative** and **exudative**. Transudative effusions are a result of Starling forces, in which fluid filtration exceeds reabsorption and there is a net accumulation of fluid in the

Table 18-1 **Transudative Vs. Exudative Effusions**

Transudate	Exudate
CHF	Infections
Nephrotic syndrome	Bacterial and viral pneumonia
Cirrhosis with ascites	Parapneumonic
Peritoneal dialysis	TB
Myxedema/hypothyroidism	Other infections
SVC syndrome	Malignancy
PE	Bronchogenic
	Metastatic
	Breast
	Lymphoma
	Mesothelioma
	Connective tissue disease (RA, SLE)
	Intra-abdominal disease (subphrenic abscess, pancreatitis)
	Chylothorax PE drug-induced pleural disease

Abbreviations: SVC, superior vena cava; RA, rheumatoid arthritis; SLE, systemic lupus erythematosus.

pleural space. This imbalance can be caused by increased hydrostatic pressures, as in congestive heart failure (CHF), or decreased oncotic pressures as in severe hypoalbuminemia due to nephrotic syndrome. Exudative effusions can be as simple as disruption of the vasculature resulting in a hemothorax or disruption of the thoracic duct leading to a chylothorax, but may be a more complex process caused by altered permeability of the pulmonary vessels due to inflammation of the pleurae. This is most commonly seen in malignant, infectious, or rheumatologic processes. See Table 18-1 for conditions that produce transudates versus exudates, keeping in mind that some conditions can produce either form (pulmonary embolism [PE]), and in some conditions the initial effusion will appear transudative but progress to exudative as the disease progesses.

CLINICAL PRESENTATION

Pleural effusions are often asymptomatic, but can cause chest pain or shortness of breath due to mechanical compression of the lung and irritation of the parietal pleura. The constellation of presenting symptoms often holds indications of underlying diagnosis (e.g., classic symptoms of CHF or fever suggesting an infectious process). The physical examination may show tachypnea, fever, and tachycardia, with evidence of the underlying abnormality (such as ascites). The lung examination will be characterized by decreased or absent breath sounds over the area of effusion, with decreased tactile fremitus and dullness to percussion. One might also detect egophony, crackles, and bronchial breath sounds in the area of compressed lung above the effusion.

EVALUATION

Chest x-ray will confirm the effusion (Fig. 18-1). However, effusions of <250 mL are often not seen on posterior-anterior (PA) upright chest radiographs. When seen, an effusion most often will cause blunting of the costophrenic angles. Larger effusions can cause opacities at the base, concave meniscus at the superior border of the effusion (meniscus sign), and opacification of the fissures. Lateral decubitus chest films with the effusion side down can be helpful in detecting smaller effusions or evaluating for loculation of larger effusions. Free flowing effusions will flow with gravity. Other findings on plain chest radiograph may be due to the causative etiology, for example, pulmonary edema, cardiomegaly, masses, and lymphadenopathy. **Computed tomography (CT) scan** is more sensitive for detecting small effusions and can define loculations if present. **Ultrasound** is useful for defining the size of effusions especially if small. It can also be helpful prior to thoracentesis of small or loculated effusions to mark for needle insertion.

Pleural Fluid Findings

The first step in diagnosing the cause of a pleural effusion is to ascertain whether the fluid is transudative or exudative. This is done by analysis of the fluid obtained by thoracentesis and comparison to serum (see Chap. 3). This evaluation is based on criteria defined by Light and colleagues (Light criteria). Fluid is classified as **exudative** if it meets one of these criteria:

- Pleural fluid to serum protein ratio >0.5
- Pleural fluid to serum lactate dehydrogenase (LDH) ratio >0.6
- Pleural fluid LDH greater than two-thirds of normal serum values

Recent meta-analyses suggest pleural fluid analysis alone may have sensitivity and specificity comparable to Light's criteria. Exudates have at least one of the following:

- Pleural fluid LDH >0.45 of upper limit of normal serum values
- Pleural fluid cholesterol >45 mg/dL
- Pleural fluid protein >2.9 g/dL

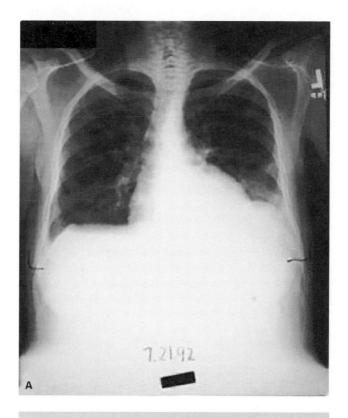

Figure 18-1 **Pleural effusion. (A) The elevation of the left hemidiaphragm may be caused by a pleural effusion at the left base. The appropriate way to determine the nature of this abnormality is to obtain a left lateral decubitus film (see B). (B) The lateral decubitus film in the same patient demonstrates a very large left pleural effusion. In looking at the upright view of the chest, it is clear that the effusion was beneath the left lung and therefore had a contour simulating that of an elevated left hemidiaphragm.** (*Courtesy of H. Goldberg.*) (*Source:* Reproduced with permission from Tierney LM, McPhee SJ, Papadakis MA, et al. *Current Medical Diagnosis & Treatment,* 2006 Online Edition. New York: McGraw-Hill, Cardiology Section-Pleural Effusion Section.)

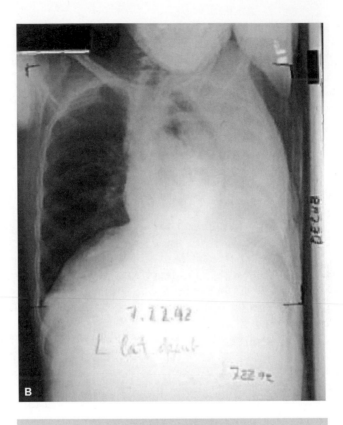

*Figure 18-1 **(Continued)***

In addition, the appearance of the fluid can be helpful. Grossly bloody fluid suggests cancer, PE, or trauma (sometimes from the thoracentesis). One can send the pleural fluid for a hematocrit. If the pleural fluid hematocrit is <1% that of the serum, this is clinically insignificant blood, likely from the procedure. A pleural fluid hematocrit 1–20% that of serum suggests cancer or PE, sometimes trauma; a pleural hematocrit >50% serum suggests hemothorax. Pleural fluid that is grossly turbid or milky could suggest a chylothorax; a pleural fluid triglyceride level >110 mg/dL confirms chylothorax, most often from trauma to the thoracic duct or from mediastinal tumors, especially lymphoma.

In addition, other studies can be helpful. These include:

- **Cell count** (the absolute cell count is less specific and useful, but the cell count differential can be helpful: if granulocyte predominance think bacterial processes or pulmonary infarction, if lymphocyte predominance think TB, fungus, or malignancy)

- **Gram stain**
- **Culture** both bacterial and fungal
- **pH**: a pleural fluid pH <7.10 suggests empyema (an infected pleural effusion)
- **Amylase** (if elevated and left-sided think pancreatitis or perforated esophagus)
- **Cytology** (if cancer is suspected; cytology will often be negative, however, requiring thoracoscopy to yield the definitive diagnosis)

MANAGEMENT

In addition to diagnostic thoracentesis, a larger amount of fluid can be removed for symptom relief (therapeutic thoracentesis). Removal of more than 1000 mL at a time greatly increases the risk of re-expansion pulmonary edema so fluid removal is generally limited to 1 L. Thoracentesis should be performed for any unexplained pleural effusion. An exception would be patients with CHF, no fever, and symmetric bilateral pleural effusions that decrease with diuresis.

The definitive management option for pleural effusion is to treat the underlying cause. If cure or long-term control of the cause is not possible or feasible then chronic measures may include intermittent therapeutic thoracentesis if the effusion is fairly slow to reaccumulate; indwelling chest tube placement (i.e., Denver drain) if quickly reaccumulating and the underlying cause is being treated; or pleurodesis if the effusion is rapidly accumulating and the underlying cause is chronic. Pleurodesis is the instillation of an irritative agent (e.g., talc, tetracycline) into the pleural space which forms fibrous adhesions between the visceral and parietal pleura, resulting in obliteration of the space and preventing reaccumulation.

Patients with empyema or complicated parapneumonic effusions will require chest tube drainage. Pleural fluid which is frank pus or fluid with a positive Gram stain for bacteria obviously needs drainage. Characteristics of the pleural fluid which might suggest the need for drainage include a low pH (<7.10), low glucose (<40–60 mg/dL), and loculation. Chest tubes remain in place until the drainage rate has fallen below 50 mL/day.

ACUTE RESPIRATORY
DISTRESS SYNDROME

Janet N. Myers
Russell C. Gilbert

KEY POINTS

- ARDS is a life-threatening disorder characterized by severe ALI that may occur in a variety of clinical settings.
- Damage to the pulmonary system may be a localized injury or a systemic process resulting in diffuse damage to the pulmonary endothelium and epithelium with increased capillary permeability.
- ARDS is characterized by the sudden onset of diffuse, bilateral, alveolar infiltrates, refractory hypoxia, and decreased lung compliance in the absence of cardiogenic failure.
- Management consists primarily of supportive therapy and treatment of the underlying disorder.
- Low volume lung ventilation improves survival.

INTRODUCTION

Acute respiratory distress syndrome (ARDS) is a complex disorder characterized by the rapid onset of diffuse bilateral pulmonary infiltrates and refractory hypoxia, without evidence of cardiogenic failure, usually in the setting of other serious acute conditions such as trauma, aspiration, or sepsis. Acute lung injury (ALI) is a similar, but less severe form of ARDS, and may progress to ARDS in many cases. Critical to the definitions of ALI and ARDS is the absence of left atrial or pulmonary capillary hypertension as the primary cause of hypoxemia in these patients. The distinction between ALI and ARDS is the degree of hypoxemia, with a PaO_2/FiO_2 ratio of <200 in

ARDS, and <300 in ALI. Both are life-threatening disorders, frequently requiring mechanical ventilation and admission to an intensive care unit (ICU) for aggressive monitoring and hemodynamic support. The incidence of ARDS is widely variable, and has been reported as high as 75/100,000 people per year, carrying a mortality of between 34 and 65%.

PATHOPHYSIOLOGY

Clinical conditions associated with ARDS are numerous (Table 19-1). Two major categories are those causing direct (primary) lung injury such as aspiration or multilobar pneumonia, and those causing a systemic (secondary) lung injury, such as sepsis, severe pancreatitis, or trauma. Underlying disorders such as chronic lung disease or alcoholism may increase the risk of developing ARDS.

The histopathologic findings found in ARDS are described as diffuse alveolar damage (DAD). DAD may be divided into two phases, the exudative phase which is followed by a fibroproliferative phase. The extent of involvement is variable. Following either direct lung injury or response to a systemic insult, neutrophils adhere to the capillary endothelium and migrate into the interstitial and alveolar spaces. Activated neutrophils may secrete numerous cytokines, such as tumor necrosis factor-alpha, which may further promote the inflammatory response. Production of oxygen radicals and proteases may further damage endothelia and alveoli. Hyaline membrane formation with intra-alveolar erythrocytes and neutrophils are characteristic. The acute injury may resolve in some patients, with full recovery of function. However, in other patients, impaired fibrinolysis may lead to capillary thrombosis and infarction. Pulmonary hypertension may be severe and progress to right heart failure. A third phase is characterized by gradual improvement in hypoxemia and partial or complete resolution of fibrosis.

Table 19-1 **Clinical Disorders Associated with ARDS**

Direct Lung Injury	Indirect Lung Injury
Aspiration of gastric contents	Severe sepsis
Thoracic trauma (lung contusion)	Trauma (long bone fractures, pelvic fracture)
Severe pneumonia (bilateral)	Pancreatitis
Toxic inhalation	Severe bleeding requiring transfusions
Near drowning	Hypovolemic shock

CLINICAL PRESENTATION

Following the inciting insult, patients may initially present with agitation and dyspnea with progressive tachypnea, tachycardia, and hypotension. Infiltrates on the chest radiograph usually will appear within 24–48 hours. The inflammatory response and alveolar damage result in **marked hypoxia, unresponsive to high levels of oxygen**. On examination, the patient may appear cyanotic and have diffuse crackles. The cardiac examination is often nonspecific and may not show evidence of cardiac failure (e.g., jugular venous distention, S_3 gallop). Extremities may or may not demonstrate edema. Pulmonary parenchymal changes lead to increased stiffness of the lungs and decreased expansion, resulting in small tidal volumes, increased respiratory rates, and increased work of breathing. Mechanically ventilated patients may demonstrate high peak and plateau airway pressures during attempts to maintain adequate tidal volumes and ventilation. The relationship of volume to pressure is known as compliance, and decreased compliance is a characteristic feature of ARDS. Laboratory studies usually find leukocytosis due to the underlying disease or to the inflammatory process associated with ARDS. Frequently, ARDS is associated with failure of other organ systems, such as the kidney or liver. Acute pulmonary arterial hypertension may occur from hypoxemia or destruction of lung tissue, which may cause distension of the right ventricle. This can result in encroachment on the left ventricle, causing heart failure to occur and compounding the problem of capillary leak in the lungs. Multiorgan system failure may eventually lead to death.

EVALUATION

Infiltrates on chest radiograph and computed tomography (CT) show **bilateral alveolar infiltrates**, predominately dependent, interspersed with normal lung (Fig. 19-1). Unlike patients with heart failure, patients with ARDS may not demonstrate pleural effusions or cardiomegaly. Arterial blood gases may reveal early respiratory alkalosis and hypoxemia followed by metabolic acidosis with progressive hypoxemia. Because the PaO_2 will be dependent on the FiO_2, the **ratio of arterial to alveolar oxygen (PaO_2/FiO_2)** is included in the definition of ARDS and ALI. The necessity of central pulmonary catheter placement is controversial, but is sometimes used if the patient's fluid status is unclear. If the patient has a central pulmonary artery catheter, pulmonary capillary wedge pressures are <18 mmHg, as higher levels would indicate the presence of heart failure. B-type natriuretic peptide (BNP) levels may be low to normal in the absence of heart failure, but this has not been well studied in ICU patients. Diagnostic evaluation includes searching for an underlying cause of ARDS, for example, amylase and lipase levels to look for pancreatitis, or cultures to look for infection. ARDS can be

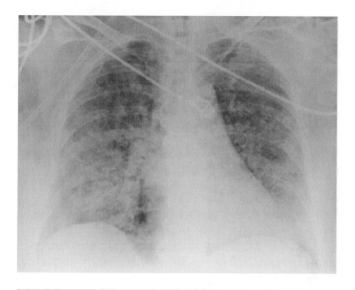

Figure 19-1 **A representative anteroposterior (AP) chest x-ray in the exudative phase of ARDS that shows diffuse interstitial and alveolar infiltrates, which can be difficult to distinguish from left ventricular failure.** (*Source:* Reproduced with permission from Kasper DL, Braunwald E, Fauci AS, et al. *Harrison's Principles of Internal Medicine*, 16th ed. New York: McGraw-Hill, 2005, Figure 251-2.)

confused with other illnesses such as congestive heart failure or pneumonia, and these conditions can coexist with ARDS.

Bronchoscopy with bronchoalveolar lavage (BAL) is useful when the cause of ARDS is unclear. The evaluation of BAL fluid is used primarily to rule out other causes of diffuse pulmonary infiltrates, such as infectious pneumonia, acute eosinophilic pneumonia, or alveolar hemorrhage syndromes.

MANAGEMENT

Aggressive, early supportive therapy and identification and treatment of the underlying cause of ARDS are critical. Thus, patients with infection are treated with broad-spectrum antibiotics until the source is known and the antibiotic regimen can be more specific. If surgical intervention is needed to remove pus or repair trauma, this is undertaken as soon as possible. In cases of pancreatitis, reversible causes such as biliary stones, obstructing tumors, or infected cysts must be treated.

When necessary, mechanical ventilation should be instituted with the goal of maintaining adequate oxygenation and minimizing ventilator-induced lung injury. Ventilator-induced lung injury is a complex process caused by repetitive stress or strain from excessive positive pressure ventilation on some areas of the lung but not others. ARDS is a heterogenous disorder, usually with involvement of dependent areas of the lung with relative sparing of other areas. Consequently, different areas of lung respond differently to the same volumes and pressures delivered by the ventilator. When attempts are made to ventilate the abnormal areas of the lung, some alveoli may be repetitively "overstretched" (volutrauma) and may literally "crack." Other units may repetitively "snap open" during inspiration and "snap close" at the end of expiration (atelectrauma), causing shearing forces that damage alveoli. The resultant damage may trigger the release of inflammatory mediators and destructive proteinases. Injury from mechanical ventilation has been shown to develop in both acutely injured lungs as well as normal lung.

Clinical markers of ventilator-induced lung injury include progressive infiltrates despite control of the primary insult or process, worsening hypoxemia, and decreased lung compliance. While the term "barotrauma" is often used to describe damage resulting in "air leaks" or air outside of the alveolar space (e.g., subcutaneous emphysema, pneumomediastinum, and pneumothorax) high ventilating pressures associated with barotrauma are also thought to contribute to ventilator injury. Pneumothorax frequently requires placement of a chest tube with suction to evacuate air from the pleural space.

Low tidal volume ventilation is recommended in patients with ALI and ARDS to help prevent lung injury. Because injured alveoli have a tendency to collapse, various strategies are used to keep lung units open in order to maintain adequate oxygenation and to prevent atelectrauma. Positive end-expiratory pressure (PEEP) is routinely used where the ventilator provides additional pressure after the patient's breath has ended, thus keeping the alveoli open. In patients with persistent hypoxemia, another approach used involves prolonging the inspiratory duration of the breathing cycle, and shortening the expiratory duration (also known as "inverse ratio" ventilation). This can improve oxygenation because it allows greater recruitment of more severely affected areas of lung which require more time to open and ventilate.

Other measures have sometimes been used in patients with persistent hypoxemia, but have yet to show a mortality benefit: prone positioning, nitric oxide, surfactant replacement, high frequency ventilation, prostacyclin, extracorporeal membrane oxygenation, and liquid ventilation.

While high-dose steroids have not been shown to be beneficial in the acute stage of ARDS, moderate doses of steroids may have a role in the late fibroproliferative phase. It is currently not clear if the benefit of steroids seen in patients with pressor-dependent severe sepsis and ARDS may be related to a relative adrenal insufficiency. Larger trials are currently ongoing. Activated Protein C has been shown to improve survival in patients with sepsis and may also be beneficial in ALI and ARDS.

Nonventilatory Supportive Care

In addition to providing ventilatory supportive care, nonventilatory supportive care is also key to the care of patients with ARDS. In addition to hemodynamic support and careful fluid management, patients require:

- Nutritional support
- Pulmonary toilet (control respiratory secretions with suctioning and postural drainage)
- Prevention of stress ulcers (gastrointestinal prophylaxis)
- Deep vein thrombosis prevention (DVT prophylaxis)
- Pain and sedation management (minimize pain without oversedating the patient)
- Attention to pharmacology (e.g., dose adjustment for renal failure or drug-drug interactions and side effects)
- Prevention of nosocomial infections (elevate the head of the bed >45°, avoid parenteral nutrition when the gut is functional, use full-barrier precautions during line placement, and simple hand washing)

PROGNOSIS

Patients with ARDS have a mortality of 35–40% overall, with most patients succumbing to nonpulmonary causes such as sepsis. Mortality in ARDS has improved in the past several years, likely due to improvements in supportive care. Factors contributing to increased mortality include advanced age, immunosuppression, and underlying liver disease. Those patients who survive generally do well, often with recovery of normal or near-normal lung function. ARDS survivors are at risk for neuropsychiatric disorders such as posttraumatic stress-like syndrome.

CHAPTER 20

PNEUMOTHORAX

Anthony Bottiggi
Andrew Bernard

KEY POINTS

- Pneumothoraces are the accumulation of air within the pleural space.
- Most are from trauma but they may be spontaneous.
- Presence of a pleural line on CXR is usually diagnostic.
- Symptomatic pneumothoraces are managed with a chest tube.
- Tension pneumothoraces require emergent needle thoracostomy.

INTRODUCTION

Pneumothoraces most commonly occur after trauma but may also be spontaneous or iatrogenic. **Spontaneous pneumothoraces** are typically classified as either primary, in a patient without underlying lung disease, or secondary, in a patient with underlying lung disease. This is a somewhat arbitrary delineation, because primary spontaneous pneumothoraces occur almost exclusively in smokers, most of whom have subclinical lung disease. Iatrogenic pneumothoraces are most commonly associated with transthoracic lung biopsies, but also occur during mechanical ventilation or following thoracentesis, central venous catheterization, or transbronchial lung biopsy.

Pneumothoraces may also be classified as simple or complex (i.e., tension pneumothorax). In a **simple pneumothorax**, air enters the pleural space on one side of the hemithorax causing unilateral lung collapse (Fig. 20-1). By contrast, in a **tension pneumothorax**, the pressure in the pleural space increases resulting in compression of the entire lung (shift of the mediastinum away from the pneumothorax; Fig. 20-2). A tension pneumothorax is a medical emergency because it causes severe respiratory and hemodynamic compromise.

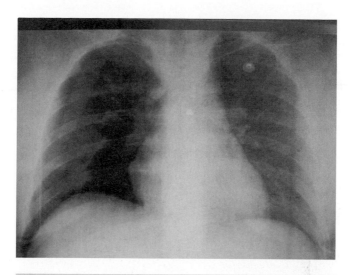

Figure 20-1 **Simple pneumothorax. The CXR demonstrates a large right pneumothorax with widening and deepening of the right costophrenic angle, also known as the deep sulcus sign. Occasionally, this sign is the only radiographic indication of a pneumothorax in a supine patient.** (*Source:* Reproduced with permission from Stone KC, Humphries RL. *Current Emergency Diagnosis & Treatment,* 5th ed. New York: McGraw-Hill, 2004, Figure 24-2.)

PATHOPHYSIOLOGY

The pleural space lies between the visceral (lining the lung) and parietal (lining the chest wall) pleura, and is normally filled with a thin layer of fluid. In a normal individual, intrapleural pressure is zero when fully exhaled. Chest wall expansion or diaphragmatic movement causes a negative pressure within the pleural space, expanding lung spaces and pulling air into the lung (negative pressure breathing). If the visceral (or parietal pleura) is damaged, air will flow from the lung (or the atmosphere) into the pleural space until the pressure difference normalizes or the communication is closed. The intrapleural pressure will become positive and the visceral and parietal pleurae will no longer be apposed, creating a pneumothorax. If the air in the pleural space is only a small amount, the lung will remain mostly expanded and symptoms will be mild. As the quantity of air increases, the lung will collapse further and the patient will usually have progressive symptoms as the pneumothorax enlarges.

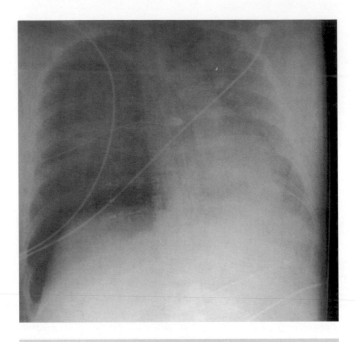

Figure 20-2 **Tension pneumothorax.** (*Source:* Reproduced with permission from Stone KC, Humphries RL. *Current Emergency Diagnosis & Treatment*, 5th ed. New York: McGraw-Hill, 2004, Figure 24-1.)

A tension pneumothorax typically develops in patients receiving mechanical ventilation, because positive pressure is necessary to force air into the pleural space under high pressure. In a breathing patient, a **one-way valve mechanism** is required, such that more air enters the pleural space on inspiration than can escape during exhalation. In either mechanism, intrapleural pressure will eventually exceed atmospheric pressure, resulting in mediastinal shift and compression of the contralateral lung, vena cavae, and heart. This is heralded by a sudden deterioration in both the respiratory and hemodynamic status of the patient. Cardiac output diminishes because of the limited venous return to the heart and hypoxia ensues from ventilation-perfusion mismatches.

Primary spontaneous pneumothoraces occur because of the **rupture of a subpleural bleb,** an area of visceral pleura (>1 cm) that lacks an epithelial lining, typically located in the apex of the lung. Sudden increases in airway pressure, such as during coughing, can rupture blebs resulting in escape of air into the pleural cavity. Secondary spontaneous pneumothoraces are also caused from the rupture of blebs, but the blebs are caused by known underlying lung pathology, most commonly chronic obstructive pulmonary disease (COPD).

CLINICAL PRESENTATION

Patients with pneumothoraces may present with a spectrum of symptoms from none to extremis. Symptomatic patients usually complain of **chest pain** that is exacerbated by respiration. They also have **dyspnea**, which varies in severity depending on the size of the pneumothorax and the patient's underlying cardiopulmonary reserve. Less common symptoms include a nonproductive cough and orthopnea.

Primary spontaneous pneumothoraces occur almost exclusively in smokers. They also occur more frequently in tall thin individuals and are characteristically men. The most common underlying lung pathology in individuals with secondary spontaneous pneumothoraces is COPD, but they can occur with any lung disease. Other conditions with a high incidence of pneumothorax include cystic fibrosis, lymphangioleiomyomatosis, and Langerhans cell granulomatosis.

Symptomatic patients will have varying degrees of respiratory distress, including tachypnea, accessory muscle use, and decreased oxygen saturation. The classic physical examination findings on lung examination are decreased or absent breath sounds and hyperresonance to percussion over the side of the pneumothorax. However, **lung examination is often normal when the pneumothorax occupies <25% of the hemithorax**. Less commonly, some patients may have subcutaneous emphysema on chest wall palpation.

When a tension pneumothorax develops, the patient's clinical status will abruptly change. They develop marked respiratory distress with labored respirations, cyanosis and diaphoresis, and poor hemodynamics characterized by marked tachycardia and hypotension. The trachea may be deviated away from the pneumothorax as the mediastinum shifts but this is a late and insensitive physical examination finding. Likewise, jugular venous distention occurs as the vena cava is compressed but again this is an inconsistent finding.

EVALUATION

Chest radiography is diagnostic. Increased radiolucency along the parietal pleura may be noted due to the presence of air in the pleural space and the margin of the visceral pleura can usually be seen separated from the parietal pleura (**pleural line**). Large pneumothoraces are also associated with collapse of the ipsilateral lung, seen as increased density of the lung parenchyma on chest x-ray (CXR). Although the best view is an upright film, this is often not possible in patients who have had trauma or are critically ill. Supine x-rays present a significant challenge to diagnosing a pneumothorax, because air in the pleural space will move anteriorly and the pneumothorax may not be visualized.

If a tension pneumothorax is suspected, immediate treatment with a needle thoracostomy (see "Management," below) should be instituted prior to obtaining a CXR. The presence of a tension pneumothorax is confirmed if air escapes from the thoracostomy. X-ray evidence of a tension pneumothorax includes mediastinal shift, tracheal deviation, and depression of the diaphragm.

MANAGEMENT

Patients with hypoxia should be given 100% oxygen by face mask (as long as other contraindications do not exist). It has been proposed that high-flow oxygen promotes absorption of small pneumothoraces but supportive clinical data are scant. A suspected tension pneumothorax should be immediately managed with **needle thoracostomy**. A large-bore (14- to 16-gauge) catheter with needle (Angiocath, BD Medical, Sandy, Utah) should be inserted into the second anterior intercostal space along the midclavicular line. After insertion into the chest, the needle is removed and a large syringe containing a few milliliters of sterile saline is attached to the catheter. The plunger is then removed from the syringe to allow equalization of intrapleural and atmospheric pressure. If air bubbles through the saline, the diagnosis of tension pneumothorax is established.

Small pneumothoraces (usually <15–20% lung collapse) can be managed without a chest tube if the patient is asymptomatic and the pneumothorax is stable on sequential CXRs. As a general rule, a small pneumothorax only has air in the pleural space visible on upright x-ray at the apex in the first two or three rib spaces. A pneumothorax will spontaneously reabsorb about 1% of the total volume of the pleural space every 24 hours.

Definitive management of a pneumothorax is evacuation of the air in the pleural space allowing re-expansion the lung. This can be accomplished in a number of ways. Simple aspiration of air has been associated with a 50–80% success rate but is usually reserved for iatrogenic pneumothoraces not associated with mechanical ventilation. **Tube thoracostomy** (chest tube placement) and underwater seal drainage is the most common modality for managing a pneumothorax. The typical location for a chest tube is through the fourth, fifth, or sixth intercostal space in the mid-to-anterior axillary line. Once inserted, the chest tube is connected to a three-chambered closed drainage system (Fig. 20-3). Although different varieties exist, the first chamber is always for collection of fluid or blood, the second chamber is the water-seal chamber (visualizes of air escaping from the pleural space), and the third chamber controls the amount of suction in the circuit. Typically, an adult patient is initially placed on a suction pressure of -20 cmH$_2$O but higher pressures may be used for recalcitrant pneumothoraces.

The chest tube should be left on suction until there is no evidence of air escaping the chest (the presence of bubbles in the water chamber). When the suction is stopped, the patient is considered to be "on water seal" because the chest tube is effectively under water, allowing air to escape the chest but

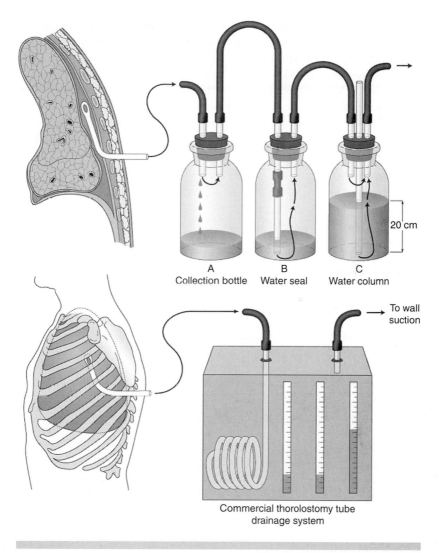

20 cm

A
Collection bottle

B
Water seal

C
Water column

To wall suction

Commercial thorolostomy tube
drainage system

Figure 20-3 **Closed suction drainage system.** (*Source:* Reproduced with permission from Dunphy JE, Way LW, eds. *Current Surgical Diagnosis & Treatment*, 5th ed. New York: Appleton & Lange, 1981.)

preventing air from entering the chest. Water seal is then maintained for 6–24 hours during which time the clinician follows the patient's symptoms and signs, including the presence or absence of an air leak during coughing. If there is no air leak after a period of water seal and the lung is expanded on CXR, then the chest tube may be removed and the exit site covered with an occlusive dressing (usually petroleum covered gauze).

One special consideration for spontaneous pneumothoraces (whether primary or secondary) involves the high rate of recurrence, approaching 20–40% after an initial pneumothorax. Surgical intervention is generally recommended after the second episode. This typically involves resection of the diseased portion of lung (the bleb or bulla) combined with pleurodesis. **Pleurodesis** consists of mechanically or chemically irritating the pleurae such that inflammation and adhesion formation between the lung and the chest wall ensue, obliterating the pleural space and preventing future episodes of pneumothorax.

CHEST X-RAY

INTERPRETATION

Eric Bensadoun

KEY POINTS

- A systematic approach is crucial to the interpretation of chest x-rays.
- Start with verification of the patient information, type of chest x-ray, and quality of the image.
- Perform a thorough visual survey of the frontal and lateral chest x-ray.
- Localize any abnormalities and determine the radiographic pattern that best describes those abnormalities.
- Formulate a differential diagnosis based on the radiographic pattern.

CHEST RADIOGRAPH INTERPRETATION

When evaluating chest radiographs (chest x-rays), it is important to develop a systematic approach. The following represents an outline for this type of stepwise approach.

Step 1: First Things First

Locate the name, medical number, and date on the x-ray to be sure you have the right film. If available, always obtain old films for comparison. The standard chest x-ray examination consists of a **posterior-anterior (PA) projection** and a **left lateral radiograph,** both obtained in a standing patient at full inspiration. The **anterior-posterior (AP)**, or "portable" chest x-ray is another common type of chest x-ray examination, which is usually performed at the bedside. The AP chest x-ray must be interpreted with some caution as the AP film technique may magnify the heart and superior mediastinum up to 15–20%, may accentuate lung markings (mimicking interstitial lung disease) because of the variable levels of inspiration on AP films, and may cause vascular redistribution (mimicking venous hypertension) because of the supine position of the patient.

Step 2: Image Quality Assessment

The diagnostic accuracy of the chest radiograph can be greatly affected by the quality of the images themselves. To assess the quality of the radiographic image one must assess patient positioning, inspiratory effort, and exposure. **Patient positioning** must be such that the x-ray beam is properly centered and the patient is not rotated. On properly centered films the medial ends of the clavicles are equidistant from the spinous processes of the spine, which are considered to represent the midline (unless there is scoliosis). Poorly centered films can give the false impression of mediastinal shift, hilar prominence, or a hyperlucent hemithorax. A chest radiograph should be taken at **full inspiration**, with, the right midhemidiaphragm reaching the level of the 9th to 10th rib posteriorly or the 6th to 7th rib anteriorly. A less than full inspiration can give the false impression of volume loss, increased interstitial markings, or cardiomegaly. On a PA chest radiograph, **film exposure** is optimal when it allows for faint identification of the intervertebral discs of the midthoracic spine while still allowing for clear visualization of the lung markings behind the heart.

Step 3: The Visual Survey

Begin the process of interpretation by performing a systematic visual survey of the frontal and lateral chest radiograph.

PA OR AP CHEST RADIOGRAPH

Examine the **extrathoracic soft tissues** which include the neck, supraclavicular fossa, soft tissues of the lateral chest wall, pectoralis muscles, and breast shadows (Fig. 21-1C). Note any masses, swelling, calcifications, air, or foreign bodies. Then examine the **extrathoracic bony structures** which include the clavicle, the scapula, the humerus, the acromioclavicular joint, and the glenohumeral joint. Note any fractures, lytic/blastic lesions, or arthritic changes.

Survey the structures that constitute the **thoracic cage**. Start with the **ribs** (Fig. 21-1), making sure to examine the anterior (Fig. 21-1B) and posterior portions of each rib (Fig. 21-1A), as well as, the lateral portions along the lateral chest wall. Note any fractures, lytic/blastic lesions, rib notching, or costal cartilage calcifications. Then inspect the **vertebral column** (Fig. 21-1K) with attention to the spinous processes, pedicles, transverse processes and height of each vertebra. Note any osteophytes, lytic/blastic lesions, fractures, kyphosis, or scoliosis.

The **diaphragm** constitutes the inferior border of the thoracic cage. Inspect the area below the diaphragm, the gastric air bubble may be seen on the left (Fig. 21-1J). The distance from the top of the bubble to the dome of the diaphragm is usually <1–2 cm; a greater distance may suggest a subpulmonic pleural effusion. Inspect the upper abdomen for a spleen or liver shadow, air in the colon, or free air under the diaphragm. Then examine the diaphragm

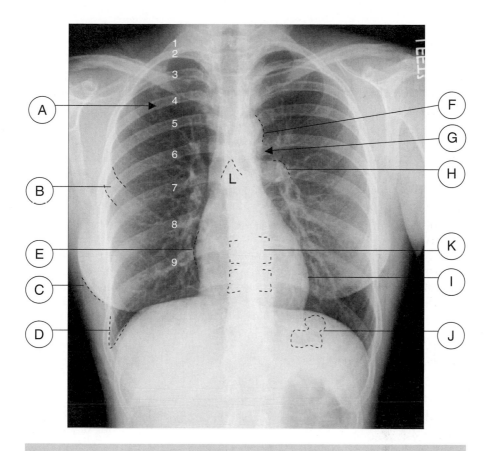

Figure 21-1 **PA chest radiograph: A: posterior portion of 4th rib, B: anterior portion of 4th rib, C: right breast shadow, D: right costophrenic angle, E: right atrium, F: aortic arch, G: aortopulmonary window, H: left main pulmonary artery, I: left ventricle, J: gastric air bubble, K: vertebral bodies, L: carinal angle. Numbers 1–9 correspond to the posterior portions of the right ribs.**

itself. Normally, the diaphragm is dome-shaped with its peak near its mid-point and the right diaphragm is higher than the left, but by no more then 1 rib interspace or 1.5 cm.

The examination of the **intrathoracic structures** begins with the **pleura**. The parietal pleura coats the diaphragm and the inner surface of the chest wall. The diaphragm and the lateral chest wall are inspected for pleural thickening or calcifications. The **costophrenic angle** (Fig. 21-1D) is examined for blunting or medial displacement, which may indicate the presence of pleural fluid or scarring. The pleural space and the visceral pleura are usually not seen except in cases of pleural effusions or pneumothorax. The minor fissure can sometimes be seen on a PA film as a thin line extending from the right hilum to the lateral chest wall at the level of the axillary portion of the fifth or sixth rib.

Examination of the **mediastinum** starts with overall position of the mediastinum, which should lie in the center of the chest. It may be deviated to one side as a result of a pleural effusion, pneumothorax, or atelectasis. Then, follow the tracheal air column by starting at the top and tracing the normal narrowing of the trachea at the level of the vocal cords and the slight deviation to the right at the level of the arch of the aorta. Any abnormal narrowing or deviation should be noted. The trachea bifurcates into the right and left mainstem bronchi at the level of the main carina. Note that the right mainstem has a more vertical descent than the left. The normal **carinal angle** (Fig. 21-1L) is about 60° (range of 45–75°); however, abnormal widening can be seen if there is left atrial enlargement or subcarinal adenopathy. Examine the contours of the mediastinum. On the left, the first bump is the **aortic arch** (Fig. 21-1F), which is followed by a concavity called the **aortopulmonary window** (Fig. 21-1G). The loss of this concavity should raise the suspicion of mediastinal adenopathy. The next protuberances are the **left pulmonary artery** (Fig. 21-1H) and then the left heart border (Fig. 21-1I), which represents the left atrial appendage and the left ventricle. On the right, the superior vena cava makes up the superior lateral border of the mediastinum and inferiorly is the right pulmonary artery followed by the right heart border, which represents the right atrium. The **cardiac silhouette** should be examined for shape and size. The normal heart usually spans <50% of the total transverse diameter of the chest.

The **hila** lie just lateral to the mediastinum. The hilar shadows contain the pulmonary arteries, pulmonary veins, lymph nodes, and bronchial walls; however, the normal density of the hila is primarily the result of the pulmonary vessels. Note the shape, density, size, symmetry, and position of the hila. Normally, the right hilum is found at the level of the anterior third rib and the left hilum is higher by less than 1 rib interspace or 2 cm. The hila may become enlarged if there is adenopathy present or if the pulmonary arteries are enlarged as in pulmonary hypertension.

Finally, examine the **lung parenchyma**. Compare corresponding areas of the right and left lungs, looking for asymmetry due to an increased or decreased density. Also examine the apices, the retrocardiac area, and portion of the lungs that projects below the diaphragm. Normally, there are fine linear opacities that can be seen throughout the lung parenchyma representing the blood vessels which gradually taper as they extend toward the periphery up to 1–2 cm from the visceral pleura. If the lung markings are seen beyond this point, it may be indicative of interstitial lung disease.

LATERAL CHEST RADIOGRAPH

The lateral chest x-ray is very useful to confirm and localize abnormalities as well as detect lesions in areas that may not be well visualized on the PA film.

The review of the lateral film also starts with the soft tissues and the bones. The **vertebral column** should become more lucent (darker) as they are traced down the column. Absence of this normal increase in lucency may indicate an overlying mass or infiltrate.

Then examine the **diaphragms** noting their contour and the sharpness of the posterior costophrenic angle where fluid can accumulate. One should be able to distinguish the right (Fig. 21-2H) from the left diaphragm (Fig. 21-2G) by using the following observations: the right is usually higher than the left, the gastric bubble lies under the left, and most reliably, the right diaphragm can be seen extending from anterior to posterior chest wall while the anterior portion of the left diaphragm is not seen because of the overlying heart.

Next examine the **mediastinum** and trace the tracheal air column (Fig. 21-2A) down to the right upper lobe bronchus and then the **left upper lobe bronchus** (Fig. 21-2C) immediately below it. Note the **right pulmonary artery** (Fig. 21-2F) anterior to the left upper lobe bronchus and the descending **left pulmonary artery** (Fig. 21-2E) posterior to it. Above the left pulmonary

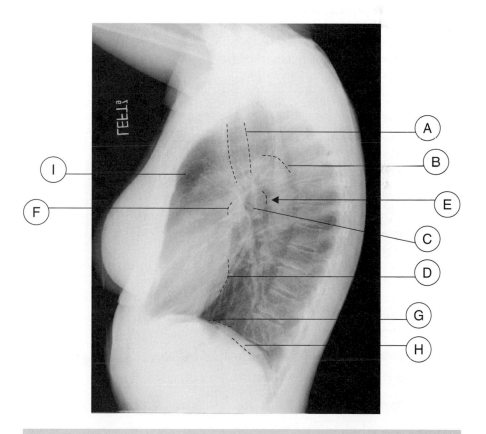

Figure 21-2 **Lateral chest radiograph: A: trachea, B: aortic arch, C: left upper lobe bronchus, D: left atrium, E: descending left pulmonary artery, F: right main pulmonary artery, G: left diaphragm, H: right diaphragm, I: retrosternal air space.**

artery is the **arch of the aorta** (Fig. 21-2B). The **retrosternal space** (Fig. 21-2I) is above and anterior to the anterior heart border. This space can be opacified when there is enlargement of the right ventricle or when an anterior mediastinal mass is present. The posterior heart border (Fig. 21-2D) represents the outline of the left ventricle and left atrium. At the inferior portion of the posterior heart border one can often see the inferior vena cava.

Last, examine the parenchyma including the **retrocardiac area** and the **fissures**. The right major fissure is usually not seen on a PA film; however, on the lateral film it can be seen extending obliquely from the fifth vertebrae toward the anterior chest wall at the level of the diaphragm (the anterior costophrenic angle). The left major fissure is usually slightly higher than the right. The minor fissure is usually seen extending horizontally from the hilum to the anterior chest wall.

Step 4: Pattern Recognition and Differential Diagnosis

Once an abnormality has been identified, it should be localized to the pleura, the mediastinum, the hilum, the chest wall, or the parenchyma. Next determine the radiographic pattern that best describes the abnormality. Then based on the anatomic location and the pattern of radiographic findings formulate a differential diagnosis for the radiographic abnormality.

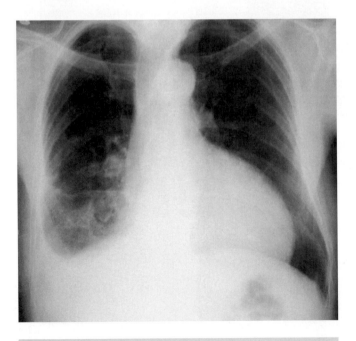

Figure 21-3 **Right pleural effusion. Note blunting of right costophrenic angle.**

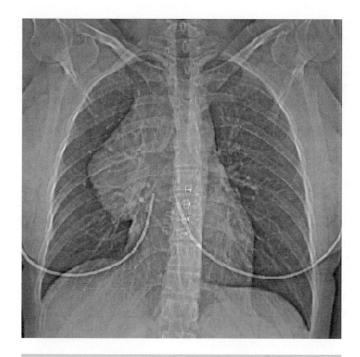

Figure 21-4 **Anterior mediastinal mass due to lymphoma.**

Pleura: Pleural effusions are often first detected by the presence of blunting of the costophrenic angle (Fig. 21-3). Pneumothorax (see Chap. 20) can be detected by the absence of lung markings in the periphery of the lung, and the presence of a line demarcating the surface of the lung from free air around the lung.

Mediastinum: Mediastinal widening can be seen with aortic dissection or mediastinal masses (Fig. 21-4). The latter can be further differentiated based on their location within the mediastinum (assessed on lateral chest x-ray):

- Anterior compartment: thymoma, lymphoma, teratoma, and retrosternal thyroid
- Middle compartment: adenopathy, mediastinal cyst, esophageal masses, and lesions of the aorta
- Posterior compartment: neurogenic tumors

Hilum: Enlarged hila can be due to adenopathy or enlarged pulmonary arteries (Fig. 21-5). Adenopathy usually has a lobulated contour and is commonly due to sarcoidosis, cancer, and tuberculosis. Enlarged pulmonary arteries usually have a smooth contour and are usually due to pulmonary hypertension.

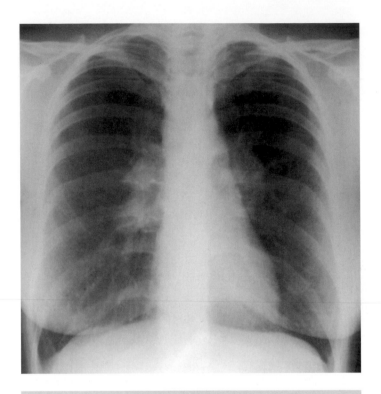

Figure 21-5 **Bilateral hilar adenopathy due to sarcoidosis.
Note the lobulated contour of the hilar enlargement.**

Parenchyma: The main radiographic patterns of parenchymal abnormalities are air space disease, interstitial disease, nodules/masses, atelectasis, and hyperlucency of the lungs.

Air space disease pattern (Fig. 21-6) can be diffuse or focal in distribution and represent pulmonary edema, pneumonia, hemorrhage, and inflammatory conditions of lung such as BOOP (bronchiolitis obliterans with organizing pneumonia). Air space disease is recognized by the following characteristics:

- One or more homogenous opacities obscuring the underlying pulmonary vessels
- Poorly defined margins unless abutting the pleura or fissures
- "Air bronchogram sign": a lucent branching shadow of the airways, often seen within the area of opacification
- Usually no volume loss

Interstitial disease patterns are linear (reticular), nodular opacities, or combinations of both. A **reticular pattern** (Fig. 21-7) consists of interlacing

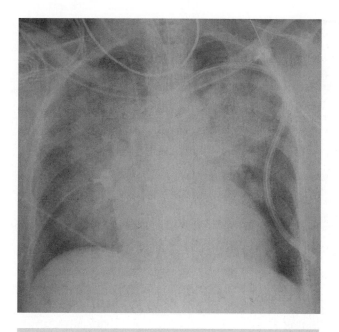

Figure 21-6 **Bilateral airspace disease secondary to pulmonary edema.**

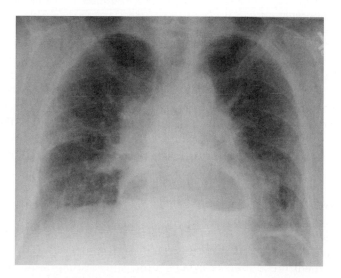

Figure 21-7 **Diffuse reticular pattern due to idiopathic pulmonary fibrosis. Also note the large hiatal hernia (lucency behind the heart).**

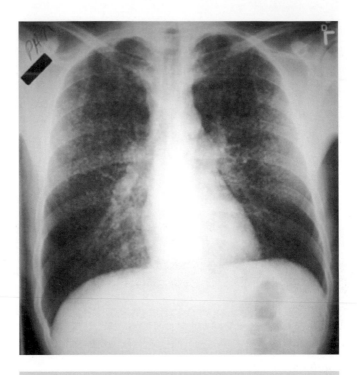

Figure 21-8 **Diffuse nodular pattern secondary to miliary tuberculosis.**

lines creating the appearance of a mesh. Examples of reticular patterns include pulmonary edema, idiopathic pulmonary fibrosis, and asbestosis. Kerley B lines or septal lines are a specific type of reticular marking, which are 1–2 cm in length, <1 mm thick, nonbranching, and located in the periphery of the lung abutting and perpendicular to the pleura. These are found in pulmonary edema and less commonly in lymphangitic carcinoma. The **nodular pattern** (Fig. 21-8) consists of rounded opacities which are homogenous, well circumscribed, and <1 cm in diameter. Causes of this pattern include disseminated infection (miliary tuberculosis), silicosis, coal workers' pneumoconioses, and sarcoidosis.

Nodules and masses (Figs. 21-9 and 21-10) are well circumscribed, more or less rounded opacities that can be either single or multiple. A solitary pulmonary nodule is most often caused by lung cancer or a granuloma from an infection such as tuberculosis or histoplasmosis. A nodule that is >3 cm in diameter is called a mass and is most likely to be a primary lung cancer. Multiple pulmonary nodules (>1 cm in diameter) are most commonly due to metastatic disease to the lungs.

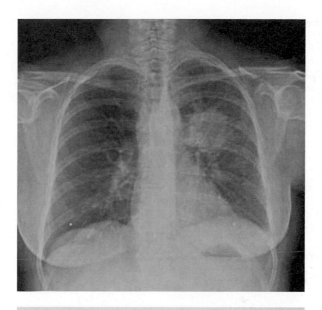

Figure 21-9 **Left upper lobe mass diagnosed as adenocarcinoma of the lung.** (*Courtesy of Janet Myers, MD.*)

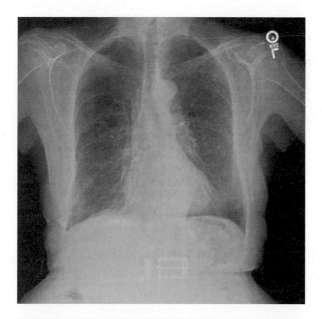

Figure 21-10 **Right lower lobe solitary pulmonary nodule.** (*Courtesy of Janet Myers, MD.*)

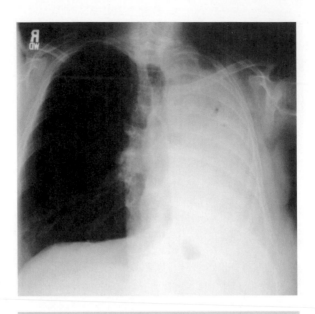

Figure 21-11 **Complete left lung atelectasis due to lung cancer obstructing the left mainstem bronchus.**

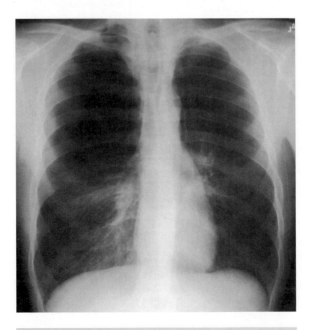

Figure 21-12 **Focal hyperlucency in right upper lung zone secondary to a large bulla.**

Atelectasis or collapse (Fig. 21-11) is most often due to endobronchial obstruction (e.g., lung cancer). There are usually signs of volume loss on the side of the atelectasis, and a characteristic opacity can be seen which varies in appearance and location based on the atelectatic lobe or lobes.

Hyperlucency of the lung (Fig. 21-12) can be seen with emphysema (diffuse hyperlucency) and bullae (focal hyperlucency).

GASTROINTESTINAL

ABDOMINAL PAIN

Carol D. Spears
Bernard R. Boulanger
Shushanth Reddy

KEY POINTS

- Acute abdominal pain requires prompt evaluation, diagnosis, and management.
- Pain may be vague or referred and may not correlate directly to the area of pathology.
- Acute onset of severe abdominal pain should raise concern for perforated hollow viscus, acute mesenteric embolus, volvulus, ruptured AAA, or other intra-abdominal emergency.
- Some patients require immediate operative exploration and should have early surgical involvement without an extensive workup.
- One should consider gynecologic causes of abdominal pain in women (e.g., ectopic pregnancy, ovarian torsion).

INTRODUCTION

Acute abdominal pain is one of the more commonly encountered patient presentations in the emergency room, the inpatient setting, and in the ambulatory setting. The various underlying causes of the pain range from benign processes to life-threatening conditions. Dr. Zachary Cope in the classic text *Cope's Early Diagnosis of the Acute Abdomen* reminds us that "the general rule can be laid down that the majority of severe abdominal pains that ensue in patients who have been previously fairly well, and that last as long as 6 hours, are caused by conditions of surgical import." Therefore, the "acute abdomen" requires urgent evaluation and treatment to discern the etiology, with a low threshold for surgical consultation.

PATHOPHYSIOLOGY

Acute abdominal pain is usually the result of inflammation of the peritoneum, distention of a hollow viscus, or contraction against obstruction (e.g., biliary colic). The abdominal viscera have autonomic innervation. The abdominal wall and parietal peritoneum have somatic innervation. Because of the complex dual visceral and parietal sensory network innervating the abdominal area, and the overall sparse innervation of the viscera in particular, abdominal pain is often nonspecific and difficult to localize. Nevertheless, some patterns emerge. For example, the visceral peritoneum is innervated by C fibers, which are slow transmitters. Therefore, visceral pain is often dull and crampy, of insidious onset, and poorly localized. In contrast, the parietal peritoneum, the skin, and muscles are innervated not only by C fibers, but also by fast transmitting A delta nerve fibers, which result in sharp pain, often of acute onset, and better localized. Pain that localizes after having started centrally usually indicates progression of disease from visceral peritoneal irritation to inflammation of the parietal peritoneum in the specific region (e.g., appendicitis, diverticulitis, and cholecystitis). The embryologic origin of the abdominal structures may help determine the clinical pain location. For example, the distal esophagus, stomach, proximal duodenum, liver, biliary tree, and pancreas originate in the foregut, and pain is perceived in the midepigastrium. The small intestine, appendix, and the proximal two-thirds of the transverse colon arise from the midgut, with pain perceived periumbilically. The distal one-third of the transverse colon, the descending colon, and the rectosigmoid arise from the hindgut, with pain perceived between the umbilicus and pubis.

CLINICAL PRESENTATION

Much can be learned from the onset, symptom complex, and nature of abdominal pain (Table 22-1). The **character** of the pain can aid in diagnosis. Crampy or colicky pain may be due to vigorous intestinal contractions as in obstruction or gastroenteritis, biliary colic due to cholelithiasis, or renal colic due to a ureteral stone. Severe, diffuse pain may indicate perforated viscus or intestinal ischemia. Beware that epigastric pain or pressure may be of cardiac origin. A patient may have **referred pain**, for example, right shoulder pain from cholecystitis, or left shoulder pain from a splenic abscess, or abdominal pain from lower lobe pneumonia. Pain that **radiates** from the back, around the flank into the groin can be associated with kidney stones. Acute onset of abdominal pain may indicate volvulus or perforated viscus. Gradual onset may be associated with an inflammatory process such as appendicitis, diverticulitis, obstruction, or ischemia. Timing of **other symptoms** becomes important. It is common for nausea and vomiting to follow the onset of pain in

Table 22-1 *Classic Presentations of Various Causes of Abdominal Pain by Location*

Location	Diagnosis	Character of Pain	Associated Sign/Symptom
Diffuse	Acute Mesenteric Ischemia	Rapid onset of severe pain out of proportion to examination and worse with eating	Abdominal examination usually benign
	Chronic Mesenteric Ischemia	Dull, crampy postprandial pain occurring within 1 h of eating	Weight loss secondary to food aversion
	Peritonitis	Marked localized pain with palpation and movement with rebound tenderness	Systemically ill with fever and hypotension
			Ascites is common
	Intestinal obstruction	Crampy pain worse with eating	Abdominal distention, vomiting, inability to pass flatus, high-pitched bowel sounds
Epigastric	Pancreatitis	Boring or stabbing pain radiating to the back and worse with eating	Almost always associated with nausea and vomiting
	Peptic ulcer disease	Constant, gnawing pain improved (duodenal) or worsened (gastric) by eating	No other symptoms evident
RUQ	Biliary colic	Constant pain radiating to right shoulder or back and worse after eating fatty foods	Nausea, vomiting, and anorexia
	Cholangitis	Pain radiating to right shoulder or back	Fever, jaundice, confusion, and hypotension
LUQ	Splenic abscess/rupture	Fullness or discomfort radiating to the left shoulder	Early satiety (compression of the stomach)
			Splenomegaly

(Continued)

Table 22-1 Classic Presentations of Various Causes of Abdominal Pain by Location (Continued)

Location	Diagnosis	Character of Pain	Associated Sign/Symptom
RLQ	Appendicitis	Periumbilical pain which then localizes to the RLQ	Nausea, vomiting, anorexia Occasional fever
LLQ	Diverticulitis	Aching pain which progressively worsens over several days	Fever, blood in stool
LLQ or RLQ	Ectopic pregnancy	Sudden onset of intermittent pelvic pain	Amenorrhea Acute onset of vaginal bleeding
	Pelvic inflammatory disease	Lower abdominal pain with onset during or after menses, and worse with coitus	Abnormal uterine bleeding Vaginal discharge
	Testicular torsion	Sudden onset of pain after mild or severe testicular trauma	Asymmetric high-riding testes
Flank	Renal colic	Paroxysmal aching pain radiating into the groin	Gross or microscopic hematuria

obstruction or inflammation. However, anorexia, nausea, and vomiting that precede pain do not usually indicate a surgical disease process. The absence of flatus suggests obstruction. Fever and chills may be due to intra-abdominal infection and possible bacteremia. A menstrual history is crucial to the diagnosis of ectopic pregnancy and other gynecologic causes of abdominal pain (endometriosis, ruptured ovarian cyst). Vaginal discharge could suggest pelvic inflammatory disease. **Aggravating or alleviating factors** also give insight as to the pathology. A patient with the colicky pain of a kidney stone will be unable to lie still and will be sitting up and fidgeting. Conversely, a patient with peritonitis will lie perfectly still and any slight movement will cause increased pain. Pain from peptic ulcer disease may be relieved by food while food may exacerbate symptomatic cholelithiasis. If this is a regularly occurring pain, it may require different consideration than if this is the first episode; for example, right lower quadrant (RLQ) pain in a young woman that occurs monthly at the midpoint of the menstrual cycle is more likely to be associated with ovulation and less likely to be appendicitis—but an appropriate evaluation is always warranted.

Location of the pain can be very helpful in narrowing down diagnostic possibilities.

Several conditions cause **diffuse abdominal pain. Mesenteric ischemia** can occur from one of three pathways: intra-arterial embolus or thrombus (two of three vessels occluded—celiac, superior mesenteric artery [SMA], inferior mesenteric artery [IMA]); venous (venous congestion leads to extra-arterial compression and ischemia); or nonocclusive or "low flow" (seen after MI or in sepsis). The classic finding of mesenteric ischemia is "**pain out of proportion to exam**," indicating the patient will exhibit evidence of severe pain, but the abdominal examination is usually benign.

A **ruptured abdominal aortic aneurysm (AAA)** may present with sudden back pain and hypotension. **Obstruction** can be of the small or large intestine from a variety of sources. Mechanical causes of small bowel obstruction include adhesions and hernia.

Large bowel obstruction occurs from tumor, benign stricture, hernia, or volvulus. Adhesions do not cause large bowel obstruction. Functional causes of obstruction include ileus, colonic pseudoobstruction, and toxic megacolon (from severe colitis, especially in ulcerative colitis and *Clostridium difficile* colitis). Ileus can also be caused by electrolyte imbalance (especially hypokalemia), narcotic use, immobilization, intra-abdominal inflammation/infection, and infection (e.g., urinary tract infection [UTI], pneumonia). In addition, diffuse abdominal pain can be caused by **bacterial peritonitis, gastroenteritis, sickle cell crisis, and diabetic ketoacidosis. Midepigastric abdominal pain** suggests pancreatitis or perforated peptic or gastric ulcer. **Right upper quadrant (RUQ) pain** suggests gallbladder disease (biliary colic, cholecystitis, cholangitis), hepatitis, and less commonly, peptic ulcer disease, and pneumonia. **RLQ pain** is seen in appendicitis and terminal/regional ileitis. **Left lower quadrant (LLQ)**

pain in an older person suggests **diverticulitis**. **Ovarian pathology** (ruptured cyst, ovarian torsion, tubo-ovarian abscess), ectopic pregnancy, psoas abscess, inflammatory bowel disease, Mittelschmerz, endometriosis, and renal or ureteral calculi are causes of **either right or LLQ pain**. Isolated **left upper quadrant (LUQ) pain** is an unusual presentation. In such a case, consider extra-abdominal causes such as angina, pneumonia, and pleuritis. Splenic processes (rupture, infarction, aneurysm, abscess) are rarer causes.

EVALUATION

Physical examination by an experienced physician is essential to evaluating a patient with abdominal pain, ideally before the administration of narcotic pain medications which may mask signs. First, it is important to determine if the patient "looks sick." Is the patient able to move freely and communicate well? Is the patient pale and lying absolutely still? Does the patient appear to be dehydrated? Is there jaundice?

A complete head-to-toe physical examination should be performed. For the abdominal examination, the patient should be lying supine with adequate exposure. **Inspection** of the abdomen determines distention, scars, skin and subcutaneous tissue changes, or waves of peristalsis (seen in a thin person). **Auscultation** determines the presence of bowel signs and may indicate the high-pitched tones of obstruction. Contrary to popular belief, the presence or absence of bowel sounds is not conclusive of disease. **Percussion** may indicate rebound tenderness, a fluid wave of ascites, or tympany of distended bowel. **Palpation** begins away from the area of pain and is conducted systematically, moving to the area of concern. Some clinicians begin palpation with but one finger, to localize pain more precisely. Remember to observe the patient's face and reactions to palpation, partly to be cognizant of patient comfort, but also some stoic patients may not complain of pain as they are being examined, even as they are obviously grimacing. Voluntary guarding is noted when the patient tenses the abdominal muscles in preparation for palpation. Involuntary guarding is noted with the spontaneous contracting of muscles during palpation. Rebound tenderness is noted if the pain of releasing pressure is worse than the pain of deep palpation. The degree of tenderness and the presence of findings such as involuntary guarding may determine the need for immediate surgical exploration. For example, muscle rigidity is evidence of generalized peritoneal inflammation and may indicate the need for surgical intervention. In general, a patient is deemed to have "peritonitis" when the abdominal examination includes involuntary guarding, rebound tenderness, tenderness to percussion, or a rigid abdomen.

In addition, a rectal examination is important in patients with abdominal pain to assess for masses, localized pain during examination, and evidence of gross blood. A **pelvic examination** is indicated in women patients, with cervical motion tenderness suggesting pelvic inflammatory disease, and adnexal pain or mass suggesting tubo-ovarian abscess or ectopic pregnancy.

Several other clinical signs and maneuvers can aid in diagnosis. **McBurney's point** is classically the area of greatest tenderness in appendicitis, located 5 cm from the right anterior superior iliac spine on a line running to the umbilicus. The **psoas sign** is elicited by either (1) extending the patient's right leg at the hip when they are in the left lateral decubitus position; or (2) with the patient in the supine position, have that patient lift the thigh against your hand placed just above the knee. Increased pain with either maneuver suggests irritation of the psoas muscle by an inflamed appendix. The **obturator sign** is elicited by passively flexing the right hip and knee and internally rotating the leg at the hip, stretching the obturator muscle, with increased pain suggesting local irritation of the obturator muscle, as in appendicitis. **Rovsing's sign** is pain in the RLQ on palpation of the LLQ, suggesting appendicitis. **Murphy's sign** tests for a large inflamed gall bladder, and is elicited by exerting pressure in the RUQ, then asking the patient to take a deep breath. Inspiration will cause the gall bladder to descend; when the inflamed gall bladder strikes the examining fingers, the patient will experience pain and abruptly stop the inspiratory effort. **Carnett's sign** entails identifying an area of localized tenderness, then asking the patient to contract the abdominal musculature, such as by raising the head. With the patient in this position, the tender area is palpated again. If the pain is more visceral, the contracted abdominal wall should diminish the tenderness by protecting the underlying viscera. If the pain and inflammation involves the abdominal wall, the pain will be just as severe and perhaps increased.

Laboratory studies include serum electrolytes and a complete blood count (**CBC**); leukocytosis could suggest microperforation and infection, such as in appendicitis or diverticulitis. If diffuse abdominal pain is present or if the history indicates an alcohol binge, a **lipase** and **amylase** are indicated, for possible pancreatitis. If cholelithiasis is suspected or jaundice is present, **liver function tests** should be obtained, which include the hepatic transaminases and total bilirubin. An elevated **lactate** may be seen in a patient with mesenteric ischemia. **A serum B-HCG (human chorionic gonadotrophin)** should be ordered in women of reproductive age with abdominal pain. The urinalysis may show red blood cells with nephrolithiasis.

An **acute abdominal series (AAS)** includes an upright chest x-ray (CXR), and flat and upright abdominal x-rays. An abdominal x-ray is also referred to as a KUB which stands for kidneys, ureter, bladder. The AAS includes imaging of the rectum. The upright CXR may show "free air" under the diaphragm. This free air, or pneumoperitoneum, is indicative of a perforated hollow viscus. Air throughout the small bowel is an abnormal finding and indicates that the bowel is distended with air possibly secondary to obstruction or ileus. A distended colon is seen with a distal obstruction and it is important to determine if there is air in the rectum (which is a sign that air is passing through and suggests that obstruction is only partial). With sigmoid volvulus, there is a massively dilated colon that has twisted and has a point, or beak, pointing to the LLQ.

Air fluid levels are lines that are visible on the upright abdominal film where fluid settles and air rises. This finding may be present in small bowel obstruction.

For a patient with suspected gallbladder pathology, jaundice, or abnormal liver enzymes, a **RUQ ultrasound (U/S)** is the initial test of choice. This imaging modality is inexpensive, readily available, and noninvasive. The U/S will evaluate the gallbladder wall for thickening, the common bile duct for enlargement, the intrahepatic biliary system for enlargement, the area around the gallbladder for pericholecystic fluid, and will visualize the pancreas, kidneys, and liver.

Computed tomography (CT) scan provides a tremendous amount of information about the viscera, vasculature, soft tissue, bones, and retroperitoneum, and is necessary in a patient with abdominal pain that does not have an obvious etiology or when the pain could result from several causes. For example, a young woman with abdominal pain in the RLQ may require a CT scan to evaluate for appendicitis versus ovarian pathology. **CT angiography** (CTA) is useful for evaluation of potential vascular pathology, such as mesenteric ischemia.

MANAGEMENT

A comprehensive discussion of therapies for all the various cause of acute abdominal pain is beyond the scope of this chapter. Surgery is obviously indicated in such situations as ruptured viscous, ruptured AAA, bowel infarction, and appendicitis. Details of the management of several causes of abdominal pain can be found in the chapters on cholecystitis/cholangitis, pancreatitis, gastrointestinal (GI) bleed, and inflammatory bowel disease.

Mechanical bowel obstruction requires laparotomy if the obstruction is complete.

Partial obstruction (e.g., small bowel obstruction secondary to adhesions with intermittent passage of stool and/or flatus) may be observed initially and may resolve with bowel rest and decompression (NPO and nasogastric tube to suction). Obstruction from an incarcerated inguinal, ventral, or parastomal hernia may be relieved with reduction of the hernia, although one should not reduce a hernia when there is concern that the incarcerated bowel is not viable. If a tumor is discovered when a patient presents with obstruction, an ostomy is often required because of the emergent nature of surgery. Sigmoid volvulus is often reduced with flexible sigmoidoscopy. Resection is then done electively to prevent recurrence. Cecal volvulus and transverse colon volvulus and small bowel volvulus are very rare and usually require laparotomy.

Diverticulitis usually resolves with bowel rest and broad-spectrum antibiotics with anaerobic activity. Surgery is indicated for generalized peritonitis, lack of resolution of attack, or repeated attacks. Surgery consists of sigmoid colon resection with colostomy or anastomosis.

NAUSEA AND VOMITING

IN THE HOSPITALIZED

PATIENT

Lisbeth Selby

KEY POINTS

- N/V are common symptoms associated with wide variety of disorders.
- The evaluation of N/V should be directed by a detailed history and physical examination.
- Antiemetic treatment should be directed toward the suspected underlying problem.

INTRODUCTION

Nausea is defined as the sensation that one is about to vomit and vomiting as the forceful expulsion of the gastric and/or proximal small bowel contents via the mouth. Nausea frequently precedes vomiting, hence the common association of the two terms. The etiologies of nausea and vomiting (N/V) are numerous and require a directed evaluation. Sequelae of N/V, such as dehydration, electrolyte imbalance, and malnutrition, frequently require hospital admission. The direct and indirect costs associated with inpatient management of N/V are impressive, considering the number of hospitalizations for N/V during pregnancy, associated with gastroparesis, and occurring postoperative.

PATHOPHYSIOLOGY

Nausea is a subjective sensation which is difficult to study, leaving much still unknown about its etiology. However, recent studies of motion sickness suggest that physiologic interactions between gastric motility and neuroendocrine responses mediate the sensation. Subjects who develop nausea have gastric rhythm abnormalities and increases in cortisol, norepinephrine, and epinephrine prior to their feelings of nausea. Although nausea typically results in vomiting, it can occur alone, particularly in disorders such as functional dyspepsia and gastroparesis.

By contrast, the mechanisms of vomiting have been better elucidated. Vomiting is mediated by a "**vomiting center**" located in the medulla, which receives stimuli from sympathetic and vagal nerves, and from the chemoreceptor trigger zone also located in the medulla. **Vagal** and **sympathetic** stimuli arise mainly from the gastrointestinal system, but can occur from virtually any system, including the vestibular system, pharynx, peritoneum, and higher central nervous system (CNS) centers. The **chemoreceptor trigger zone** lacks a blood-brain barrier and is susceptible to a wide variety of humoral stimuli (e.g., hormones, toxins, and drugs). The gastrointestinal afferents seem to activate 5-hydroxytryptamine$_3$ (5-HT$_3$) receptors, stimuli from the vestibular system stimulate muscarinic (M$_1$) and histamine (H$_1$) receptors, and the chemoreceptor trigger zone activates 5-HT$_3$, M$_1$, H$_1$, and dopamine (D$_2$) receptors. An understanding of these receptors is essential to planning appropriate antiemetic therapy.

Regardless of the stimuli, the vomiting center induces a well-coordinated response including forceful abdominal wall contractions and relaxation of the lower and upper esophageal sphincters to cause the retrograde propulsion of the antral and small bowel contents. Vomiting must be differentiated from other conditions, which may also result in the expulsion of gastric contents. Vomiting is always accompanied by strong abdominal wall contractions, which distinguishes it from regurgitation (e.g., esophageal reflux) and rumination (effortless regurgitation of a recent meal into the mouth followed by rechewing and reswallowing).

CLINICAL PRESENTATION

The history should focus first on establishing whether the patient is actually vomiting (see above). This is usually straightforward; however, patients can mistake emesis for other actions, such as expectoration of sputum, expectoration of posterior epistaxis, and coughing out ingested food which has entered the respiratory tract. Once vomiting is confirmed, the clinician should look for historic clues to the etiology of the vomiting. Given the wide variety of stimuli (both neural and humoral) that can result in vomiting, a review of the basic differential diagnosis of N/V prior to the patient interview will

Table 23-1 **Causes of N/V**

Gastrointestinal obstruction	Gastric outlet obstruction
	Small bowel obstruction
	Colonic obstruction
Gastrointestinal motility	Gastroparesis
	Gastroesophageal reflux
	Small bowel dysmotility
Gastrointestinal irritation	Nonsteroidal anti-inflammatory drugs (NSAIDs)
	Alcohol
	Antibiotics
	Viral gastroenteritis (Norwalk, rotavirus)
	Toxins (*Staphylococcus aureus, Bacillus cereus*)
	Hepatitis A or B
	Abdominal irradiation
Peritoneal irritation	Intestinal perforation
	Spontaneous bacterial peritonitis
	Appendicitis
Hepatobiliary	Cholecystitis
	Pancreatitis
CNS disorders	Meningitis
	Encephalitis
	Increased ICP
	Migraine
Vestibular	Labyrinthitis
	Motion sickness
	Ménière's disease
Drugs affecting the chemoreceptor trigger zone	Calcium channel blockers
	Opioids
	Anticonvulsants
	Nicotine
	Digoxin
Systemic disorders affecting the chemoreceptor trigger zone	Diabetic ketoacidosis
	Uremia
	Adrenal crisis
	Hypothyroidism
	Pregnancy
	Sepsis
	Postoperative vomiting
Psychogenic	Cyclic vomiting
	Anticipatory vomiting
	Bulimia

prove useful (Table 23-1). Key features to determine are the duration and onset of the N/V. Acute and chronic (>1 month) etiologies are often considerably different with regard to differential diagnosis, workup, and management. An insidious onset suggests chronic disorders such as functional dyspepsia, metabolic disorders, or pregnancy.

Characterization of the vomiting episodes should include the time of day and the substance of the vomitus. **Morning N/V** is classic in pregnancy, for example, but also characteristic of patients with diverse disorders such as increased intracranial pressure (ICP), uremia, and alcohol ingestion (nausea may not precede emesis in cases of increased ICP). Emesis which occurs over 1 hour after eating suggests gastroparesis or gastric outlet obstruction. Food that is not mixed with stomach acid strongly suggests regurgitation from the esophagus, as opposed to vomiting, has occurred, such as in achalasia or from a Zenker's diverticulum. Nonbilious but acidified vomitus suggests either functional or mechanical gastric outlet obstruction. Bilious vomitus is associated with small bowel obstruction. Vomitus with a foul, fecal-like odor is termed **feculent** and suggests obstruction with resultant stagnation and bacterial overgrowth.

Symptoms commonly associated with N/V should be sought since they often suggest an etiology. These would include abdominal or chest pain, fever, diarrhea, headache, vertigo, or neurologic deficits. A careful medication history, including prescribed, over-the-counter, herbal preparations and supplements, should be obtained. A prior history of similar episodes can be found in numerous conditions including chronic intestinal pseudo-obstruction, Crohn's disease, peptic ulcer disease, and gastroparesis.

The physical examination should be directed at assessing complications of N/V and looking for clues to the etiology. Complications of N/V chiefly include dehydration, electrolyte imbalances, and malnutrition. Vital signs should be scrutinized as volume depletion is suggested by tachycardia, hypotension, or orthostasis. Table 23-2 lists some physical findings and

Table 23-2 **Physical Examination Findings**

Jaundice	Hepatitis, cholangitis, gallstone pancreatitis
Lymphadenopathy	Malignancy, HIV, infectious etiologies
Abdominal mass	Malignancy, pregnancy, benign mechanical obstruction
Succussion splash	Functional or mechanical gastric outlet obstruction
Distended abdomen	Mechanical or functional bowel obstruction (e.g., ileus)
Papilledema	Increased ICP
RUQ tenderness	Hepatitis, cholecystitis, cholangitis, biliary colic
RLQ tenderness	Appendicitis, Crohn's disease, PID, ectopic pregnancy
LLQ tenderness	Diverticulitis, colitis, PID, ectopic pregnancy

Abbreviations: RLQ, right lower quadrant; LLQ, left lower quadrant; PID, pelvic inflammatory disease.

conditions they suggest. Although the site of abdominal tenderness suggests the site of intra-abdominal pathology, there is considerable variability in this regard. For example, gallbladder disorders such as biliary colic and cholecystitis can present with epigastric pain and tenderness instead of the classic right upper quadrant (RUQ) location.

EVALUATION

The initial step in the evaluation should focus on addressing any complications. Vomitus is rich in sodium, hydrochloric acid, and potassium; therefore, prolonged N/V will generally result in hypovolemia and hypokalemic metabolic alkalosis. Serum **electrolytes** and **renal function** should be assessed to evaluate for volume status, acid-base abnormalities, and electrolyte imbalances. A less immediate goal is to address malnutrition if present. Checking albumin and prealbumin levels can approximate the patient's current protein stores. Although one might expect malnutrition to be more of an issue in chronic N/V, acute N/V can pose a nutritional risk in the critically ill with increased metabolic demands.

The next step in the evaluation is to complete an investigation for the cause of the symptoms. In acute N/V, if no clues to an etiology exist after a thorough history and physical, a period of observation and empiric antiemetic treatment is appropriate. Diagnostic testing is usually reserved if N/V are prolonged, result in complications, or fail empiric treatment. Three caveats always apply to the diagnostic evaluation of N/V. First, any female of childbearing age, regardless of the type of contraception used, should be evaluated for pregnancy. Second, drug toxicity should always be considered. Finally, psychological or psychiatric etiologies, such as bulimia nervosa, should be diagnoses of exclusion. A discussion of the workup for every disorder is beyond the scope of this chapter, but diagnostic testing should be specifically directed by the patient's history and physical.

MANAGEMENT

Initially, patients should be resuscitated with fluids for any signs of volume depletion and any complications, particularly electrolyte abnormalities, should be addressed. Ultimately, the underlying disorder must be corrected, but suppression of N/V should occur during the diagnostic process. As noted above, suppression may be all that is required in the acute setting. Several different classes of medications are effective for N/V depending on the etiology (Table 23-3).

Table 23-3 **Commonly Used Antiemetic Classes**

Class	Drugs	Indications
Anticholinergic (block M_1 receptors)	Scopolamine	Motion sickness
Antihistamines (block H_1 receptors)	Diphenhydramine Meclizine	Motion sickness Vestibular disturbances Migraine
Butyrophenones (block D_2 receptors)	Droperidol Haloperidol	Chemotherapy-induced Postoperative
Cannabinoids	Dronabinol	Chemotherapy-induced
Phenothiazines (block D_2 receptors)	Prochlorperazine Promethazine Chlorpromazine	Drug-induced (via the chemoreceptor trigger zone) Gastroenteritis Vestibular disturbances Migraine
5-HT_3 antagonists	Ondansetron Granisetron	Chemotherapy-induced Drug-induced (via the chemoreceptor trigger zone) Postoperative
Prokinetic agents	Metoclopramide Erythromycin	Gastroesophageal reflux Gastroparesis

GASTROINTESTINAL HEMORRHAGE

Misha Rhodes

KEY POINTS

- Differentiate between upper and lower sources of bleeding by performing nasogastric lavage and rectal examination.
- Maintain an active type and cross at all times on patients with a GI bleed.
- Maintain IV access with two large bore IVs (18–20 gauge) as the larger bore allows for the delivery of more fluids at a faster rate if at all necessary during the patient's hospital course.
- Perform a thorough history and physical examination as the history can help to define the location of the blood loss in the majority of cases.

INTRODUCTION

Gastrointestinal (GI) bleeding is commonly divided into two categories: upper GI bleed (UGIB; occurring above the ligament of Treitz) and lower GI bleed (LGIB; distal to the ligament of Treitz). Clinically, patients are usually separated into the upper versus lower categories based on symptoms. Most commonly, **UGIBs** may present with **hematemesis**, which is emesis consisting of frank red blood or "coffee-grounds" (old blood), and/or **melena**. **LGIBs** may present with frank bleeding, known as **hematochezia**, or can be more occult with the only detection made by a positive stool hemoccult test. While GI bleeds are fairly common admissions, each should be approached with the appropriate amount of caution, because mortality can reach 10% during each episode. It is important to not only understand the physiology but also the management of acute GI bleeding.

UPPER GASTROINTESTINAL HEMORRHAGE

Although patients presenting with hematemesis or melena are considered to have an UGIB, a small percentage of patients presenting with melena will have a lower GI source. The most common causes are listed in Table 24-1. In general, patients are usually separated into variceal versus nonvariceal bleeds, because the management and complications differ significantly (see Chap. 28). This section will concentrate on the presentation and management of nonvariceal UGIBs.

Pathophysiology

Peptic ulcer disease is responsible for the majority of UGIBs. Ulcers usually occur as a result of *Helicobacter pylori* infection or **nonsteroidal anti-inflammatory drug (NSAID)** use, but may also occur from chronic steroid use, stress (associated with life-threatening illnesses), and excessive gastric acid. *H. pylori* is a gram-negative bacillus which is highly adapted to the acidic environment of the stomach. *H. pylori* attaches to gastric mucosa and liberates toxins which cause mucosal damage and stimulate an inflammatory response. Most patients with *H. pylori* infection develop a chronic gastritis, but only 10–15% will develop ulcers. Ulcer formation is most likely related to the production of certain toxins which cause greater mucosal damage and induce a greater inflammatory response, or patients have other factors also involved (e.g., NSAIDs, stress). NSAIDs block cyclooxygenase, thus preventing the production of protective prostaglandins in the stomach. Patients will frequently have more than one inciting event. For example, many patients with peptic ulcer bleeds have *H. pylori* infection and frequently take NSAIDs.

Table 24-1 **Most Common Causes of Upper and Lower GI Hemorrhage**

UGIB	LGIB
Gastric or duodenal ulcers: 55%	Diverticulosis: 33%
Esophageal/gastric varices: 14%	AVMs: 20–30%
AVMs: 6%	Colon cancer: 19%
Mallory-Weiss tear: 5%	Inflammatory bowel disease: 18%
Gastric/esophageal cancer: 4%	Unknown: 16%
Dieulafoy's lesion: 1%	Hemorrhoids: 4%
Esophageal perforation	Anal fissure: 4%
Esophagitis	UGIB
Gastritis	Colonic ischemia
	Meckel's diverticulum

A **Mallory-Weiss tear** is a longitudinal laceration of the esophageal or proximal gastric mucosa occurring secondary to a sudden increase in intraabdominal pressure. It is typically associated with forceful vomiting or retching.

Angiodysplasias or vascular ectasias can form in any part of the GI tract. They are most commonly sporadic, but may occur as a result of genetic disease (e.g., hereditary hemorrhagic telangiectasia), chronic renal failure, or collagen vascular disease, especially scleroderma.

Dieulafoy's lesion is a congenital aberrant submucosal arteriole which is abnormally large and runs immediately beneath the mucosa. This large dilated vessel erodes the overlying mucosa in the absence of a primary ulcer. The majority are located near the gastroesophageal junction in the lesser curvature. Because this is an arteriole, bleeding can be sudden, massive, and frequently recurrent.

Evaluation

The initial history and physical examination should be directed at determining the severity of the bleed as well as possible etiologies. History should be directed toward signs of hypotension, such as dizziness or generalized weakness, especially on standing. On physical examination, patients presenting with tachycardia, hypotension, or orthostasis should be presumed to have a significant GI bleed. Although not definitively diagnostic, a thorough history and physical examination will often yield clues as to the etiology of the bleed. Patients with peptic ulcer disease frequently report dyspepsia, a burning or gnawing epigastric pain. Classically, patients with gastric ulcers will report pain with food and patients with duodenal ulcers will report pain several hours after eating. On physical examination, patients may have epigastric tenderness. Peritoneal signs on examination suggest ulcer perforation. Gastric cancer is difficult to differentiate from peptic ulcer disease on history and physical, because of similar presentations. Patients with a Mallory-Weiss tear should have a history of prolonged vomiting or retching prior to hematemesis or melena. Alcoholism is also frequently associated with Mallory-Weiss tears.

Laboratory evaluation should evaluate the degree of blood loss, any comorbidities, and possible etiologies. A complete blood count is essential to document the degree of anemia; however, in patients with an acute bleed, the hemoglobin may remain normal for several hours until equilabration occurs. Evaluation of platelets and coagulation studies (prothrombin time [PT] and partial thromboplastin time [PTT]) is essential as abnormalities will need to be corrected to control the bleeding. Renal and liver function should also be evaluated as both may increase the risk of bleeding or suggest certain etiologies. Last, although not specific, *H. pylori* antibodies may suggest a reason for peptic ulcers.

Management

Immediate resuscitation is always paramount in the management of UGIBs. **Two large bore (18 gauge) peripheral IVs** are essential to adequate volume resuscitation. Normal saline should be administered immediately to any patient with hypotension, tachycardia, or orthostasis. **Packed red blood cells (PRBCs)** should be administered to maintain a hematocrit of >30 for high-risk patients (multiple medical problems) or >20 for lower-risk patients.

Nasogastric lavage should be performed in every patient presenting with a suspected UGIB. Lavage can localize the cause to the stomach or esophagus if blood or coffee-ground material is present. Further, patients with frank blood that does not clear after multiple lavages should be considered to have an ongoing bleed and managed more aggressively.

All patients should receive acid suppression therapy with **high dose proton pump inhibitors (PPIs)**. These can be administered orally in patients who are no longer bleeding and are stable, but should otherwise be given intravenously. PPIs have been shown to decrease the risk of rebleeding and the need for further transfusions. H_2-blockers are generally not recommended because they have not been shown to decrease the risk of rebleeding.

Esophagogastroduodenoscopy (EGD) is essential for both diagnosis and perhaps therapy. Most etiologies of an UGIB can be ascertained by an endoscopy that extends into the first part of the duodenum. Further, hemostasis can be obtained through either cautery or injection of epinephrine via the EGD. Any gastric ulcers visible on EGD should be biopsied for diagnosis. Gastric ulcers can rarely be definitively diagnosed by inspection alone, so pathologic analysis is important. In addition, the best test for *H. pylori* is urease testing of a gastric mucosa biopsy. Endoscopy also has prognostic importance (Table 24-2).

Patients who have no apparent source of bleeding after EGD should have a colonoscopy because the source may be from the lower GI tract. Other modalities that may be helpful include angiography and tagged red cell scans; however, both of these are only useful if the patient is actively bleeding.

Once hemostasis is achieved, further management depends on the underlying etiology. Patients with peptic ulcer disease should all receive acid-suppression therapy and testing for *H. pylori*. If patients are infected

Table 24-2 **Risk of Rebleeding from a Peptic Ulcer Based on Endoscopic Findings**

Endoscopic Finding	Risk of Rebleeding (%)
Active bleeding	55–90
Pigmented protuberance (visible vessel)	43–50
Adherent clot	12–33
Clean ulcer base	3–5

with *H. pylori*, a multidrug regimen is necessary to eradicate. Patients should also be counseled to avoid NSAIDs and aspirin as these will impair healing and promote further ulcers (see Chap. 21 in the *First Exposure to Internal Medicine: Ambulatory Medicine*).

LOWER GASTROINTESTINAL HEMORRHAGE

Patients presenting with hematochezia are considered to have a lower GI etiology or bleeding, but brisk upper GI blood loss can also result in maroon or even bright red blood in the stools. The most common causes of LGIBs are listed in Table 24-1.

Pathophysiology

Diverticulosis is the most common cause of hematochezia and the incidence increases with age. A diverticulum is produced when increased intraluminal pressure in the colon causes the herniation of colonic mucosa through the muscularis layer. These sac-like projections often cause the supplying arteriole to become draped over the dome of the diverticulum. Over time, vessel injury leads to weakness of the arteriole wall and a propensity to rupture. Although diverticular disease tends to be predominantly left-sided, most diverticular bleeding (50–90%) is from the right colon.

Angiodysplasias (also known as **arteriovenous malformations [AVMs]**) were discussed in the UGIB section but note that the colon is the most common site for AVMs.

Any cause of **colitis** can lead to mucosal injury and resultant bleeding. Common causes include infectious, ischemic, and inflammatory (inflammatory bowel disease). Ischemic colitis is caused by a transient ischemia to the colon, usually related to hypotension, heart failure, or occasionally arrhythmias. The ischemia is typically left-sided in the splenic flexure, which is a watershed area with blood supply from both the superior mesenteric and inferior mesenteric arteries.

Meckel's diverticulum is an occasional cause of LGIB. It is a congenital abnormality resulting from the incomplete obliteration of the vitelline duct. Rule of 2's: incidence is 2% in the population, male:female ratio 2:1, within 2 ft of ileocecal valve, measures 2 in. long.

Evaluation

Similar to upper GI bleed, the evaluation should focus on determining the extent of bleeding and potential etiologies. History and physical examination are usually not sufficient to determining the etiology, but will often provide some important clues.

Diverticular disease is most common in the older population, present in over a third of adults over the age 60. However, only 5–15% will experience bleeding. Classically, patients present with the abrupt onset of painless rectal bleeding. It is usually self-limited (75%), but may be sudden and massive.

Infectious colitis is most commonly due to *Salmonella, Shigella,* and *Campylobacter.* A history of acute diarrhea associated with fever and abdominal pain is typical.

Inflammatory bowel disease has a bimodal distribution for age of onset, with peaks at 20 and 50 years of age (see Chap. 26). Ulcerative colitis typically presents with frank rectal bleeding, whereas Crohn's disease can occasionally cause bloody stool but more frequently presents with mucoid or watery stools. Patients will frequently have abdominal pain, tenesmus, or fecal urgency.

Colon cancer most commonly presents as chronic or occult blood loss, but has been associated with ~10% of acute LGIBs. The incidence increases with age with a significant rise after age 40. Risk factors include family history, inflammatory bowel disease, and tobacco use. Presenting signs and symptoms can include abdominal pain, change in bowel habits, melena, and new-onset microcytic anemia in men and in postmenopausal women.

Anorectal disease is the most common cause of LGIBs in young individuals. Hemorrhoids typically present with small amounts of bright red blood on toilet paper or streaked in the stool and rarely cause significant hemorrhage. Anal fissures are usually associated with constipation and present with pain and bleeding during bowel movements.

Ischemic colitis occurs in the elderly population with risk factors for reduced blood flow, such as hypotension, heart failure, or arrhythmias. Patients present with postprandial abdominal pain out of proportion to examination findings and hematochezia.

Laboratory evaluation is the same for UGIBs, with the possible addition of a lactic acid, which can be elevated in individuals with ischemic colitis. Diagnosis is made by serum lactate level, abdominal x-ray, computed tomography (CT) scan, colonoscopy, barium enema, or angiography.

Management

As with an UGIB assessment of the patient is critical. Patients with hemodynamic instability should be managed in the ICU. Fluid resuscitation with intravenous fluids, blood products or both is also important. Guidelines for transfusion are the same as those for UGIB. Maintain good IV access at all times. As with UGIB, nasogastric lavage is useful as a brisk UGIB can present as hematochezia. If the nasogastric lavage demonstrates blood or coffee-ground material, an EGD should be the first test performed. Otherwise, a colonoscopy should be performed to localize and potentially treat the site of bleeding. Patients with active bleeding who are unstable should be considered for an emergent unprepped colonoscopy. However, this is only necessary if the patient is having significant bleeding and hemostasis is urgent. Otherwise, the patient should have a bowel prep (usually GoLytely) prior to colonoscopy to provide adequate visualization. Other options to localize the site of bleeding include angiography or a tagged red cell scan; however, these are only useful if the patient is actively bleeding. If the colonoscopy does not reveal a source of bleeding, an EGD should be pursued. Most causes of LGIBs will end on their own and do not require further therapy.

Treatment is dependent on the severity and etiology. For example, patients with known diverticulosis and classic hematochezia who are stable and no longer bleeding may only require observation and often don't require colonoscopy. By contrast, patients with ischemic colitis may require urgent surgical intervention. In general, management requires colonoscopy with possible cauterization or injection to control bleeding. If source of bleeding is not seen then tagged red cell scans and angiography can be utilized. If bleeding recurs more than three times in a year surgery is considered an option.

PSEUDOMEMBRANOUS COLITIS

Christine Yasuko Todd

KEY POINTS

- CDAD should be considered in any patient currently or recently on antibiotics, especially in the hospital setting.
- Classic symptoms are fever, leukocytosis, crampy abdominal pain, and watery diarrhea, although not every patient exhibits all symptoms, even diarrhea.
- ELISA and latex agglutination tests for *C. difficile* toxin are the most commonly used methods of diagnosis.
- Oral metronidazole is the preferred agent for CDAD, although recurrence is common and requires extended treatment.
- *C. difficile* is easily spread within the hospital environment and can occur in hospital-wide epidemics. Hand washing of staff prevents transmission between patients.

INTRODUCTION

Intestinal disease caused by *Clostridium difficile* is encountered frequently by any doctor who works with hospitalized patients. It is one of the most common nosocomial infections and causes a significant amount of morbidity and mortality, especially among elderly and immunocompromised patients. *C. difficile* causes a spectrum of intestinal diseases, ranging from a clinically asymptomatic carrier state (playing an important role in epidemics in hospitals) to toxic megacolon, intestinal perforation, and death. This range of disease causes some confusion in regards to nomenclature—**pseudomembranous colitis, antibiotic-associated diarrhea**, and *C. difficile*

colitis are used interchangeably by clinicians. For the purposes of this discussion, we will use the term *C. difficile* **associated disease (CDAD)**.

PATHOPHYSIOLOGY

C. difficile is a fairly ubiquitous organism, found quite commonly in soil. Infants become colonized with *C. difficile* within weeks of being born but remain well because their colonic mucosa has not yet developed receptors for *C. difficile's* enteric toxins. Infants develop antibodies to *C. difficile* and either eradicate it or become an asymptomatic carrier. In carriers, the population of this bacterium is held in check during health by competing communities of colonic bacteria. Alteration of this balance of bacterial competition and intact host immunity by the administration of antibiotics or an immunocompromising condition (or, frequently, both) results in the growth of the colony of *C. difficile* and elaboration of its two toxins, toxins A and B. Patients without *C. difficile* in their colons can acquire it when hospitalized, as *C. difficile* can live for weeks on fomites such as stethoscopes, bathroom surfaces, and the unwashed hands of hospital staff. When a patient on broad-spectrum antibiotics is exposed to *C. difficile*, CDAD is a likely result, especially if an amnestic immunologic response to *C. difficile* (from infant exposure) is lacking or weak.

As it proliferates, *C. difficile* (so called because it is difficult to grow in culture) produces two toxins—toxin A and toxin B. Both toxins adhere to colonic receptors and cause necrosis and shedding of the brush boarder into the lumen of the intestine. Toxin A, in particular, has been shown in animal experiments to cause an acute inflammatory diarrhea. Unlike other known intestinal toxins, such as cholera toxin, *C. difficile* toxins do not affect second messengers such as cyclic adenosine monophosphate (AMP) or guanosine monophosphate (GMP) to cause cell death. Instead, the toxins appear to inactivate actin filaments, causing detachment of damaged cells from the basement membrane. Be aware that C. *difficile* does not penetrate into the gut wall but remains in the lumen of the gut.

CLINICAL PRESENTATION

As mentioned, CDAD encompasses a spectrum of disease, ranging from an asymptomatic carrier state, through a mild hospital-acquired diarrhea, to a severe illness accompanied by massive intestinal inflammation, dilation ("toxic megacolon"), intestinal perforation, and death from sepsis. Because CDAD is so common, one should have a low threshold for pursuing its diagnosis and instituting therapy. Be alert to the classic symptoms of CDAD: **fever, leukocytosis, watery diarrhea**, and **crampy lower abdominal pain**. Any patient with a **recent history of antibiotic use** (and it can be **as recent**

as 1 day prior or up to 8 weeks prior) who develops suspicious symptoms should be evaluated for CDAD. **Hospitalized patients** on (or recently on) antibiotics who develop symptoms should be particularly suspect, and **should be considered for empiric therapy for CDAD** while a diagnosis is pursued. It is important to be aware that hospitalized patients who develop diarrhea after 72 hours in house are rarely shown to have any enteropathogen other than *C. difficile*.

It is important to remember that patients often do not exhibit the entire constellation of symptoms. In fact, **diarrhea,** which one might erroneously consider a necessary symptom for the diagnosis, **can be absent** in patients with CDAD. The absence of diarrhea, in fact, can be seen in severe, advanced cases of CDAD where a toxic megacolon has caused atony and a functional obstruction of the bowel.

The development of a **profound leukocytosis** (20,000–100,000) is commonly associated with CDAD. Fever is usually low grade, and the abdominal pain is usually of a crampy or colicky nature, with relief after episodes of diarrhea. The diarrhea rarely contains blood or a melanotic component, but can occur in excess of 10 times a day. Through the process of this diarrhea, a significant amount of protein can be lost. The protein-losing enteropathy accompanying CDAD can result in a rapid decline in serum albumin and significant edema.

EVALUATION

There are a number of ways to establish a diagnosis of CDAD, each with its advantages and drawbacks. Stool cultures for the presence of *C. difficile* can be done, but as noted before, *C. difficile* is a difficult bacterium to successfully culture and the time and expense it takes to perform a culture are significant disadvantages. In addition, the presence of *C. difficile* does not prove it is the source of a patient's illness, as the patient could be an asymptomatic carrier and the abdominal complaints could be from another cause. The presence of *C. difficile* toxins A and B can be shown by their toxic effects on a tissue culture of fibroblasts. This method is considered the "Gold Standard" test for the presence of *C. difficile* toxins but is expensive and takes a number of days to complete, a major disadvantage in a disease that can have a rapid and toxic course. Most practitioners use an **enzyme-linked immunosorbent assay (ELISA) or latex agglutination method** to detect the presence of *C. difficile* **toxin** or toxin-related chemicals. These tests are fast and cheap, but can result in a higher rate of false positives than tissue culture. To increase the specificity of these tests, three samples taken on three different days are submitted for testing, of which at least two should be positive in patients with CDAD.

The presence of **fecal leucocytes** can be found quickly by performing a Wright's stain on a fecal sample. This test, if positive, points toward an inflammatory/infectious cause for diarrhea. If negative, however, it does not rule out these diagnoses. **Abdominal imaging** can be helpful in assessing the severity of CDAD. "Thumb printing" on a KUB (kidney, ureter, and bladder) signifies significant intestinal mucosal inflammation. Similar findings can be found on computed tomography (CT) of these patients. KUB or CT findings are not necessary for the diagnosis of CDAD. The most rapid, accurate way to establish a diagnosis of CDAD is through direct visualization of the colonic mucosa through **sigmoidoscopy** or colonoscopy. The sloughing of intestinal cells causes a patchy yellow-white appearance to the mucosa, the "pseudomembranes" with which the disease is pathognomonically associated (see Fig. 25-1). Not all patients with CDAD develop pseudomembranes,

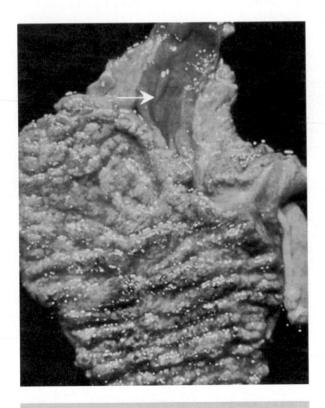

Figure 25-1 **Autopsy specimen showing confluent pseudomembranes covering the cecum of a patient with pseudomembranous colitis. Note the sparing of the terminal ileum (arrow).** (*Source:* Reproduced with permission from Kasper DL, Braunwald E, Fauci AS, et al. *Harrison's Principles of Internal Medicine,* 16th ed. New York: McGraw-Hill, 2005, Figure 114-1.)

however, and the inflammation of the mucosa makes it friable and prone to perforation. Thus, endoscopy for the diagnosis of CDAD is rarely done.

MANAGEMENT

In patients with mild disease, discontinuation of the offending antibiotics results in cure. In more compromised patients, however, a number of approaches can be used to ameliorate the disease.

Antibiotics active against *C. difficile* can be used—**metronidazole** and **vancomycin** are the drugs used in the United States for this purpose. Oral versions of these antibiotics are superior to parenteral versions, as they afford better contact of the antibiotic treatment with the *C. difficile* within the gut lumen. Metronidazole is preferred over vancomycin as the use of oral vancomycin is the chief driver in the development of vancomycin-resistant *Enterococcus*. In addition, oral vancomycin is very expensive. These antibiotics are also effective when given by retention enema. **IV vancomycin is ineffective** against *C. difficile*, as it doesn't penetrate the gut wall and move into the gut lumen, where the pathogen is. Antibiotics against *C. difficile* are usually given for 14 days in patients for whom the offending antibiotics can be stopped. If a full course of the offending antibiotics must be given, treatment antibiotics for CDAD should be continued at least 7 days after the course of the offending antibiotics is over.

Cholestyramine has been shown to bind *C. difficile* toxin and can be added to a regimen of metronidazole. Some sources have shown that cholestyramine may also bind metronidazole, reducing its effectiveness. The probiotic agents *Lactobacillus* and *Saccharomyces boulardii* taken orally in capsule form have been used to reestablish "good" bacterial flora in the gut after treatment for CDAD. Probiotic treatment has met with some success in clinical trials.

Unfortunately, **CDAD recurs frequently**—in up to 35% of patients who initially respond to metronidazole or vancomycin. **Recurrence is rarely due to resistance** to these antibiotics but instead due to the immunocompromised nature of the patients and the continued use of necessary broad-spectrum antibiotics. Repeated and lengthy (up to 6 weeks) courses of metronidazole or vancomycin are sometimes required. Surgical intervention (colectomy) is sometimes necessary for patients who develop toxic megacolon.

INFLAMMATORY

BOWEL DISEASE

Douglas Bazil Tzanetos

KEY POINTS

- UC is limited to the colon, and classically presents with bloody diarrhea.
- Crohn's disease most commonly involves the terminal ileum, but can affect any portion of the GI tract, and is characterized by "skip" lesions and transmural inflammation (with subsequent stricture and fistula formation).
- Both UC and Crohn's are associated with extraintestinal manifestations, such as pyoderma gangrenosum, erythema nodosum, uveitis, arthritis, and PSC.
- Both conditions are associated with an increased risk of colon cancer, mandating surveillance colonoscopy on a regular basis.

INTRODUCTION

The term inflammatory bowel disease (IBD) can refer to Crohn's disease or ulcerative colitis (UC). These two conditions are chronic, relapsing diseases which can involve both gastrointestinal (GI) and systemic symptoms, but they differ in their presentations and associated complications. The incidence of IBD is on the order of 10 per 100,000 people in the United States, and UC is about twice as common as Crohn's. IBD is typically a disease of young adults, and most people are diagnosed between the ages of 15 and 40. There is no gender difference in the prevalence of IBD. Risk for development of IBD is at least partially genetic, with a 10–25% chance of affected patients having an affected family member. Type of diet is not a risk factor for IBD, and there are few clear risk factors for IBD. Some studies suggest that smoking may actually reduce the risk of developing UC, but it can increase the risk of Crohn's disease. Although morbidity can be significant, studies suggest that IBD confers only a slightly increased risk of mortality. Therefore, with careful evaluation, treatment, and monitoring, patients with IBD can usually lead full, active lives.

PATHOPHYSIOLOGY

The ultimate cause of IBD is unknown; however, it has been posited to result from a chaotic immune response to unknown environmental triggers in genetically predisposed individuals. There is some evidence to suggest an imbalance in activity between proinflammatory cytokines (e.g., interleukin (IL)-1B, tumor necrosis factor) and anti-inflammatory cytokines (e.g., IL-1 receptor antagonist, IL-10, and certain prostaglandins).

Crohn's disease can involve any portion of the GI tract **from the mouth to the anus**. Crohn's is typified by **transmural inflammation** (involving the entire thickness of the bowel wall). The most commonly involved area is the small bowel (80% of patients), especially the **distal ileum**. However, some patients have both large and small bowel involvement, some only large bowel involvement, while others have predominance of disease in the oral, esophageal, or gastroduodenal areas. On gross examination, bowel in Crohn's disease is visually distinct from normal, healthy bowel and can be friable, ulcerated, and swollen. The bowel in Crohn's also has fat along the wall in unusual locations. Usually fat is on the mesenteric side of normal bowel, but in bowel affected by Crohn's disease, the fat is often on the antimesenteric side (**creeping fat**). The inflammation in Crohn's disease causes mucosal damage to the bowel and is typified by the presence of **non-caseating granulomas** (nonnecrotic nodular inflammatory lesions containing phagocytes). This inflammation often leads to the formation of **fissures** in the bowel which, if they deepen, can lead to **fistulas**. A fistula is an abnormal sinus tract between two different areas such as bowel and the outside skin, a blind cavity, or another region of bowel. Another hallmark of Crohn's is the sharp demarcations between normal and inflamed bowel; when multiple areas of diseased and nondiseased bowel are adjacent, these areas are called **skip lesions**. **Mucosal ulcers** on the bowel can lead to a **cobblestoned appearance**. The mucosal inflammation involves an infiltration of neutrophils into the intestinal crypts forming a histologic feature of Crohn's, the **crypt abscess**. The chronic, relapsing inflammation in Crohn's can result in significant bowel edema, fibrosis, and narrowing (or frank obstruction) of the lumen of the bowel. This can be evidenced on a small bowel follow-through as a **string sign** in which a thin stream of barium can be seen passing through diseased bowel segments. One-third of patients with Crohn's

Table 26-1 **Distinctions between Crohn's and UC**

	Crohn's Disease	**UC**
Location	Anywhere in GI tract	Colon only
Distribution	Skip lesions	Continuous/diffuse
Bowel inflammation	Transmural (full thickness)	Mucosa only
Ulcers	Deep	Superficial
Fibrosis/stricture	Marked	Mild
Granulomas	Yes (50%)	No
Fistulae	Yes	No
Bloody diarrhea	Sometimes	Often/usually
Surgery can cure	No	Yes

disease will also evidence perianal disease. These patients can have **perianal abscesses**, anal fissures, and fistulous tracts involving the anus.

UC differs from Crohn's disease in several important anatomic and physiologic distinctions. First, UC **almost always involves the rectum** and can but does not always extend up the entire colon. It never involves small bowel. The inflammation in UC is not transmural but is instead **confined to the colonic mucosa**. Unlike in Crohn's disease, the involvement of diseased bowel is always continuous (i.e., there are no skip lesions). As in Crohn's, the hallmark feature of UC is recurring, chronic inflammation of affected bowel. **Hemorrhage** is much more common in UC than in Crohn's (Table 26-1).

CLINICAL PRESENTATION

Crohn's disease has a more variable clinical presentation than UC because of the variable extent and location of the disease. Classic Crohn's is characterized by **diarrhea, fever, weight loss, abdominal pain**, and loss of appetite. Crohn's can be active during acute episodes (flares) and then dormant for long periods in which the patient may be asymptomatic or have only mild symptoms. The diarrhea is most often nonbloody but can be bloody. Patients may have multiple bowel movements, sometimes in excess of 10 per day. Bowel movements may be painful. The transmural inflammation in Crohn's can cause first narrowing, then **strictures** (a narrowing of a lumen secondary to fibrosis and scarring), then sometimes frank **bowel obstruction** develop which can manifest as abdominal pain. The ulcers and fistulas can lead to bowel wall perforation and the formation of abscesses in the abdomen or near the anus. **Perianal disease** is more common in Crohn's than in UC and can manifest as anal fissures, perianal abscesses, or rectoanal fistulae. Oral aphthous ulcers can occur. Small bowel involvement can lead to fat malabsorption.

UC is characterized by **bloody diarrhea**. The patient often has multiple, sometimes painful bowel movements. Bowel movements also may be associated with passage of mucus. Alternating constipation and diarrhea can occur. As in Crohn's, fever, weight loss, and abdominal pain can occur. In severe UC, blood loss can be significant enough to warrant transfusion. As in Crohn's disease, the patient may experience flares of disease activity followed by long periods of general good health and disease dormancy.

Extraintestinal or systemic manifestations of Crohn's and UC can also occur in about 10% of patients, presumably from the chronic, recurrent inflammation. These include eye findings such as **uveitis**, an inflammation of the posterior, pigmented part of the iris which can also affect the cornea and retina. Uveitis is characterized by pain, photophobia, and a "ciliary flush," which is dilation of the fine capillaries around the corneal border, with redness of the eye confined to that area rather than diffuse redness. Skin findings can occur and include **erythema nodosum** (tender red nodules usually on the shins) and **pyoderma gangrenosum** (necrotic skin ulcers with purple-red borders; Figs. 26-1 and 26-2). **Arthritis** involving large joints and **ankylosing spondylitis** can also occur. Ankylosing spondylitis is a type of arthritis which involves the spine and the sacroiliac joints which can result in stiffness and rigidity and produce "bamboo spine" deformities. Finally, **primary sclerosing cholangitis (PSC)** can develop which is fibrosis and stricture formation of the intra- and extrahepatic bile ducts, classically presenting as progressive obstructive jaundice, with symptoms of malaise, pruritus, and anorexia. Ten percent of patients with PSC eventually develop cholangiocarcinoma.

In very ill patients with IBD, the inflammation may extend beyond the colonic mucosa into the muscle layers causing impaired motility, dilatation, and ultimately perforation, a condition known as **toxic megacolon**. Toxic megacolon essentially is a nonobstructive dilatation of the colon accompanied by systemic symptoms (e.g., fever, anemia, tachycardia, and abnormal electrolytes). Toxic megacolon occurs in fewer than 5% of patients with Crohn's and UC. It is a more common complication of UC than of Crohn's.

Finally, patients with IBD are at an **increased risk of colon cancer**. This risk has been more clearly defined in patients with UC. In patients with UC, 10 years after initial presentation, there is a 1% per year risk of developing colorectal cancer. While it was once thought that the risk of developing colon cancer was greater in UC than in Crohn's, in actuality, for long-standing Crohn's disease involving the colon, the risk is probably similar.

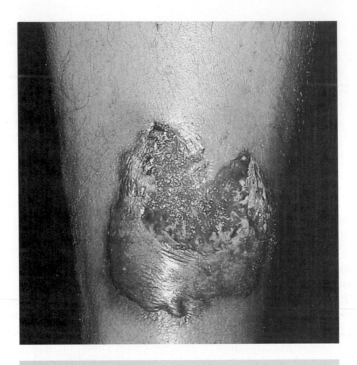

Figure 26-1 **Pyoderma gangrenosum: early. This extremely painful, boggy ulcer developed from a hemorrhagic pustule in the course of only 3 days. The patient had UC and had experienced similar lesions previously. Note the dusky peripheral rim; the bullous detachment of epidermis at the lower margin; and the irregular, undermined border with pustules on top. Pus is also seen at the base of the ulcer.** (*Source:* Reproduced with permission from Wolff K, Johnson RA, Suurmond R, et al. *Fitzpatrick's Color Atlas & Synopsis of Clinical Dermatology,* 5th ed. New York: McGraw-Hill, 2005, Figure 7-28.)

EVALUATION

Because of the variety of presentations that Crohn's can take and the often nonspecific symptoms of IBD early in the disease course, the differential diagnosis can be broad. Generally speaking, for patients with chronic diarrhea, abdominal pain, and nonspecific symptoms, the following should be considered: infectious enterocolitis (especially *Yersinia, Salmonella, Shigella, Escherichia coli,* and *Campylobacter*), irritable bowel syndrome, lactose intolerance, malabsorption syndromes, appendicitis, diverticulitis, ischemic colitis,

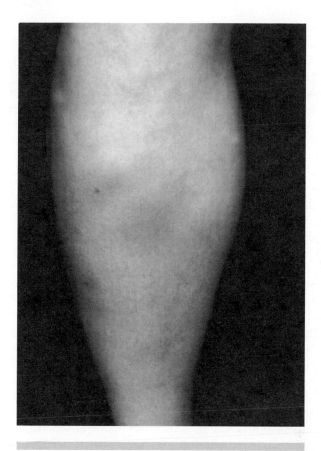

Figure 26-2 **Erythema nodosum. Indurated, very tender inflammatory nodules mostly in the pretibial region. Lesions are seen as red, ill-defined erythemas but palpated as deep-seated nodules, hence the designation.** (*Source:* Reproduced with permission from Wolff K, Johnson RA, Suurmond R, et al. *Fitzpatrick's Color Atlas & Synopsis of Clinical Dermatology*, 5th ed. New York: McGraw-Hill, 2005, Figure 7-25.)

and GI cancers (colon cancer, lymphoma, or carcinoma in particular). The presence of certain symptoms such as fever and bloody diarrhea (hematochezia) can help narrow the differential; for example, it would exclude such entities as irritable bowel syndrome, lactose intolerance, and simple malabsorption syndromes.

The diagnosis of IBD is usually established by supportive endoscopy (**colonoscopy**) findings in a patient with a compatible clinical history.

Colonoscopy should generally not be done during acute flares of disease, however, to avoid perforation. Endoscopic findings of friable colon with uniform, superficial inflammatory changes extending from the rectum proximally through the colon support the diagnosis of UC. In contrast, the presence of terminal ileum disease (supportive but not required), focal ulcerations adjacent to normal colonic mucosa (skip areas), noncaseating granulomas, and a cobblestoned appearance of the mucosa due to ulcerations all are more consistent with Crohn's disease. Biopsies usually confirm rather than make the diagnosis. In up to 10% of patients with IBD, endoscopic findings may be so nonspecific as to not allow the distinction between Crohn's and UC, and therefore the patient may be diagnosed with "indeterminate colitis."

Helpful lab tests include an erythrocyte sedimentation rate (ESR) or C-reactive protein (CRP) to document the presence of systemic inflammation, a complete blood count (CBC) to evaluate for anemia, hemoccult cards for occult GI bleeding, and certain antibody tests. *Anti-Saccharomyces cerevisiae* antibodies (ASCA, interestingly an antibody to the yeast which when fermented produces beer) are positive in over 60% of patients with Crohn's. In contrast, perinuclear antineutrophil cytoplasmic antibody (p-ANCA) is positive in up to 75% of patients with UC. ASCA is not usually positive in patients with UC, and p-ANCA is not usually positive in patients with Crohn's, therefore these tests are relatively specific but only moderately sensitive. These are helpful antibody tests but alone do not make the diagnosis; they must be interpreted in context of clinical history and endoscopy results. Other laboratory findings could include low albumin (from malnutrition) and low vitamin B_{12} (in Crohn's patients with terminal ileum involvement, with concomitant neurologic and hematologic findings of B_{12} deficiency). Finally, adjunct tests may include abdominal x-ray (look for abdominal perforation or the colonic dilatation of toxic megacolon). An upper GI series may help reveal extent of disease, and barium enema may reveal bowel strictures, the "string sign" as described above, and can also help evaluate disease extent. However, a barium enema should not be performed during acute disease flares.

MANAGEMENT

Inflammatory bowel disease is best managed by a team of primary care physicians working in conjunction with specialty consultants such as gastroenterologists and surgeons. The classes of drugs used for IBD are **aminosalicylates** (e.g., sulfasalazine), **steroids** (e.g., prednisone, hydrocortisone enemas), **immunomodulating agents** (e.g., azathioprine, 6-mercaptopurine or 6-MP, and methotrexate), **antibiotics** (e.g., metronidazole), and the newer **biologic agents** (e.g., infliximab). The chief drugs used are the aminosalicylates and steroids. Many of these drugs have occasional serious side effects such as bone marrow suppression, immune suppression leading to infection, hepatic dysfunction, and the host of side effects associated with prolonged steroid use (e.g., hypertension, diabetes, and obesity). Therefore, these drugs are often used in a stepwise fashion, first starting with less toxic regimens.

Crohn's Disease

In general, the medications used include **aminosalicylates**, **corticosteroids**, immunomodulating drugs, antibiotics, and the new biologic agents (infliximab).

Treatment of patients with Crohn's is directed by the clinical manifestation of their Crohn's disease. Crohn's disease with the chief manifestations of fibrosis and stenosis is often treated with 5-ASA (5-aminosalicylic acid, a component of sulfasalazine). Predominately, inflammatory Crohn's is treated with 5-ASA, steroids, 6-MP, methotrexate, infliximab, or surgery. Finally, those with fistulizing disease respond to 6-MP, metronidazole, and infliximab. **Sulfasalazine** is often the initial drug used in **mild** Crohn's disease. It is only helpful for colonic disease, and not small bowel disease. Many of the side effects of sulfasalazine (severe allergic reactions, hepatitis, and bone marrow suppression) are caused primarily by an inactive sulfa moiety, rather than the active 5-aminosalicylate portion (also known as mesalamine). Newer forms of this drug consist of 5-ASA dimers (olsalazine) and coated 5-ASA that are not degraded in the proximal bowel, as well as mesalamine delivered in enema form. **Antibiotics** such as metronidazole (Flagyl) are especially helpful **for patients with fistulae and perianal disease**, and sometimes are tried in those who do not respond well to sulfasalazine. In patients who fail both of these, steroids are often the next choice. **Steroids** are used often **during acute flares** but because of an extensive side effect profile should **not be used to maintain disease remission**. **Azathioprine** or **6-MP** should be used for **maintenance therapy** for those with frequent relapses (with toxicities of bone marrow suppression and pancreatitis of which to be aware). Finally, **infliximab**, a synthetic antibody to tumor necrosis factor-alpha has more recently been used to treat Crohn's disease, especially with fistulae formation. In general, azathioprine, 6-MP, methotrexate, and infliximab are used with more severe or refractory disease.

Periodic colonoscopies with biopsies every 1–2 years should be done on patients who have had Crohn's disease with extensive colitis for at least 8 years as surveillance for colon cancer. If dysplasia (abnormal cellular morphology) or precancerous lesions or cancer are found, colectomy should be considered. Other indications for surgery are disease refractory to medical therapy, steroid dependence, and complicated disease (e.g., multiple strictures). It should be noted that surgery is not curative in Crohn's disease, because Crohn's can affect any portion of the GI tract, even after a diseased colon is removed.

Ulcerative Colitis

Mild disease (less than four bowel movements a day with absence of systemic symptoms) is treated with 5-ASA. Moderate disease (four to six bowel movements a day, some systemic symptoms) is treated with 5-ASA, steroids, and 6-MP. Severe disease (more than six bowel movements a day with many systemic symptoms) is treated with IV steroids, cyclosporine, an immuno-suppressive agent, and sometimes with surgery. Enema preparations of 5-ASA or hydrocortisone are often needed. For refractory disease, or disease with serious complications such as toxic megacolon, colectomy is often consid-ered. Unlike in Crohn's disease, **colectomy** may be curative in UC. As in Crohn's with extensive colitis, periodic surveillance colonoscopies should be done, especially in patients who have had UC for over 8 years.

EVALUATION AND

MANAGEMENT OF

ASCITES

Michelle L. Rossi

KEY POINTS

- Fluid accumulates in the peritoneal cavity by two primary mechanisms: increased portal pressure or primary peritoneal disease.
- The most common cause of ascites is cirrhotic liver disease.
- The serum-to-ascites albumin gradient (SAAG) is critical to making an accurate diagnosis.
- Spontaneous bacterial peritonitis (SBP) should be considered in any patient with ascites and worsening symptoms.

INTRODUCTION

Ascites is an accumulation of fluid in the peritoneal cavity. The predominant cause of ascites in the United States is **cirrhotic liver disease, which accounts for ~80% of all cases**. Ascites may also result from other systemic diseases, such as heart failure (cardiac ascites) and nephrotic syndrome, or from primary peritoneal pathology, such as peritoneal carcinomatosis or tuberculosis. The presence of ascites is often suspected based on the history and physical examination—which will often give clues to the etiology and therefore the treatment.

PATHOPHYSIOLOGY

In general, edema results from one of three main mechanisms: decreased plasma oncotic pressure, increased vascular hydrostatic pressure, or increased capillary permeability. Ascites from cirrhotic liver disease is actually the result of all three mechanisms via a complex interaction of neurohumoral cascades and vascular changes (Fig. 27-1). The first step in the development of ascites is **portal hypertension**, which results in the local production of vasodilators, predominantly nitric oxide (NO). As NO production increases, **splanchnic vessel dilatation** becomes so pronounced that pooling of blood in the splanchnic circulation effectively decreases arterial blood volume and pressure. As arterial pressure decreases the **sympathetic nervous**

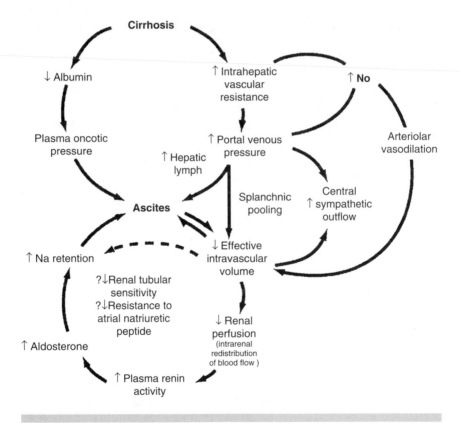

Figure 27-1 **Pathophysiologic mechanisms for the formation of ascites.** (*Source:* Reproduced with permission from Kasper DL, Braunwald E, Fauci AS, et al. *Harrison's Principles of Internal Medicine,* 16th ed. New York: McGraw-Hill, 2005, Figure 289-2.)

and the renin-angiotensin systems are activated. The resulting sodium and water retention maintain arterial pressure, but also further contribute to ascites formation by increasing capillary hydrostatic pressure. The portal hypertension and splanchnic pooling **alter capillary permeability**, allowing further fluid leak into the abdominal cavity. Last, patients with cirrhosis tend to be hypoalbuminemic, and since albumin is responsible for the majority of plasma oncotic pressure, they have decreased plasma oncotic pressure. Therefore, all three of the major factors that contribute to the development of edema can be present in patients with cirrhotic liver disease.

Ascites can also complicate heart failure and nephrotic syndrome. As in cirrhosis, decreased effective arterial blood volume plays a primary role in the pathogenesis of ascites in both conditions. The diminished arterial pressure activates the vasopressin, renin-aldosterone, and sympathetic nervous systems. These compensatory mechanisms lead to renal vasoconstriction as well as sodium and water retention. Fluid retention results in increased pressure within the hepatic sinusoids and portal vein, which allows fluid to collect in the abdominal cavity.

Primary peritoneal diseases such as peritoneal carcinomatosis and tuberculosis cause ascites through the production of proteinaceous material within the peritoneum. This increased oncotic pressure forces extracellular fluid into the peritoneal cavity to re-establish the oncotic balance.

Last, any disease which obstructs the portal vein will cause fluid accumulation. This occurs with massive liver metastases or occlusion of the portal vein from tumor or thrombosis.

CLINICAL PRESENTATION

Patients often don't seek medical attention until the ascites become clinically evident. They are often bothered by practical things and will say that "my clothes don't fit" or "my belly is getting big." **Symptoms typically do not develop until the end-stage of the underlying disease**, because the peritoneal space can accumulate large amounts of fluid and <500 mL of fluid is generally undetectable by physical examination. Symptoms are typically more attributable to the underlying disease process, such as cirrhosis, heart failure, and nephrotic syndrome. Symptoms associated with ascites include generalized discomfort—the abdomen is reported to feel bloated and stretched. Fluid accumulation is also associated with early satiety, heartburn, and sometimes nausea. When patients have significant ascites, they may report shortness of breath secondary to a limitation in diaphragmatic excursion.

The initial evaluation of a patient with suspected ascites should concentrate on confirming the presence of ascites and identifying any contributory underlying diseases. The history and physical examination are important steps in determining both the presence of ascites and possible etiologies, particularly cirrhosis (Fig. 27-2). However, every patient will ultimately require a **paracentesis** to determine the etiology. As the most common etiology for ascites is cirrhosis, history should also be directed at the risk factors and other manifestations of the various causes of cirrhosis (Table 27-1). In the United States, **the majority of all cases of cirrhosis are as a result of alcohol or chronic viral hepatitis**.

Signs of ascites on physical examination are often difficult to elicit, especially if the patient is obese. Bulging flanks are occasionally noticed when the patient reclines on the examination table and result from the pooling of fluid

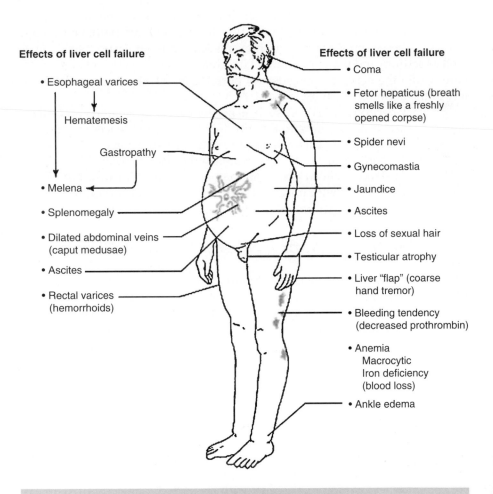

Effects of liver cell failure

- Esophageal varices
  ↓
  Hematemesis

  Gastropathy

- Melena
- Splenomegaly
- Dilated abdominal veins (caput medusae)
- Ascites
- Rectal varices (hemorrhoids)

Effects of liver cell failure

- Coma
- Fetor hepaticus (breath smells like a freshly opened corpse)
- Spider nevi
- Gynecomastia
- Jaundice
- Ascites
- Loss of sexual hair
- Testicular atrophy
- Liver "flap" (coarse hand tremor)
- Bleeding tendency (decreased prothrombin)
- Anemia
  Macrocytic
  Iron deficiency
  (blood loss)
- Ankle edema

Figure 27-2 ***Clinical manifestations of cirrhosis.*** (*Source:* Reproduced with permission from Chandrasoma P, Taylor CE. *Concise Pathology*, 3rd ed. Originally published by Appleton & Lange. Copyright1998 by The McGraw-Hill Companies.)

Table 27-1 **Most Common Causes of Cirrhosis with Key Diagnostic Tests**

Cause	Key Diagnostic Test
Alcohol	History of alcohol abuse
	AST 2× greater than ALT
Chronic hepatitis C	HCV antibodies, PCR for HCV RNA
Chronic hepatitis B	HBsAg, PCR for HBV DNA
Nonalcoholic fatty liver disease	History of obesity, diabetes, and hyperlipidemia
	Negligible alcohol consumption
Primary biliary cirrhosis	Alkaline phosphatase significantly elevated
	Antimitochondrial antibodies
Primary sclerosing cholangitis	History of inflammatory bowel disease
	ANA, antismooth muscle antibody
Wilson's disease	Ceruloplasmin, urinary copper excretion
Hemochromatosis	Ferritin, transferrin saturation, HFE genotype
α1-Antitrypsin deficiency	Serum α1-antitrypsin levels
Hepatic vein thrombosis	Presence of a hypercoagulable state
(Budd-Chiari syndrome)	Doppler ultrasonography
Autoimmune chronic hepatitis	ANA, antismooth muscle antibodies, anti-liver–kidney microsomal antibody (LKM), ANCA

Abbreviations: AST, aspartate aminotransferase; ALT, alanine transaminase; HCV, hepatitis C virus; PCR, polymerase chain reaction; HBV, hepatitis B virus; ANA, antinuclear antibody; HFE, hemochromatosis gene test; ANCA, antineutrophil cytoplasmic antibodies.

in the peritoneum. On inspection, the umbilicus may evert or an umbilical hernia may be present. Some patients will jokingly refer to it as a "pressure valve" indicating continued development of ascites. The classic findings for ascites are a fluid wave and shifting dullness. The **fluid wave** is difficult for one person to perform, and may require the patient to act as an assistant. The assistant places the ulnar aspect of their hand firmly across the patient's midabdomen. The examiner then taps the patient's flank while placing the other hand on the patient's other flank. If the impulse is noted on the receiving side, a positive fluid wave is noted. Intraperitoneal fluid will conduct the impulse, whereas fat or other solid tissue will dampen the impulse. **Shifting dullness** is performed by percussing the abdomen with the patient lying flat.

Note the location where percussion changes from dull to tympanitic. Next, ask the patient to roll on one side, wait about a minute, and then repeat the percussion, noting again where the dullness is present. If the dullness has "shifted," ascitic fluid is present and is layering out according to gravity and patient position. The test for shifting dullness is considered less sensitive than the fluid wave, particularly in the obese patient.

EVALUATION

Any patient with new ascites must have a paracentesis performed to analyze the ascitic fluid in order to determine the etiology. It should also be performed in all patients with known cirrhosis who develop clinical deterioration (fever, abdominal pain, rapid worsening of renal function, or worsened hepatic encephalopathy) because these symptoms are associated with spontaneous bacterial peritonitis. A diagnostic paracentesis removes a small amount (50–100 mL) of fluid for analysis. A therapeutic paracentesis removes larger volumes of ascites and is performed for the patient's comfort—to relieve pressure and discomfort from distention (see Chap. 3).

Important tests of ascitic fluid to consider include:

- Albumin is essential to determining the cause of ascites
  - Serum-to-ascites albumin gradient (SAAG) is used to determine whether the ascites resulted from portal hypertension (Table 27-2)
  - SAAG = serum albumin-ascitic fluid albumin
- Total protein (see "Spontaneous Bacterial Peritonitis," below)
- WBC count and differential (see "Spontaneous Bacterial Peritonitis," below)
- Gram stain and culture should be done whenever infection is considered

Table 27-2 **Most Common Diagnoses Associated with a High Vs. Low SAAG**

High SAAG (≥1.1) (Presence of Portal Hypertension)	Low SAAG (<1.1) (Absence of Portal Hypertension)
Cirrhosis	Nephrotic syndrome
Congestive heart failure	Peritoneal carcinomatosis
Constrictive pericarditis	Peritoneal tuberculosis
Veno-occlusive disease	Pancreatitis
Budd-Chiari syndrome	
Inferior vena cava (IVC) obstruction	

- Glucose and LDH will both be low in secondary peritonitis and malignancy
- Acid-fast bacillus staining and culture if tuberculous peritonitis is suspected
- Amylase over half the serum amylase value suggests pancreatitis or bowel perforation
- Cytology examination if malignancy is suspected (more fluid provides better yield)
- Appearance may suggest further testing
  - Milky fluid suggest chylous ascites and a triglyceride level is confirmatory (>200 mg/dL)
  - Brown ascites suggests biliary tree perforation and a bilirubin level is confirmatory

MANAGEMENT

Treatment options are extensive and varied depending on the underlying etiology of the ascites, and beyond the scope of this chapter. Frequently, treatment goals include management of symptoms, prevention/treatment of complications, and correction of underlying pathophysiology.

Treatment for ascites secondary to cirrhosis ranges from simple bedrest, to pharmacologic interventions, to liver transplantation depending on the severity of the ascites and the underlying liver disease. Avoidance of hepatotoxins is critical in the treatment of cirrhosis, so patients should completely abstain from alcohol.

Bed rest can help to return fluid to the central circulation. Although impractical long-term, this can be useful for hospitalized patients. The renin-angiotensin system is activated in patients with ascites, and lying recumbent decreases this activity. As such, many patients undergo spontaneous natriuresis with bedrest. A negative sodium balance is essential to prevent the further accumulation of ascitic fluid. Sodium restriction can be tailored to the degree of ascites, and a standard "no added salt" diet (<2 g) is a good starting place.

One of two strategies is generally recommended for patients with ascites. First, increasing doses of the diuretics **spironolactone and/or furosemide** can be used to remove ascitic fluid. Spironolactone is considered the diuretic of choice, because spironolactone actually results in better natriuresis than loop diuretics such as furosemide. Loop diuretics are often combined with spironolactone, as there is a synergistic natriuretic effect. A good rule of thumb is if peripheral edema is also present, then loop diuretics are also necessary. In patients with cirrhosis, the doses are usually higher than those used for patients without ascites: spironolactone is generally started at 100 mg once per day and furosemide is started at 40 mg once per day. Doses can be increased to induce natriuresis to maximums of 400 mg of spironolactone and 160 mg of furosemide daily. The limitations of diuretic therapy include hyponatremia, prerenal azotemia, encephalopathy, and electrolyte imbalances.

The second option is **therapeutic (large-volume) paracentesis** to alleviate symptoms. In patients with voluminous ascites, paracentesis is the method of choice, because it is faster, more effective, and associated with fewer adverse events. However, large-volume paracentesis can reduce effective arterial blood volume and result in further activation of vasoconstrictor and antinatriuretic factors. This hypovolemia is associated with hepatorenal syndrome (HRS), dilutional hyponatremia, and shortened survival. Plasma expanders must be used to if more than a liter of fluid is to be removed. Albumin is superior to other options in preventing complications after paracentesis.

Refractory ascites is defined as a lack of a response to high-dose diuretic therapy. In these cases, either repeated large-volume paracentesis must be performed or a transjugular intrahepatic portosystemic shunt (TIPS) should be placed. A TIPS consists of a stent placed within the liver between the hepatic vein and the portal vein. The TIPS achieves portal venous decompression and prevents the reaccumulation of ascites. Further, it has also been shown to decrease sodium retention and improve the renal response to diuretics. The main disadvantages of this procedure are the high rate of shunt stenosis and worsening of hepatic encephalopathy.

Spontaneous Bacterial Peritonitis

Spontaneous bacterial peritonitis (SBP) develops primarily in individuals with preexisting ascites from cirrhosis, although it has also been reported with ascites associated with malignancy and congestive heart failure (CHF). The most likely cause of SBP seems to be hematogenous spread of organisms which is made possible because liver dysfunction and altered portal circulation reduce the usual filtration functions. Ascitic fluid is a good medium for bacterial growth because it has low counts of complement proteins and antibodies. In fact a risk factor for SBP is a total protein level in the ascitic fluid of <1 g/dL.

The clinical manifestations of SBP can be quite subtle. Although fever and abdominal pain are the most common symptoms, patients may also present with worsening hepatic encephalopathy, worsening hepatic function, worsening renal function, or unexplained persistent leukocytosis. The key to diagnosis is finding **>250 polymorphonuclear cells (PMNs) per cubic millimeter** in the ascitic fluid. Blood culture bottles should also be inoculated with ascitic fluid at the bedside to attempt to isolate an organism. However, even in the best circumstances, an organism is isolated only about 50% of the time.

Given the difficulty in isolating an organism, empiric therapy is recommended against the most common causative organisms, gram-negative enterics (such as *Escherichia coli* and *Klebsiella pneumoniae*) and *Streptococcus pneumoniae*. Recommended antibiotics include third-generation cephalosporins, fluoroquinolones, or ampicillin/sulbactam for 5 days of total therapy. Another consideration is the 20% risk of type 1 HRS associated with SBP (see Chap. 28). Prophylaxis against HRS with albumin replacement should be considered for patients admitted with SBP. In a randomized-controlled trial, administration of albumin 1.5 g/kg at diagnosis and 1 g/kg infused 48 hours later was shown to decrease the incidence of HRS and improve survival from SBP.

After a single episode of SBP, 70% of patients will have a recurrence. Thus, prophylaxis is recommended for patients at high risk. Recommended regimens include either daily fluoroquinolone or sulfamethoxazole/ trimethoprim.

COMPLICATIONS OF

PORTAL HYPERTENSION

Alexander I. Reiss

KEY POINTS

- Major clinical complications of portal hypertension include GI bleeding, HE, ascites, and HRS. Often, more than one complication occurs simultaneously and a high index of suspicion of coexisting complications is advisable.
- Variceal bleeding may be rapid and devastating; early action and intervention with EGD is essential.
- HE is usually reversible and triggers such as SBP and GI bleeding should be ruled out.
- HRS implies a very poor prognosis. It resembles prerenal azotemia except that there is no response to fluid challenge.

INTRODUCTION

Portal hypertension results from a wide variety of conditions that increase the usually low pressure of the portal venous circulation. Portal hypertension may be caused by prehepatic, intrahepatic, and posthepatic conditions (Table 28-1). The most common cause of portal hypertension in the United States is **cirrhosis**. Although portal hypertension by itself causes few symptoms, patients with portal hypertension can present with unique and potentially disastrous complications. The major complications include gastrointestinal (GI) bleeding, altered mental status, and azotemia.

Table 28-1 **Major Causes of Portal Hypertension**

Prehepatic	Intrahepatic	Posthepatic
Massive splenomegaly	Schistosomiasis	Extrahepatic Budd-Chiari
Arterial-portal venous	Infiltrative conditions	syndrome
fistula	Sarcoidosis	IVC obstruction superior
Portal vein thrombosis	Myeloproliferative	to the junction of the
Splenic vein thrombosis	disorders	hepatic vein and IVC
	Primary biliary cirrhosis	Constrictive pericarditis
	Sclerosing cholangitis	Right-sided congestive
	Cirrhosis	heart failure
	Alcoholic hepatitis	Severe tricuspid
	Hepatic vein thrombosis	regurgitation
	(Budd-Chiari syndrome)	

PATHOPHYSIOLOGY

The liver receives dual blood supply from the hepatic artery (one-third) and the portal vein (two-thirds). The portal circulation is a low pressure (usually 7–10 mmHg) venous circulation that drains the GI tract, gallbladder, spleen, and pancreas. Flow from the splenic, superior, and inferior mesenteric veins converges into the portal vein which enters the liver at the porta hepatis. It branches into a vast network of functional channels (sinusoids) before reconverging into the hepatic veins that drain the liver into the inferior vena cava (IVC). Portal hypertension occurs with an **increase in portal blood flow** or an **increase in sinusoidal pressure** causing increased vascular resistance. For example, patients with Budd-Chiari syndrome (thrombosis of the hepatic veins) develop portal hypertension because of the increased resistance to venous return from the liver. By contrast, patients with massive splenomegaly commonly have portal hypertension secondary to increased venous return from the spleen. Cirrhosis actually causes portal hypertension by a combination of both mechanisms. In the cirrhotic liver, hepatocyte destruction, fibrosis, and regenerative nodules increase the intrahepatic resistance to portal blood flow. Further, adaptive responses by the body result in dilatation of the splanchnic circulation thus increasing the amount of blood in the portal system.

The majority of the complications from portal hypertension are related to the formation of **collaterals between the portal and systemic venous**

circulations. Such collaterals occur typically at the level of the distal esophagus (**esophageal varices**), proximal stomach (**gastric varices**), anterior abdominal wall (**caput medusae**—distended superficial veins emanating from the umbilicus), and anorectum (**rectal hemorrhoids**). The formation of these collaterals requires an increase in portal pressure **relative to IVC pressure**. For example, patients with cirrhosis must develop a pressure gradient of 10–15 mmHg in order for esophageal varices to develop. While increased pressure in the proximal IVC (as in congestive heart failure) can lead to portal hypertension, it also leads to systemic venous hypertension. Thus, conditions such as right heart failure and constrictive pericarditis may cause ascites (primarily a hydrostatic/oncotic pressure imbalance), but varices and encephalopathy rarely develop.

In addition to portosystemic shunting, cirrhosis produces a number of neurohormonal and metabolic changes that further complicate portal hypertension. Alterations include activation of the renin-aldosterone and sympathetic nervous systems, avid sodium and fluid retention, and decreased total systemic vascular resistance (SVR). This complex pathophysiology permits the development of ascites, GI bleeding from varices or portal gastropathy, encephalopathy, pulmonary dysfunction, splenomegaly with hypersplenism, and hepatorenal syndrome (HRS).

CLINICAL PRESENTATION

While physical examination and appropriate laboratory abnormalities are suggestive of portal hypertension, imaging is helpful in establishing the diagnosis as well as obtaining useful anatomic and physiologic information. Duplex ultrasonography with color flow Doppler of the portal system and hepatic veins is a noninvasive, relatively inexpensive study and should be obtained for all patients in whom the diagnosis is suspected. Similarly, esophagogastroduodenoscopy (EGD) should be performed in patients with portal hypertension to evaluate for presence of varices and to perform any therapeutic measures necessary. More invasive assessment of portal anatomy and hepatic venous pressure gradient (HVPG) with hepatic venous catheterization may be necessary in preparation for surgical or interventional radiology procedures such as portosystemic shunting and may guide therapeutic decisions.

Patients with portal hypertension present because of complications from their portal hypertension. The most common complications are ascites, GI hemorrhage, hepatic encephalopathy (HE), and HRS. As cirrhosis is the most common cause of portal hypertension in the United States, these complications will be discussed in relation to cirrhosis. The manifestations and management of each major complication of portal hypertension are discussed individually with the exception of ascites and spontaneous bacterial peritonitis (SBP; see Chap. 27).

Gastrointestinal Hemorrhage

Of cirrhotic patients, **90% will ultimately develop varices** and hemorrhage will occur in 25–35%. Variceal hemorrhage is associated with a high mortality rate (30–50%) and a high rate of recurrence—70% can expect further hemorrhages. Of all the sites of portosystemic collateral development, the distal esophagus/proximal stomach represent the location of highest clinical significance with esophageal varices accounting for most episodes of bleeding. In fact, the presence of gastric varices without esophageal varices should raise suspicion of splenic vein thrombosis. A thrombosed splenic vein can cause obstruction of the short gastric veins without involvement of the distal esophagus. Risk factors for an initial hemorrhage include continued alcohol use, larger variceal size, and the severity of the patient's underlying liver disease. Although technically venous, the increased pressure of varices often leads to vigorous hemorrhage and the high mortality associated with it. Compared to nonportal hypertensive forms of GI bleeding in which up to 90% stop spontaneously, **only about half of variceal hemorrhages resolve without therapy**.

The most important consideration in patients with esophageal varices is the *prevention* of an initial hemorrhage. Controlled trials support the use of **nonselective beta-blockers** such as propranolol or nadolol for **primary prevention** of bleeding in patients with varices. Nonselective beta-blockers such as propranolol or nadolol reduce portal pressure via multiple effects. Beta-1-blockade permits activation of α-adrenergic splanchnic vasoconstriction while beta-2-blockade reduces splanchnic and peripheral vasodilatation. The dose should be titrated to a resting heart rate of 55 or, preferably, to a HVPG <12 mmHg, the level considered a threshold for development of variceal bleeding. Combination therapy with nonselective beta-blockers and nitrates may be beneficial but limited by side effects and requires further study at this point. While endoscopic variceal band ligation appears to be effective in preventing initial hemorrhage, it carries significant risk, inconvenience, and expense, so it is typically reserved for patients at high risk or who are poorly tolerant of beta-blockers.

Management of active bleeding from gastroesophageal varices requires a rapid, multimodal, aggressive approach. As portal hypertension stems from a combination of resistance to outflow and increased portal inflow from splanchnic arteriolar vasodilatation, treatments for hemorrhage attempt to reduce portal pressures by either reducing resistance to portal drainage or by reducing portal venous inflow. Goals of therapy focus on hemodynamic resuscitation, cessation of bleeding, prevention of complications, and supportive care. Initial resuscitation requires transfusion of packed red blood cells and perhaps fresh frozen plasma (to replace clotting factors) and platelets. Caution must be used however to avoid over hydration. Volume expansion may increase portal pressure, so judicious use of blood products is warranted. A general goal would be to transfuse packed red blood cells to achieve a hemoglobin of 10 mg/dL. Cirrhotic patients with GI hemorrhages commonly have thrombocytopenia and elevated prothrombin times, so these must be corrected as well.

Aggressive therapy must be undertaken to stop the bleeding, usually a combination of endoscopic therapy and medications. Octreotide, a long-acting somatostatin analogue, is the most commonly used medicine in the United States Octreotide inhibits release of glucagon and other vasodilatory hormones, resulting in splanchnic vasoconstriction and decreased portal inflow. Octreotide is of marginal benefit, so is typically used as a temporizing agent until endoscopy can be performed. **Early endoscopy with sclerotherapy or band ligation** is the most effective means of controlling hemorrhage. These therapies are usually successful in achieving hemostasis in 80–90% of patients. If unsuccessful, emergent balloon tamponade may be necessary while arranging for definitive surgical intervention. Balloon tamponade is achieved by insertion of a specialized nasogastric tube (e.g., Sengstaken-Blakemore) with an inflatable balloon that applies direct pressure from within the lumen of the esophagus to the bleeding varix. Although very effective in achieving hemostasis, balloons have a high rate of complications (such as esophageal perforation) and varices usually rebleed once the balloon is deflated. If bleeding persists despite the above measures, a transjugular intrahepatic portosystemic shunt (TIPS) should be considered.

Special considerations with this form of upper GI bleeding should be taken into account, including the risk for infection, encephalopathy, and renal failure. Cirrhotic patients presenting with a GI hemorrhage have a >50% chance of having a concomitant infection. Typical infections include urinary tract infection, SBP, aspiration pneumonia, and bacteremia. The use of prophylactic antibiotics has been shown to not only improve survival, but also decrease the risk of rebleeding. Therefore, antibiotics are recommended for all patients admitted with a GI hemorrhage. Fluoroquinolones or third-generation cephalosporins are typically used to cover gram-negative bacteria. GI hemorrhage can also precipitate development of or worsening of HE. Therefore, lactulose should be given as soon as it is feasible to do so. Last, GI hemorrhage often precipitates renal failure, either as a result of volume depletion or HRS (see "Hepatorenal Syndrome," below).

The highest risk for rebleeding is in the first few days after cessation of hemorrhage. The risk of rebleeding drops considerably after the first 6 weeks following the initial hemorrhage but still remains high. The ultimate treatment for secondary prevention of variceal hemorrhage is orthotopic liver transplantation; every patient should be evaluated following a first episode. Unfortunately, transplantation often requires a substantial waiting period so intermediary measures are necessary. Strategies usually include endoscopic band ligation and medical therapy with beta-blockers with/without nitrates. Should bleeding continue to recur, consideration of TIPS or surgery is appropriate.

Hepatic Encephalopathy

An altered level of consciousness in a patient with portal hypertension should raise suspicion of this generally reversible condition. Initial hypotheses regarding pathogenesis involved the role of portosystemic shunting past the liver and decreased hepatic metabolism of ammonia. While both of these play key roles, HE is currently understood to be much more complex. The absorption of neurotoxins, including ammonia, which bypass detoxification from the liver are likely key participants. The brain also has impaired neurotransmission, particularly due to the production of false neurotransmitters and excessive levels of γ-aminobutyric acid (GABA). Finally, the brain seems particularly susceptible to these insults secondary to cerebral edema and increased blood-brain barrier permeability.

The end result is a syndrome of depressed mental status, reduced cognitive ability, and personality changes that range from the subclinical to a deeply comatose state with cerebral edema. The classic finding of **asterixis**, a "flapping" motion of the dorsiflexed hands with the arms extended forward, results from a periodic loss of tone of dorsiflexors at a rate of about every 2–3 seconds. If necessary, the examiner may hold the patient's hands lightly in the dorsiflexed position to assess the finding. A nonspecific finding, asterixis may occur in other forms of encephalopathy. As the condition progresses, diffuse upper motor neuron signs such as hyperreflexia and muscle rigidity may appear. While focal neurologic signs may also occur, they should trigger an evaluation for other causes of mental status changes.

A sudden change in the level of encephalopathy in a cirrhotic patient usually occurs from a precipitating event. Triggers of episodes of HE should be sought for all hospitalized patients (Table 28-2). The most common precipitating event in hospitalized patients is acute GI hemorrhage.

The diagnosis is made on clinical grounds in the setting of portal hypertension and absence of other forms of encephalopathy or altered mental status. Various laboratory tests are available but their applications are limited. While the role of ammonia in HE is the most established, measuring blood levels proves problematic. Arterial and venous levels both vary with meals and sample collection/handling techniques. Additionally, normal levels of ammonia do not exclude the diagnosis. Brain imaging with computed tomography (CT) or magnetic resonance imaging (MRI) are useful only to exclude other etiologies and to monitor for increased intracranial pressure/cerebral edema.

Acute management of patients with HE involves correction of the precipitating conditions and reduction of intestinal ammonia levels. A targeted workup to identify any potential triggers should exclude the presence of infections such as SBP, GI bleeding, sedatives, and hypokalemia and hypovolemia. These should be corrected urgently if found. Simultaneously, efforts to lower ammonemia should be undertaken regardless of actual serum ammonia levels. **Lactulose**, a synthetic nonabsorbable disaccharide is the

Table 28-2 **Triggers of HE**

Increase of nitrogenous substances (increased levels of ammonia)	GI bleeding
	High dietary protein
	Uremia or azotemia
	Hypokalemia
	Infections
	Metabolic alkalosis
	Constipation
Worsening of portosystemic shunting	Progression of underlying condition
	Diuretic nonadherence
	Fluid overload
	Iatrogenic (post-TIPS or surgical shunt procedure)
Central nervous system depression	Benzodiazepines and barbiturates
	Hypoglycemia
	Hypoxia
	Hypothyroidism

mainstay of treatment for HE. By directly decreasing bacterial ammonia production and by increasing fecal clearance of nitrogen, the drug reduces systemic absorption of ammonia. Additionally, after metabolism by gut bacteria to organic acids, stool pH is lowered which promotes a net movement of ammonia from the blood to the bowel lumen. It is given orally, typically 30–60 g a day to produce three to four loose, acidic (pH <6) bowel movements a day. Lactulose administration improves HE in about three-fourths of patients. For patients unable to tolerate oral administration, lactulose enemas are an acceptable alternative.

A number of agents have been utilized as "second line" for patients who fail to respond to disaccharide therapy. The use of antibiotics to decrease production of ammonia by colonic bacteria appears to attenuate HE; however, alterations in gut flora and side effects may be problematic. In particular, neomycin should be avoided because it is absorbed systemically, producing ototoxicity and nephrotoxicity. Oral vancomycin, metronidazole, and rifamaxin appear to be better tolerated. Once again, these agents should be considered second line and are inappropriate for chronic use. Another option may be the use of flumazenil. Supporting the hypothesis of excessive GABA activation in HE, 30% of patients show short-term improvement after administration of flumazenil. However, because of its short half-life and uncertain benefits, it should be reserved for patients who are concomitantly using benzodiazepines to eliminate the confounding effects of those medications.

Chronic management of HE involves chronic lactulose therapy and limitation of protein intake to 70 g/day. Protein restriction beyond this level may worsen protein calorie malnutrition.

Hepatorenal Syndrome

The development of renal dysfunction in portal hypertension portends a very poor prognosis relative to portal hypertension without azotemia. Many possible renal insults occur in the setting of portal hypertension such as hypovolemia from bleeding or overdiuresis, exposure to nephrotoxic medications or radiocontrast dyes, sepsis, and glomerulonephritis from conditions such as cryoglobulinemia in patients with hepatitis C. The development of azotemia in the absence of such situations characterizes HRS. The pathophysiology of HRS is believed to involve a dysfunctional combination of splanchnic vasodilatation and renal vasoconstriction. The initial drop in SVR with portal hypertension is primarily a result of splanchnic vasodilatation. This in turn activates both the sympathetic nervous system and the renin-angiotensin system resulting in vasoconstriction (at sites such as the extremities, brain, skeletal muscle, spleen, and renal arteries) and avid sodium and fluid retention. Despite this, production of local vasodilators such as nitric oxide maintains splanchnic vasodilatation, keeping the overall SVR low. Renal arterial dilators become overwhelmed and intense renal vasoconstriction occurs. The result is a decrease in renal perfusion and glomerular filtration. The role of liver but not renal dysfunction as the etiology of HRS is supported by the fact that after liver transplant, renal function returns to normal. Similarly when kidneys of patients with HRS are transplanted into normal patients, they function well.

HRS develops in patients with advanced cirrhosis, who have both portal hypertension and ascites. Clinically, the typical patient has a rise in creatinine and oliguria (urine output of 400–800 mL/day), a picture resembling prerenal azotemia. However, unlike prerenal azotemia, they are not volume depleted and do not respond to fluid therapy. Two variations of HRS are recognized. Type 1 manifests as a rapid deterioration in renal function and, if untreated, is typically fatal within several weeks. Type 2 is more gradual and occurs in patients with preserved hepatic function but often refractory ascites. Survival is reduced but is usually measured in months to a year.

The diagnosis of HRS should be considered when plasma creatinine concentration exceeds 1.5 mg/dL and progresses over days to weeks. By definition, evaluation must verify absence of intrinsic renal conditions. For example, urinary sediment should not have evidence of glomerular (RBC casts, dysmorphic RBCs, or protein) or tubular (muddy brown casts) injury. The essential step in diagnosis is to exclude prerenal azotemia as an etiology. Thus, serum creatinine concentration should not improve following the **discontinuation of diuretics** and a **fluid challenge** of 1.5 L of isotonic saline. **Urine sodium is typically <5 meq/dL** secondary to the renal vasoconstriction and decreased glomerular flow.

Treatment of HRS is often unsuccessful, so prevention of HRS is of critical importance. HRS frequently follows GI hemorrhage, SBP, or large-volume paracentesis for ascites without the use of concomitant albumin replacement. Acute management of GI hemorrhage should include prompt volume resuscitation. In the setting of SBP, as many as 20% of patients will develop type 1 HRS. Because of this high risk, albumin replacement should be considered for patients admitted with SBP. Similarly, intravenous albumin should be given following large-volume paracentesis to prevent HRS, at a dose of 10 g of albumin/L of fluid removed.

Early recognition of HRS, elimination of nephrotoxic medications, and treatment of the underlying cause of portal hypertension are essential. Unfortunately, with the exception of acute viral and alcoholic hepatitis, most etiologies are irreversible. Hepatic transplantation is the ultimate treatment for cases without potential for improvement in hepatic function. Short of these definitive options, therapy involves treatment of portal hypertension by splanchnic vasoconstrictors (such as vasopressin analogues or the combination of octreotide and the α-adrenergic agonist, midodrine) with albumin and control of ascites with diuretics, particularly aldosterone antagonists. Additional options include portosystemic shunts such as TIPS. Unfortunately, the success of these pharmacologic therapies and procedures are limited to case reports. Hemodialysis should be reserved for those patients awaiting hepatic transplantation.

ACUTE AND CHRONIC
PANCREATITIS

Kristy S. Deep

KEY POINTS

- The most common causes of acute pancreatitis in the United States are gallstones and alcohol.
- The diagnosis is confirmed by elevated levels of serum amylase and lipase.
- All patients presenting with a first episode of acute pancreatitis should have a RUQ US, measurement of calcium and triglyceride levels, and a review of all medications in search of a cause.
- Pancreatic complications (infected pancreatic necrosis, pseudocyst, abscess, phlegmon) should be suspected if the patient has persistent pain, fever, or lack of clinical improvement; CT should then be performed.
- Chronic pancreatitis is a separate entity, characterized by persistent severe pain, pancreatic insufficiency (steatorrhea), normal amylase and lipase levels, generally attributable to alcohol.

ACUTE PANCREATITIS

Introduction

Acute pancreatitis involves inflammation and destruction of the pancreatic tissue with subsequent leakage of pancreatic enzymes. The incidence ranges from 1-5/10,000, which varies depending on the population studied as there are numerous lifestyle factors that contribute to the underlying etiology. It may be mild with a self-limited bout of abdominal pain or severe with hemodynamic collapse and death.

Pathophysiology

The pancreas plays a key role in digestion via the secretion of proteolytic and lipolytic enzymes into the lumen of the small intestines. Under normal circumstances, pancreatic proenzymes are inactive until modified by a kinase in the brush border of the small intestine. In acute pancreatitis the exact inciting event is unclear but leads to the premature activation of enzymes (such as trypsinogen) within the acinar cell. Because they obtain their proteolytic function early and in the wrong location these enzymes damage the surrounding pancreatic tissue triggering an inflammatory cascade. Cytokine release stimulates infiltration of neutrophils and macrophages, the release of proteases and hydrolases leading to increased vascular permeability and edema in the pancreas.

Clinical Presentation

The clinical presentation of acute pancreatitis is usually not subtle. It is characterized nearly universally by **abdominal pain**. Typically, a patient will describe a deep visceral pain, often poorly localized but more prominent in the epigastrium and left upper quadrant. The pain can be quite severe and lead one to moan or writhe. It frequently **radiates to the back**. **Nausea and vomiting** are seen in over three-fourths of patients. They will commonly be unable to tolerate any oral intake of food or fluids. On physical examination, patients will often have a low-grade temperature elevation from the inflammatory cascade described above. Tachycardia is common and multifactorial— pain and intravascular volume depletion from poor oral intake being the leading causes. Hypotension is an ominous sign caused by both dehydration and intra-abdominal fluid sequestration around the pancreas. If severe, patients will have evidence of systemic inflammatory response syndrome (SIRS). Other important physical examination findings include scleral icterus or mild jaundice from biliary obstruction (gallstone or swollen pancreatic head obstructing biliary drainage); pleural effusion caused by transdiaphragmatic fluid shift from the pancreas—more often left sided; and an abdomen that is frequently distended, with hypoactive or absent bowel sounds; exquisite tenderness to palpation with guarding; often tympanic to percussion if significant ileus present. Rare findings seen in severe hemorrhagic or necrotizing pancreatitis include ecchymoses around the umbilicus (Cullen's sign) or about the flanks (Grey Turner's sign).

Elevation of serum amylase and lipase is the hallmark of acute pancreatitis. The presence of elevated levels of these enzymes in the blood is evidence of pancreatic cellular leakage. Amylase has two main sources—the salivary glands and the pancreas. Beware of an isolated amylase elevation as this is not specific for pancreatitis. Amylase begins to rise within a few hours of onset of symptoms but also falls first, often normalizing within 24 hours. Lipase starts to go up later but stays elevated longer. Lipase is generally thought to be the more specific of the two. An elevated white blood cell count is commonly seen signifying the demargination of neutrophils caused by inflammatory mediators rather than infection. Platelet count may also be high as an acute phase reactant. Beware of low hemoglobin as this may herald the uncommon complication of hemorrhagic pancreatitis. If the symptoms have been present for some time, one may exhibit multiple electrolyte disturbances including an elevated blood urea nitrogen (BUN)/creatinine ratio from decreased intravascular volume, an anion gap metabolic acidosis from starvation ketosis (especially in an alcoholic), or a metabolic alkalosis and hypokalemia from intractable vomiting.

Evaluation

Assessing a patient with acute pancreatitis involves determining the etiology. Alcohol use and gallstones are by far the most common accounting for 75% of cases. Other recognized causes will also be discussed below. However, a sizable percentage of cases remain "idiopathic" after a reasonable workup.

Gallstones are the most common cause of acute pancreatitis. The exact mechanism is unclear—a stone passing through the common bile duct can cause a transient obstruction leading to either reflux of bile into the pancreas or disallows the pancreas to drain properly. Thus, eliciting a history of gallstones or symptoms of biliary colic is crucial to the evaluation. The test of choice is a **right upper quadrant ultrasound (RUQ US)** to look for gallstones and evidence of biliary ductal dilatation (distal obstructing stone). Other markers of recent biliary stone passage include an elevation of **elevated alkaline phosphatase and bilirubin**.

Alcohol use is a common cause of pancreatitis. Again, no clear causative mechanism is known. Alcohol-related acute pancreatitis is typically found in heavy drinkers 2–3 days after a binge or after they have stopped drinking. History is very important—no biochemical markers distinguish one etiology from another. The serum ethanol level may be elevated but often is undetectable, as patients may have been unable to consume alcohol in the preceding days secondary to pain. Alcoholics are also prone to chronic pancreatitis.

Drugs frequently are implicated in pancreatitis. The list is extensive but specific medications most frequently implicated include **azathioprine, didanosine (ddI), furosemide, thiazide diuretics, metronidazole, and valproic acid. Severe hypertriglyceridemia (serum values >1000 mg/dL)** is another etiology to suspect, especially in patients with diabetes or obesity. Note that serum amylase can be normal in this setting. Consider checking for **hypercalcemia** as this may be a potentially reversible metabolic cause of pancreatitis (e.g., hyperparathyroidism). Other causes include **trauma, hereditary pancreatitis, and pancreatic cancer**. A frequently encountered iatrogenic cause is **endoscopic retrograde cholangiopancreatography (ERCP)**. This procedure utilizes a radiopaque dye injected into to ampulla to visualize the biliary tree. Ironically, it is also used in the evaluation and treatment of pancreatitis. Favorite esoteric causes sometimes the subject of student query on rounds include **mumps, ascaris** (through duct obstruction), and of course, **scorpion stings**.

In about one-third of cases, an etiology is not apparent even after an appropriate evaluation. Some believe that many of these patients have microlithiasis (gallbladder sludge or "sand") that can irritate the ampulla in much the same way a biliary stone. The vast majority of patients with one episode of idiopathic acute pancreatitis will never have another one and arguably need no further workup. For those with **recurrent idiopathic acute pancreatitis**, a more specialized evaluation including **ERCP, endoscopic US**, or **sphincter of Oddi manometry may be indicated**.

Management

No matter what the cause, acute pancreatitis is initially treated in the same manner. The patient is made NPO to minimize the stimulation of pancreatic activity. As the pain can be quite severe, parenteral analgesia is administered as needed. There is a theoretical contraindication to morphine as it has been claimed to cause sphincter of Oddi spasm thus worsening the patient's pain. The clinical relevance of this is questionable. For those with severe nausea and vomiting an antiemetic like promethazine is useful. If refractory nausea, vomiting, or pain ensues, decompression of the stomach with a nasogastric (NG) tube aids in removing the gastric secretions.

As a patient with acute pancreatitis is often volume depleted at presentation, a mainstay of therapy is intravenous fluid resuscitation. Provide rapid crystalloid infusions (normal saline or lactated Ringer's) until they appear euvolemic—no longer orthostatic with heart rate and blood pressure normalized. Fluid sequestration in and around the pancreas can be massive so a patient may require several liters of fluid. Once resuscitated, the patient will need maintenance IV fluids while NPO (5% dextrose + $1/2$ NS +/− potassium if vomiting or NG suction). Once the abdominal pain has subsided and the patient starts to feel hungry again, a diet of clear liquids may be started. If pain or vomiting returns, cease enteral feeding and try another day. Once tolerating clear liquids, advance to a bland low-fat diet as this will minimize stimulation of pancreatic juices.

In gallstone pancreatitis, the presence of persistent obstruction must be determined. Patients with rising bilirubin or evidence of biliary sepsis (rising WBC, worsening pain, fevers) need urgent decompression with ERCP and sphincterotomy to remove the stone. Others will need a cholecystectomy as soon as their acute illness has resolved—within 1–3 weeks depending on the severity of their pancreatitis.

Specific treatments for other types of pancreatitis are somewhat obvious. If there is an offending medication causing the pancreatitis, it should be stopped. If alcohol is thought to be involved they should be strongly urged to stop drinking as the recurrence rate is quite high. If hypercalcemic, identify and treat the underlying cause. If due to hypertriglyceridemia (especially in diabetics), administer insulin to lower triglycerides acutely and start gemfi-brozil concomitantly. Mild acute pancreatitis is often a self-limited disease. The patient will typically be able to resume oral intake in 3–5 days and suf-fer no serious sequelae.

Severe Pancreatitis and Complications

Complicated, severe, acute pancreatitis is associated with significant morbidity and mortality. Clinical evidence of severe pancreatitis includes shock, respira-tory distress, peritonitis, or organ dysfunction (renal failure, encephalopathy). There are also numerous scoring systems used to identify these patients. The most accurate is the APACHE II (Acute Physiology and Chronic Health Evaluation II) which is based on criteria used to assess severity of illness in ICU patients; however, it is cumbersome to calculate. The most common prognostic criteria asked about on ward rounds are the Ranson criteria. Patients exhibiting three or more of these criteria have a greatly increased risk of death, approaching 100% mortality if seven to eight criteria are pre-sent (see Table 29-1).

Local complications of pancreatitis are not uncommon. **Infected pancre-atic necrosis**, which is a diffuse bacterial infection of the inflamed organ, typically occurring within the first 1–2 weeks of the onset of pancreatitis. For patients with clinical or APACHE II evidence of severe pancreatitis or who are deteriorating despite maximal supportive care, **image the pancreas with computed tomography (CT)** to assess for the degree of necrosis. If >30% necrotic, consider broad-spectrum antibiotics such as imipenem or meropenem. Many of these patients will require surgical debridement or CT-guided aspiration and drainage. **Pancreatic pseudocysts** are nonepithelial-ized collections of fluid and tissue debris which form in 15% of patients over a span of 1–4 weeks (Fig. 29-1). The natural history varies—one-third will spontaneously resolve, sometimes taking more than 6 weeks. Watchful wait-ing is the best course in small pseudocysts that are asymptomatic. If >5 cm,

Table 29-1 **Ranson's Criteria: Indicators of Severity in Acute Pancreatitis**

At Presentation	In First 48 Hours
Age >55	Drop in Hct ≥10%
WBC >16,000/μL	Fluid sequestration >6 L
Hyperglycemia >200 mg/dL	Hypocalcemia (<8 mg/dL)
LDH >350 IU/L	Hypoxemia (PO2 <60 mmHg)
Serum AST >250 IU/L	Increase in BUN >5 mg/dL
	Base deficit >4 meq/L

Abbreviations: Hct, hematocrit; LDH, lactate dehydrogenase; AST, aspartate aminotransferase.

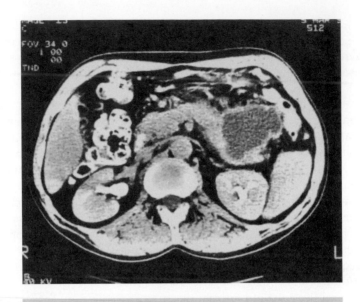

Figure 29-1 **Pancreatic pseudocyst. There is a well-defined encapsulated fluid collection arising from the pancreatic tail.** (*Source:* Reproduced with permission from Bongard FS, Sue DY, eds. *Current Critical Care Diagnosis & Treatment.* Originally published by Appleton & Lange. Copyright by The McGraw-Hill Companies, 1994.)

>6 weeks, causing symptoms such as pain or obstruction, consider US or CT-guided drainage. Pseudocyst complications include rupture, infection, and hemorrhage.

CHRONIC PANCREATITIS

Introduction

Chronic pancreatitis is a very different disease. As the name implies, it is a chronic inflammatory state of the pancreas commonly leading to exocrine insufficiency. The causes are many and overlap with acute pancreatitis. One can develop chronic pancreatitis de novo or following multiple bouts of acute pancreatitis. A distinction should be made between patients with recurrent episodes of acute pancreatitis and the separate entity of chronic pancreatitis.

Pathophysiology

Although largely unknown, it is thought to be related to chronic pancreatic inflammation, scarring, and fibrosis. In the case of alcoholic pancreatitis, a

direct toxic effect of alcohol on the gland is likely. Precipitation and inspis-
sation of pancreatic secretions leads to ductal obstruction, dilation, and atrophy of the acinar cells. Over time, the gland becomes fibrotic and the protein
plugs become calcified. Once a majority of the pancreas is affected, the organ
fails to produce and secrete the lipases and proteases necessary for fat and
protein digestion.

Alcohol is the most common cause of chronic pancreatitis accounting for
three-quarters of all cases. It does appear to have a dose-dependent relationship as the risk increases with increasing total exposure to alcohol. The next
most common subclass is idiopathic—a diagnosis of exclusion. Other etiologies are hereditary, autoimmune, and cystic fibrosis (CF). Even heterozy-
gotes for the mutation in the cystic fibrosis transmembrane conductance reg-
ulator (CFTR) channel experience chronic pancreatitis despite normal sweat
chloride tests and no pulmonary disease. This mutation leads to thickened
pancreatic secretions which cause ductal obstruction.

Clinical Presentation

The main feature of chronic pancreatitis is **abdominal pain**. The character is
typically gnawing with **radiation to the back**. It can be constant with superimposed exacerbations or only in an episodic nature. A small percentage will
have malabsorption without accompanying pain. The pain can be quite
severe at times requiring admission to the hospital for symptom control.
Notably, patients will not appear as toxic as patients with acute pancreatitis.
Alcohol consumption or a large fatty meal may exacerbate the disease.
Malabsorption is the other primary manifestation. The patient may have
foul-smelling fatty stool (steatorrhea) and weight loss. Clinically apparent
deficiencies of fat-soluble vitamins, however, are not commonly seen. The
examination of patients with chronic pancreatitis is usually unremarkable.
Reported **pain is often out of proportion to the examination**. The abdomen
will often be tender but with no peritoneal signs. The patient may appear
thin or malnourished.

In contrast with acute pancreatitis, **amylase and lipase values will typically be normal**. One may find a cholestatic pattern with mildly elevated
bilirubin and alkaline phosphatase when there is compression of the bile duct
by inflammation or fibrosis at the head of the pancreas. Exocrine function is
evaluated with the Sudan stain, a qualitative examination for fecal fat. To quantify fecal fat, the patient must eat a diet with 100 g fat per day for 72 hours.
A 24-hour fecal fat of >7 g is elevated, but will frequently be >20 g/day if due
to pancreatic insufficiency. However, due to the cumbersome nature of this
test, clinical suspicion is probably sufficient.

Evaluation

If chronic pancreatitis is suspected, pancreatic imaging is helpful to confirm
the diagnosis and establish an etiology not apparent by history. Patients

should have a CT or MRI of the pancreas to exclude pseudocysts and pancreatic cancer as the cause of their symptoms. Imaging studies will reveal **pancreatic calcification** in 30% of patients (Fig. 29-2). These can be seen on MRI, CT, and even plain radiographs. Alcohol is the most common etiology leading to calcifications, whereas they are rare in idiopathic chronic pancreatitis. If these studies are negative, an ERCP may be indicated to locate and treat strictures of the pancreatic duct.

Management

Since the two major manifestations are pain and malabsorption, treatment is primarily directed at these problems. Nonpharmacologic treatment measures

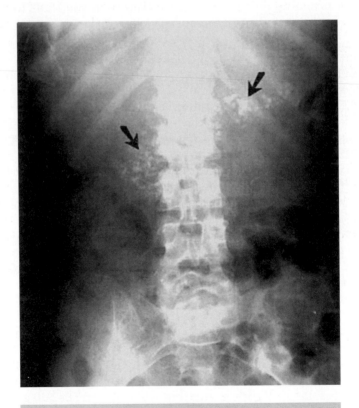

Figure 29-2 **Pancreatic calcifications. A plain film of the abdomen shows calcifications in the region of the pancreas (arrows).** (*Source:* Reproduced with permission from Krebs CA, Giyanani VL, Eisenberg RL. *Ultrasound Atlas of Disease Processes.* Originally published by Appleton & Lange. Copyright by The McGraw-Hill Companies, 1993.)

include complete abstinence from alcohol and a low-fat diet. Pancreatic enzyme supplementation reduces pain, especially in nonalcoholic chronic pancreatitis, theoretically by blocking the stimulation of cholecystokinin stimulation. Pancreatic enzymes also reliably reverse cobalamin deficiency. Narcotic analgesia is necessary for patients with severe pain. If refractory to therapy, nerve blocks of the celiac plexus can be attempted for relief but only last a few months. If a patient has a proximal pancreatic duct stricture, an endoscopic approach including dilation and stenting can alleviate pain in the majority of cases. For those with a dilated pancreatic duct, surgery may be of benefit. The modified Puestow procedure wherein the dilated duct is splayed open and anastomosed with the jejunum relieves pain in about half of patients.

In malabsorption, the mainstay of treatment is pancreatic enzyme replacement. At least 30,000 units of lipase are necessary for adequate digestion necessitating numerous pills with each meal. This will ensure adequate nutrition and decrease steatorrhea.

Progressive pancreatic failure can lead to **endocrine failure** secondary to islet cell damage—both the insulin secreting β cells and the glucagon secreting δ cells. Although many patients with chronic pancreatitis have glucose intolerance, ketoacidosis and end-organ diabetic disease is uncommon. In severe endocrine failure, glucose control is complicated by sensitivity to exogenous insulin coupled with hypoglycemia without normal glucagon secretion.

Patients with chronic pancreatitis are also at increased risk for pancreatic carcinoma and effusions containing high amylase in the pleural, pericardial, or peritoneal space. Another common problem facing patients with chronic pancreatitis is narcotic dependence. Patients who adhere to dietary modifications, abstain from alcohol, and use enzyme replacement can expect to do reasonably well.

CHOLELITHIASIS,

PCHOLECYSTITIS, AND

CHOLANGITIS

Phillip K. Chang
Richard Schwartz

KEY POINTS

- Most gallstones do not cause symptoms.
- Ultrasound is the best test to evaluate for gallstones and complications.
- Acute cholangitis requires immediate drainage; ERCP is the procedure of choice.
- Patients with acute cholecystitis or cholangitis ultimately require cholecystectomy.

INTRODUCTION

Approximately 10–20% of the general U.S. population will eventually develop gallstones. Gallstones are especially prevalent in women, persons who are obese, and diabetics. In addition, many Native Americans have extremely high rates of gallstones; for example, 75% or more Pima Indians will develop stones. The prevalence is also increased in persons of Hispanic or western European ancestry. Nevertheless, most gallstones do not cause symptoms and the majority of these people will not contract gallbladder-related illness. However, some do, and depending on the where the stones become lodged in the biliary tract, a variety of clinical problems may result. The most common presentations of gallstones are symptomatic cholelithiasis,

234

cholecystitis (inflammation of the gallbladder), cholangitis (bacterial infection of the bile duct), and gallstone pancreatitis (see Chap. 29).

PATHOPHYSIOLOGY

One of the normal functions of the liver is detoxification and excretion of endogenous waste products through the formation of bile. Bile principally consists of water, electrolytes, and dissolved organic solutes, mostly conjugated bile salts, lecithin, and cholesterol. Bile is formed by the hepatocytes and secreted into a complex network of canaliculi which coalesce to form intrahepatic bile ducts and, ultimately, the right and left hepatic ducts, which unite creating the common hepatic duct. The common bile duct (CBD) is formed where the common hepatic duct meets the cystic duct of the gallbladder, and enters the duodenum through the ampulla of Vater (Fig. 30-1). The gallbladder serves as a reservoir for bile, but also serves to concentrate bile by reabsorbing water.

Gallstones are formed when the normal substances, typically either cholesterol or bile pigment (calcium bilirubinate) form concretions in the biliary tract. Cholesterol stones comprise the majority (80%) of gallstones and are formed either because of **supersaturation** of bile with cholesterol or from **gallbladder hypomobility**. As the concentration of cholesterol in bile increases, biliary stasis leads to the formation of sludge (microlithiasis) and

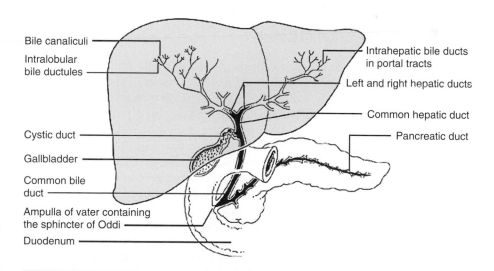

Figure 30-1 **Biliary tract anatomy.** (*Source:* Reproduced with permission from Chandrasoma P, Taylor CE. *Concise Pathology*, 3rd ed. Originally published by Appleton & Lange. Copyright by The McGraw-Hill Companies, 1998, Figure 44-1.)

stones. Bile becomes supersaturated with cholesterol secondary to genetic factors or dietary factors (high cholesterol and high caloric diets) which increase biliary cholesterol secretion. Because much of the concentration of bile occurs within the gallbladder, poor emptying of the gallbladder is generally necessary for cholesterol stones to form. Pigment stones form mostly in relation to chronic hemolytic states or increased bilirubin enterohepatic circulation (cirrhosis, cystic fibrosis, Gilbert's syndrome).

Most gallstones pass through the biliary system without difficulty; however, gallstones can become lodged in any position throughout the biliary tree. Common locations include the neck of the gallbladder, juncture of the CBD and cystic duct, and at the ampulla of Vater. If stones at the neck of the gallbladder impede bile outflow, patients may develop **symptomatic cholelithiasis**. If the obstruction is complete, normal gallbladder bacteria can proliferate causing inflammation of the gallbladder, **acute calculous cholecystitis**. Alternatively, gallstones can pass the cystic duct and become lodged in the CBD (**choledocholithiasis**). A stone at this level creates a stagnant column of fluid that has the potential to become infected (**acute cholangitis**). Obstruction of the CBD increases intraductal pressure and allows bacteria to invade the systemic circulation via the hepatic sinusoids.

The syndrome of **acalculous cholecystitis** is occasionally encountered (~5% of all cases of cholecystitis). This represents gallbladder inflammation arising secondary to gallbladder stasis and ischemia. Most patients with this condition have undergone prolonged fasts, have hemodynamic instability, and/or have atherosclerotic disease.

CLINICAL PRESENTATION

Most gallstones do not cause symptoms; indeed, many gallstones are discovered incidentally when evaluating for other disease processes (e.g., an incidental finding on ultrasound). However, symptoms referable to the gallbladder will eventually develop in only 10–25% of those patients. The classic symptoms of "biliary colic" (symptomatic cholelithiasis) consist of right upper quadrant abdominal pain that lasts for a few minutes to hours. The description as colic is actually a misnomer as most patients have constant pain rather than intermittent. The pain typically radiates to the region of the right scapular tip or right shoulder and occurs postprandially, especially after fatty meals. Patients often have associated nausea and vomiting.

Patients with acute cholecystitis present with typical biliary colic at first, with some 75% noting previous biliary colic attacks. However, the pain caused by cholecystitis tends to be constant and persistent, often >5 hours. Patients usually have nausea and vomiting as well as low-grade fever. On physical examination, there is right upper quadrant tenderness and a "**Murphy's sign**," which is the sudden cessation of an instructed deep inspiration when the examiner palpates at the right subcostal region.

Around 70% of the patients with ascending cholangitis present with the classic "**Charcot's triad**," fever, jaundice, and right upper quadrant abdominal pain. If the obstruction is not relieved, the patients can progress to develop "Reynold's pentad," which adds circulatory shock and altered mental status.

EVALUATION

An **ultrasound of the gallbladder** is the initial test of choice. It is important to look for the presence of stones, thickness of the gallbladder wall, diameter of CBD (>10 mm suggests distal obstruction), and the presence of pericholecystic fluid. Symptomatic cholelithiasis is characterized only by the presence of stone, all other findings should be normal. For acute cholecystitis, ultrasound should show gallstones or sludge, thickened gallbladder wall, pericholecystic fluid, and a normal-sized CBD. If ultrasound findings are normal and acute cholecystitis still suspected, a radionucleotide scan, **hepatobiliary iminodiacetic acid (HIDA) scan**, should be performed because of its superior sensitivity. HIDA scans may also be useful in suspected cases of acalculous cholecystitis. Findings suggestive of acute cholecystitis include good uptake of the radionucleotides in the liver with visualization of the radionucleotide in the CBD and small intestines; however, the radionucleotide fails to fill the gallbladder, which would suggest an obstruction of the cystic duct. For acute cholangitis, choledocholithiasis is rarely seen on ultrasound but the presence of CBD dilatation usually implies the presence of stones in the CBD. A normal ultrasound does not exclude acute cholangitis and suspicious cases should undergo further workup. CT scans of the abdomen are considered more sensitive for choledocholithiasis, but ultimately patients should undergo **endoscopic retrograde cholangiopancreatography (ERCP)**, which can be both diagnostic and therapeutic.

Laboratory data can also be helpful particularly in patients with suspected acute cholecystitis or cholangitis. Laboratory findings are typically normal in symptomatic cholelithiasis. Patients with acute cholecystitis typically have mild leukocytosis (<15,000/μL) and mild elevations of hepatic transaminases and bilirubin. Higher leukocyte count or bilirubin level should alarm the physician to consider cholangitis. Acute cholangitis has the typical findings of leukocytosis, elevated bilirubin level, and elevated alkaline phosphatase level (from irritation of the lining of the biliary tree) in addition to mild elevations of transaminases.

MANAGEMENT

Identification of stones, combined with the clinical findings, support definitive treatment of symptomatic cholelithiasis, which is surgical removal of the gallbladder (cholecystectomy). Today, most cholecystectomies are performed in a laparoscopic fashion, which has the advantages of decreased pain and shorter course of recovery. Medical therapies such as dissolution of cholesterol stones with ursodiol and lithotripsy have been shown to be ineffective, with slow dissolution time and high recurrence rate.

The treatment of acute cholecystitis begins with supportive measures, including NPO, initiation of IV fluids, placement of a nasogastric tube, and IV antibiotics. Recommended antibiotics should cover gram-negative enteric organisms, such as monotherapy with a third- or fourth-generation cephalosporin. For the majority of patients, these measures alone will result in resolution of acute cholecystitis. Lack of improvement can be a sign of a complication such as gangrenous cholecystitis, empyema, perforation, or cholecystenteric fistula. Any of these complications require immediate cholecystectomy. If surgery is too high-risk, placement of a percutaneous cholecystostomy tube should be considered. Any patient with an episode of acute cholecystitis should have a cholecystectomy performed within a few days to prevent recurrence and complications unless medical comorbidities preclude an operation.

Management of ascending cholangitis depends on the severity of the disease process. All patients with cholangitis should be aggressively managed with IV hydration and IV antibiotics. The antibiotics should cover the presumed organism in bile, including gram-negative enteric organisms, pseudomonas, enterococci, and anaerobes. Recommended regimens include piperacillin/tazobactam or a third- or fourth-generation cephalosporin plus metronidazole. The ultimate therapy requires biliary tract drainage with removal of the obstruction. Patients who are deteriorating clinically or who fail to respond to conservative therapy within 24 hours require urgent decompression. All others should have a procedure performed within 72 hours. The preferred procedure is an ERCP with retrieval of the stone and sphincterotomy (division of sphincter of Oddi). This has a >90% success rate. Other options for drainage include surgical exploration or percutaneous drainage of the CBD, but both are associated with significant morbidity and mortality. Similar to acute cholecystitis, all patients with acute cholangitis will ultimately need cholecystectomy to prevent recurrence and complications.

EVALUATION OF

JAUNDICE

L. Chad Hood

- Jaundice is a yellowish discoloration due to bilirubin accumulation.
- Bilirubin accumulates either due to excessive heme breakdown (hemolysis), an inability of the liver to conjugate or excrete bilirubin (congenital conditions or liver disease), or obstruction (intrinsic or extrinsic) in the bile ducts.
- Indirect hyperbilirubinemia = hemolysis or impaired liver conjugation.
- Direct hyperbilirubinemia = impaired liver excretion or biliary blockage.
- Most primary liver disorders present with elevations of both indirect and direct hyperbilirubinemia.

INTRODUCTION

Synonymous with the term icterus, jaundice refers to an abnormal yellow coloring of the sclera, mucous membranes, and skin. It specifically implies a discoloration due to the deposition of bile pigment from excess circulating blood levels of bilirubin. The discoloration of the sclera and mucous membranes distinguishes jaundice from other causes of yellowish skin discoloration (such as beta-carotene consumption or Addison's disease) which tend to be limited to the skin.

PATHOPHYSIOLOGY

An accumulation of serum bilirubin to levels >2.5–3.0 mg/dL is usually sufficient to cause jaundice. The degree of jaundice generally correlates to the level of bilirubin. The majority of bilirubin is produced by the degradation of heme molecules from circulating red blood cells. The form of bilirubin produced is referred to as unconjugated bilirubin and is not water-soluble, so must be bound to albumin to enter the bloodstream. Once transported to the liver, unconjugated bilirubin is taken up by hepatocytes. In the liver, bilirubin uridine-diphosphate (UDP) glucuronosyltransferase conjugates bilirubin with glucuronic acid, making a water-soluble compound. The conjugated bilirubin can now be secreted into the biliary system where, as a component of bile, it may be stored in the gallbladder or released through the biliary tree into the duodenum. Once in the gastrointestinal (GI) tract, conjugated bilirubin cannot be reabsorbed by intestinal epithelium. However, bacterial enzymes in the colon will convert conjugated bilirubin to urobilinogen and finally to stercobilinogen. Urobilinogen can be reabsorbed by the colonic mucosa and is then either excreted in bile again or can be excreted in urine. Stercobilinogen is the pigment which gives stool its color, thus in complete biliary obstruction with no excretion of bilirubin into the GI tract, clay-colored stools can be found.

Any condition which increases bilirubin production (hemolysis) or decreases the conjugation of bilirubin by the liver will result in an elevation of predominantly **indirect (unconjugated) bilirubin**. Liver conjugation is usually impaired by drugs or a genetic syndrome. Gilbert's syndrome is found in 7% of the population and is caused by a reduction in the amount of UDP glucuronyltransferase produced in the liver, resulting in elevation in unconjugated bilirubin. Crigler-Najjar syndrome is caused by either the absence or aberrant production of UDP glucuronyltransferase and results in greater elevations of unconjugated bilirubin. Any condition interfering with the excretion of conjugated bilirubin will result in an elevation of predominantly **direct (conjugated) bilirubin**. For example, the inherited conditions such as Dubin-Johnson syndrome and Rotor syndrome impair hepatocyte secretion of conjugated bilirubin into bile ducts. Patients with either intrahepatic or extrahepatic biliary obstruction will also develop primarily conjugated hyperbilirubinemia. Biliary obstruction ultimately results in the inability to excrete conjugated bilirubin into the biliary tree and the accumulation of bilirubin in hepatocytes. As conjugated bilirubin collects in the hepatocytes, it spills over into the bloodstream and may reverse glucuronidation increasing the amount of unconjugated bilirubin, which also diffuses into the bloodstream. Thus, biliary obstruction may present with a mixed hyperbilirubinemia. In most primary liver disorders, such as hepatitis and cirrhosis, injury or destruction of the hepatocytes impairs both bilirubin conjugation and secretion of bilirubin into the biliary ducts. Thus, these disorders can present with high amounts of direct bilirubin, indirect bilirubin, or both (Table 31-1).

Table 31-1 **Three Possible Mechanisms for Abnormal Accumulation of Bilirubin, Possible Causes, and Characteristic Clinical Findings**

	Causes	Clinical Finding
Hemolysis	Extravascular	↑ indirect bilirubin
	Autoimmune	Spherocytes on smear
	Glucose-6-phosphate dehydrogenase deficiency	
	Intravascular	↑ indirect bilirubin
	Mechanical valves	Schistocytes on smear
	Microangiopathic (TTP, DIC)	Hemoglobinuria
Hepatocellular dysfunction	Cirrhosis	↑ indirect or direct
	Hepatitis	bilirubin
	Sepsis	↑ AST/ALT
	Congestive heart failure	
	Medications	
	Toxins	
Biliary obstruction	Cholelithiasis	↑ direct bilirubin
	Stricture	↑ alkaline phosphatase
	Cholangitis	↑ pancreas enzymes
	Pancreatitis	

CLINICAL PRESENTATION

Jaundiced patients share the common pathology of bilirubin accumulation. Regardless of the etiology, they will all demonstrate the symptoms of bilirubin excess: yellow pigmentation, dark urine, pruritus at higher levels, and nausea/malaise at severe elevations. Beyond this, though, their symptoms will differ and potentially provide insight as to the cause for their jaundice.

Since the liver plays a central role in bilirubin metabolism, immediate attention to signs and symptoms from the hepatobiliary system is warranted. Patients with viral hepatitis will commonly have myalgias, malaise, nausea, vomiting, and anorexia. Acute cholangitis is associated with the classic findings of Charcot's triad—fever, jaundice, and right upper quadrant abdominal pain (Chap. 30). Signs suggestive of cirrhosis include ascites, splenomegaly, spider angiomata, and gynecomastia (Chap. 27). Right upper quadrant pain, nausea and vomiting, or a history of liver/gallbladder disease suggests a biliary origin. Complete biliary obstruction is classically associated with clay-colored stools and dark urine. Since conjugated bilirubin is water-soluble, when in excess it will be filtered by the kidneys and excreted producing dark, reddish-orange urine. Further, the metabolism of bilirubin in the GI tract results in the brown color of stool (stercobilinogen), so complete biliary obstruction will produce light-colored or clay-colored stools because of the absence of bilirubin in the GI tract. "Painless jaundice" (without abdominal pain) can be present in hemolysis, but may also be a sign of obstructive malignancy. This can be a primary biliary malignancy (most commonly pancreatic cancer), a metastatic process, or extrinsic compression of the biliary tree by a potentially malignant mass.

Patients with hemolysis often present due to complications from anemia. They generally have no GI symptoms (e.g., nausea, vomiting, abdominal pain, and anorexia), but can have splenomegaly, particularly if they have extravascular hemolysis. Patients with autoimmune hemolytic anemia may have a preceding viral infection or may have other autoimmune disorders. Valve hemolysis should be considered in any patient with a mechanical heart valve. Patients with thrombotic thrombocytopenic purpura (TTP) or disseminated intravascular coagulation (DIC) are typically quite ill and do not present primarily for jaundice.

EVALUATION

Appropriate testing should be pursued based on the history and physical. All patients should have complete liver function testing (LFT) performed, including conjugated and unconjugated bilirubin and international normalized ratio (INR), and a complete blood count. In general, greater elevations of aspartate transaminase (AST) and alanine transaminase (ALT) reflect hepatocellular etiology, whereas a greater elevation of alkaline phosphatase reflects a biliary etiology. Normal LFTs may reflect hemolysis; however, these enzymes can also begin to normalize in severe or long-standing liver disease. In the case of normal LFTs, elevation of the INR indicates that synthetic function of the liver has been impaired and is important to assess the severity of liver disease. Patients with TTP or DIC will also have elevation of the INR, but, in addition, will have elevation of the partial thromboplastin time (PTT), thrombocytopenia, and perhaps anemia. In patients who have completely normal labs and elevations of either conjugated or unconjugated bilirubin, an inherited disorder of bilirubin metabolism should be considered.

- **Hemolytic jaundice**: Hemolysis from any cause is associated with high low-density lipoprotein (LDH) levels and low haptoglobin levels. Further evaluation consists of classifying the hemolysis **by the site of**

RBC destruction, either intravascular or extravascular. Extravascular hemolysis occurs when misshapen RBCs or RBCs coated in complement are destroyed by the liver and spleen. These patients may have splenomegaly on examination and have spherocytes on the peripheral blood smear. By contrast, **intravascular hemolysis** has schistocytes or fragmented RBCs on the peripheral blood smear and causes hemoglobinemia (red to brown color of plasma) and hemoglobinuria (positive blood in the urine but no intact RBCs). Last, an echocardiogram should be ordered on any patients with a prosthetic valve to evaluate for mechanical dysfunction which may worsen hemolysis.

- **Hepatocellular jaundice**: Patients with a presentation typical for cirrhosis or hepatitis do not require an extensive workup for their jaundice unless a superimposed condition is suspected. Symptoms or lab findings suggestive of liver disease merit a workup for the cause, if not already known (Chap. 27). Ultrasound should be performed to rule out obstruction, even in patients with established liver disease due to the possibility of superimposed gallstones or other obstructive pathology.

- **Obstructive jaundice**: **Ultrasound** should be performed in any patient with suspected biliary or obstructive jaundice. It is necessary to assess for ductal dilation, and if present will provide information about the localization of the obstruction. Unfortunately, normal ducts on an ultrasound can be seen in obstructive jaundice, so the diagnosis cannot be excluded with a normal ultrasound. **Endoscopic retrograde cholangiopancreatography (ERCP)** may be performed as part of therapy (see "Management," below) or may also be performed diagnostically in cases where ductal dilation is not seen but obstructive pathology is clinically suspected. In this procedure, an endoscope is advanced through the mouth, esophagus, stomach, and duodenum, and dye is injected through the ampulla of Vater into the biliary system to assess the pancreatic and bile ducts. **Computed tomography (CT) scan of the abdomen** may be helpful in cases where ultrasound is not readily available, or when extra-biliary pathology is suspected (e.g., extrinsic mass, pancreatic disease).

MANAGEMENT

- **Hemolytic jaundice**: Treatment is of course based on the underlying condition—cessation of offending medications, valve replacement, and so forth. In autoimmune conditions, prednisone or immunotherapy is often beneficial. In chronic autoimmune conditions, splenomegaly may be warranted (Chap. 51).

- **Hepatocellular jaundice**: Management of the liver disease should be focused on the underlying cause, such as supportive care for acute hepatitis, immunotherapy for viral or autoimmune hepatitis, or consideration for liver transplant in severe cases. Alcohol cessation and avoidance of hepatotoxic medications are crucial. Gastroenterology consultation may be necessary to determine diagnosis, prognosis, or therapy.

- **Obstructive jaundice**: Resolution of the obstruction is essential. Intrahepatic cholestasis will require treatment of the underlying cause, such as stopping the offending medication, or supportive or other treatment of hepatitis. Bile acid therapy or bile acid binding resins may help relieve symptoms in chronic cases. Intrinsic obstruction from gallstones or strictures/stenosis requires early gastroenterology consultation for ERCP and in some cases biliary stent placement. Otherwise, surgery (laparoscopic or open) may be required. Empiric antibiotics are often used prophylactically and postintervention to prevent infections associated with impaired biliary drainage. Cholecystectomy is not recommended for asymptomatic gallstones. However, after an obstructive jaundice episode, cholecystectomy should be considered if there are retained stones in the gallbladder or evidence of gallbladder dysfunction. Surgery would usually be pursued after resolution of the biliary obstruction (spontaneously, via ERCP).

Extrinsic masses (including pancreatic) will usually require biopsy via ERCP, CT-guided biopsy, or abdominal surgery, followed by staging and treatment for malignancy if present. If surgical removal is not possible, endoscopic stenting or percutaneous biliary drainage catheter may be necessary if symptoms persist. As with intrinsic obstruction, empiric antibiotics may also be indicated.

Acute cholangitis is a life-threatening condition that can occur de novo or more commonly in association with an obstruction. Immediately acquire blood cultures and start empiric antibiotic therapy to cover gram-negative and anaerobic organisms. Typical regimens include a broad-spectrum cephalosporin (such as cefepime), meropenem or imipenem, or a fluoroquinolone. Anaerobic infections are uncommon, but in severely ill patients or those who are not improving the addition of metronidazole or piperacillin/tazobactam should be considered. Once again, biliary drainage is the only definitive treatment, which is typically performed using ERCP although surgical or percutaneous drains may also be used.

RENAL

ACUTE RENAL FAILURE

David W. Rudy

KEY POINTS

- ARF is generally defined as a significant elevation of Cr over baseline.
- The differential diagnosis of ARF may be categorized into prerenal, postrenal, and intrinsic renal causes.
- Most cases are related to poor kidney perfusion from either prerenal failure or ATN.

INTRODUCTION

Acute renal failure (ARF) is a common and serious condition associated with significant morbidity and mortality. Many cases of ARF if recognized early may be reversed or attenuated. Also, certain measures may be used to help prevent the onset of ARF especially in vulnerable patients. It is also imperative to recognize ARF in the earliest stages in order to rapidly treat complications and to proactively employ measures to avoid complications. ARF is a complex syndrome with a long differential diagnosis. The etiology in many cases may be multifactorial in nature. The pathophysiology is complex and not fully elucidated. Treatment options are often limited to supportive measures. In spite of these complexities, a rational approach to the patient with ARF can be developed using a classification based on the anatomy and function of the kidneys.

ARF is an abrupt decline in renal function manifested by an inability of the kidneys to excrete metabolic waste products and maintain proper fluid, electrolyte, and acid-base balance. The majority of ARF occurs in hospitalized patients due to underlying medical conditions, complications of those conditions, diagnostic studies and/or therapies. ARF affects 5–7% of all hospitalized patients including 30% of patients admitted to intensive care units (ICUs). The overall **mortality of patients with ARF is approximately 20%,** but patients with more severe ARF (serum creatinine [Cr] >3 mg/dL) and those patients requiring dialysis have mortality rates of 40–50%. ARF in the ICU setting carries a mortality rate of 50–70%. In addition, patients with ARF have increased medical complications such as infections and bleeding. Consequently, it is important to recognize patients at risk for ARF and begin therapies to actively prevent its occurrence. If renal dysfunction develops, prompt diagnosis and rapid initiation of appropriate therapy will hopefully minimize those potential complications.

PATHOPHYSIOLOGY

ARF may be classified according to primary pathophysiologic insult leading to renal dysfunction. The three main categories are: (1) prerenal ARF (approximately 55%) caused by conditions that decrease renal perfusion; (2) intrinsic renal ARF (approximately 40%) caused by insult to the renal parenchyma; and (3) postrenal ARF (approximately 5%) caused by obstruction of the urinary tract. This classification is useful in formulating a differential diagnosis as demonstrated in Table 32-1.

Prerenal ARF

Prerenal ARF is a common cause of ARF in hospitalized patients. It may be caused by any condition that leads to **decreased renal perfusion**. This includes **intravascular volume depletion** from fluid loss such as hemorrhage or GI losses, from third space losses such as pancreatitis, from conditions leading to a **decrease in effective circulating volume** such as congestive heart failure, or from intense renal vasoconstriction. Prerenal ARF ensues when the glomerular filtration rate (GFR) cannot be maintained despite the kidney's compensatory response to hypoperfusion via an activation of neurohumoral systems such as the adrenergic nervous system, the renin-angiotensin-aldosterone system, and the release of antidiuretic hormone (ADH). These compensatory mechanisms help maintain blood pressure through systemic vasoconstriction and fluid retention. GFR is further maintained by renal afferent arteriole dilation and efferent arteriole constriction. Yet if the decline in blood pressure is severe enough and/or prolonged compensation fails, ARF develops. These compensatory mechanisms may also be impaired in patients taking certain medications. For example, nonsteroidal anti-inflammatory drugs (NSAIDs) block prostaglandin production, preventing afferent dilation and angiotensin-converting enzyme (ACE) inhibitors block angiotensin II production, preventing efferent constriction. Fortunately, in prerenal ARF there is no structural damage to the kidneys and GFR can be rapidly restored with correction of the underlying condition. However, if renal hypoperfusion is severe enough or prolonged, it may lead to ischemic acute tubular necrosis (ATN).

Table 32-1 **Classification of the Major Causes of ARF**

Classification	Etiology	Evaluation
Prerenal ARF		
Hypovolemia	Hemorrhage	Tachycardia
	Vomiting	Hypotension
	Diarrhea	BUN:Cr >20:1
	Diuretics	FENa <1%
	NSAIDs	Urine osmolality >500
	ACE inhibitors	
Decreased effective	Congestive heart failure	Edema
blood volume	Cirrhosis	BUN:Cr >20:1
	Nephrotic syndrome	FENa <1%
	Sepsis	Urine osmolality >500
Intrinsic ARF		
ATN	Ischemia (see prerenal)	FENa >2%
	Aminoglycosides	Urine osmolality ~300
	Amphotericin B	Epithelial cell casts
	Radiocontrast	
	Rhabdomyolysis	
AIN	Penicillins	Fever
	Sulfonamides	Rash
	Fluoroquinolones	Eosinophilia and
		eosinophiluria
		Pyuria and WBC casts
Glomerulonephritis	Postinfectious	Dysmorphic RBCs
or vasculitis	SLE	RBC casts
	Wegener's granulomatosis	Proteinuria
	HUS/TTP	
Postrenal ARF		
Upper tract	Calculi	BUN:Cr variable
	Blood clots	FENa variable
	Papillary necrosis	Hydronephrosis on
		ultrasound
		Calcium or uric acid crystals

(Continued)

Table 32-1 **Classification of the Major Causes of ARF (Continued)**

Classification	Etiology	Evaluation
	Postrenal ARF	
Lower tract	Prostatic hypertrophy Neurogenic bladder Bladder tumor Urethral stricture	BUN:Cr variable FENa variable Hydronephrosis on ultrasound High postvoid residual bladder volume

Abbreviations: SLE, systemic lupus erythematosus; HUS, hemolytic-uremic syndrome; TTP, thrombotic thrombocytopenic purpura.

Intrinsic Renal ARF

Intrinsic renal ARF is the leading cause of renal failure in hospitalized patients and is classified according to the anatomic structures of the kidneys involved. Thus, intrinsic renal ARF may involve pathology of the renal vessels, disorders of the microcirculation or glomeruli, damage to the tubules, or abnormalities of the tubulointerstitium.

The most common form of intrinsic renal ARF is **ATN**, which is subdivided into ischemic or toxic etiologies although in many situations the etiology may be multifactorial. **Ischemic** ATN occurs when renal hypoperfusion causes tubular cell injury and is characterized by persistent renal dysfunction despite correction of hemodynamic compromise (unlike prerenal etiologies). The clinical course of ATN may be divided into three phases: initiation, maintenance, and recovery. The initiation phase represents the time when ischemic injury is evolving (and potentially reversible). The GFR declines from two essential mechanisms: the glomerular pressure is already reduced from hypoperfusion and ischemic tubular epithelial cells are sloughed into the tubular lumen causing tubular obstruction. The maintenance phase is the period of time (days to weeks) during which renal function remains depressed because of continued tubular cell dysfunction. This is followed by the recovery phase during which renal function improves as tubule cells regenerate. **Toxic** etiologies of ATN follow a similar pattern, in that the initial insult results in both intrarenal vasoconstriction and tubular epithelial cell damage.

Postrenal ARF

Obstruction may occur at any location along the urinary tract. In patients with normal renal function, a single kidney can sufficiently manage all metabolic wastes. Thus, for ARF to develop either bilateral upper tract obstruction or ureteral obstruction must occur. However, patients with preexisting renal insufficiency can develop ARF from unilateral upper tract obstruction.

Initially, with acute ureteral obstruction, there is an increase in renal blood and renal pelvic pressure. After a period of time, the increased pressure is transmitted retrograde up the nephrons back to the proximal tubules. Since hydrostatic pressure drives filtration, a reduction in this pressure reduces GFR.

CLINICAL PRESENTATION

Due to the widespread use of laboratory studies in hospitalized patients, most cases of ARF are initially detected by an asymptomatic change in serum Cr and/or blood urea nitrogen (BUN) rather than overt signs and symptoms. The symptoms associated with renal failure tend to be nonspecific and found only in a minority of patients—anorexia, nausea, vomiting, mental status changes, and edema. Some patients may note a decrease in urinary output (oliguria or anuria); however, this is most common in prerenal disease and may not be present in many other etiologies. Oliguria is defined as a 24-hour urine output between 100 and 400 mL and anuria as <100 mL. As a general rule, the minimal acceptable urine output is 0.5–1.0 mL/kg/h (approximately 1000 mL/day for an adult).

The history and physical examination may help determine the cause and/or identify possible causes of the ARF. Important historical factors include symptoms of underlying causes, comorbid diseases and current medications. The history and physical should also identify any complications of renal failure (Table 32-2). The pulse, blood pressure (including orthostatics), neck veins and skin turgor can help with assessing volume status. Also, when ARF develops in a hospitalized patient, review the patient's intake/output and daily weights to help assess volume status. Skin findings like purpura or livedo reticularis may suggest vasculitis or cholesterol emboli, respectively, while an enlarged prostate or distended bladder suggest an obstructive cause of ARF.

Table 32-2 **Complications of ARF**

Azotemia (uremia)	Encephalopathy
	Pericarditis
	Platelet dysfunction
Hematologic	Anemia—normocytic and normochromic
Metabolic	Hyperkalemia
	Hypermagnesemia
	Hyperphosphatemia
	Hypocalcemia
	Hyponatremia
	Metabolic acidosis
Volume status	Hypervolemia—pulmonary edema

EVALUATION

The initial evaluation often centers on the BUN and Cr. Making the diagnosis of ARF requires an understanding of the relationship of Cr to GFR. Cr is derived from skeletal muscle metabolism and is freely filtered by the kidney, so is often used as a marker of renal function. Serum Cr concentrations are related to body muscle mass, so tend to be lower in women and the elderly. In general, a doubling in serum Cr reflects a 50% decrease in GFR. For example, if a patient with a baseline Cr of 0.6 mg/dL develops a Cr of 1.2 mg/dL, he/she has lost half of their renal function (GFR reduced from ~120 to ~60 mL/min). Similarly, if the same patient went from a Cr of 1.2 to 2.4 mg/dL, he/she has lost half of their renal function (GFR reduced from ~60 to ~30 mL/min). However, the greatest change in the total GFR occurred when the Cr rose from 0.6 to 1.2 mg/dL, a time when many would overlook the rising Cr. BUN is a less reliable marker of renal function, because it will rise with a high protein diet, trauma, gastrointestinal hemorrhage or the use of corticosteroids. However, the ratio of BUN to Cr is useful in determining the etiology. BUN is passively reabsorbed by the proximal tubule, so when tubular flow is low (prerenal) more BUN will be reabsorbed (typical ratio of BUN:Cr >20:1). Significant elevations (>60 mg/dL) of BUN often referred to as uremia or azotemia should also be noted because of associated complications.

In determining the etiology of ARF, the **urinalysis** with microscopic evaluation of the urine sediment is essential as it can demonstrate classic patterns of renal disease (see Chap. 27 in the *First Exposure to Internal Medicine: Ambulatory Medicine*):

- Hematuria, RBC casts, proteinuria → glomerular disease or vasculitis
- Epithelial cells and epithelial cell casts (muddy brown casts) → ATN
- WBCs and WBC casts → acute interstitial nephritis (AIN) or pyelonephritis
- High specific gravity (SG) (>1.020) and hyaline casts → prerenal
- Normal → prerenal, obstruction, ATN
- Large blood but no (or few) RBCs → rhabdomyolysis

Assessment of the **fractional excretion of sodium (FENa)** will help separate prerenal failure from ATN. Prerenal failure is characterized by sodium retention, so a spot urine Na is typically <20 meq/L and the FENa is <1%. ATN results in higher sodium values because tubular damage prevents the reabsorption of sodium, thus a spot urine Na is typically >40 meq/L and the FENa is >2%. Intermediate values for spot urine Na and FENa can be seen with either disorder.

FENa = (serum Cr)(urine sodium)/(urine Cr)(serum sodium) × 100

Assessment of electrolytes including calcium, magnesium and phosphorous, and complete blood counts are also important to evaluate for complications of renal failure.

Further assessment depends on the clinical presentation and the initial laboratory evaluation. A **renal ultrasound** should be considered if the clinical scenario is unclear. Although postrenal processes account for only 5% of ARF, rapid diagnosis is essential in order to prevent permanent kidney damage. Other tests such as urine eosinophils, magnetic resonance angiography (MRA), radionucleotide renal scans, and renal biopsies are performed in certain clinical settings but are not routine.

PREVENTION

Hospitalized patients have many predisposing conditions that place them at risk to develop ARF including chronic kidney disease, diabetes mellitus, congestive heart failure, cirrhosis, vascular disease, and advanced age alone. Thus, the following preventive measures should be considered in these patients:

- Avoid dehydration and/or hypotension
- Judicious use of nephrotoxic dugs, particularly NSAIDs, ACE inhibitors, amphotericin B, aminoglycosides, and cyclosporine
- Prevent radiocontrast nephropathy in patients at risk
  - Limited use of low-osmolality contrast media
  - Hydration with 1/2 normal saline (NS) at 1 mL/kg 12 hours before and after contrast (there is some evidence that NS or bicarbonate containing fluids might be more beneficial, but hydration is the key)
  - Oral acetylcysteine 600 mg twice a day before and on the day of contrast

MANAGEMENT

Initial management of a patient with ARF focuses on both treating the underlying cause and making sure the patient does not have any life-threatening complications (Table 32-2). With the substantial number of cases due to volume depletion or ischemia, **a fluid challenge** of 500 mL of NS without potassium given over 30 minutes should be considered in most patients. Patients who are clearly hypervolemic or who have a fragile cardiorespiratory status should have hypovolemia confirmed prior to receiving fluids. General principles that should be followed in patients with ARF include: restrict potassium in the diet and in fluids (until adequate urine output is established), assure that all nephrotoxins are eliminated, and assure that necessary medications are appropriately dosed for the level of renal function. Further management depends on the cause of the renal failure.

Initially, if a urinary catheter is in place, make sure the catheter is working by irrigating with 50 mL sterile NS, using a catheter-tip syringe. The fluid should pass easily and the entire amount should be aspirated. If there is not a urinary catheter in place and obstruction is suspected, an in-and-out bladder catheterization should be performed. If a large postvoid residual is obtained, the catheter should be left in place. If a patient has very little urinary output, an indwelling catheter should be avoided due to the risk of infection.

Prerenal ARF is managed with volume replacement as noted above. Urine output is typically monitored hourly with a goal of maintaining output above 0.5 mL/kg/h.

Resolution of a urinary tract obstruction will rapidly reverse ARF, so this condition should be ruled out initially. In male patients with BPH oftentimes placement of a urinary catheter is both diagnostic and therapeutic. Ultrasound is a quick and safe means for checking for obstuction both of the upper tract as well as the bladder. Upper tract obstruction requires urologic consultation to relieve the obstruction. The consultation should be emergent if an infection is suspected in the obstructed kidney **(pyonephrosis)**. All patients should be monitored for the development of postobstructive diuresis and volume depletion. As these patients are commonly volume overloaded, the body's physiologic response to relief of obstruction can be a brisk diuresis. The usual therapy is IV maintenance fluids such as 1/2 NS initially at 75 mL/h and adjusting according to hemodynamics. Replacement of urine output with IV fluids milliliter per milliliter should be avoided.

AIN will usually respond to cessation of the offending drug.

Therapy for ATN is limited to supportive care. However, patients who are oliguric may become volume overloaded and diuretics may be required to control the patient's volume status. Traditionally, moderate- to high-dose loop diuretics (e.g., furosemide 40–80 mg) are administered intravenously and the patient should respond within an hour. If there is no response the dose can be doubled and repeated until the maximum dose is reached. Thiazide diuretics may be used synergistically with loop diuretics (e.g., metolazone 5–10 mg PO or IV chlorothiazide 500 mg infused over 30 minutes).

Rarely patients present with such severe ARF that they require emergent hemodialysis. Hemodialysis is used to treat complications of ARF, so Cr levels and urine output should not be used as reasons to undergo dialysis. In fact, some evidence suggests that hemodialysis may delay the recovery of renal function. Although no consensus exists, general indications for hemodialysis include: refractory fluid overload, hyperkalemia or rapidly rising potassium levels, metabolic acidosis, pericarditis, or mental status changes felt to be from uremia.

CHRONIC KIDNEY

DISEASE AND

COMPLICATIONS

Lisa M. Antes
Joel A. Gordon

KEY POINTS

- CKD is common and increasing in prevalence.
- Slowing the progression of CKD delays the time for initiation of maintenance renal replacement therapy.
- As renal function declines, disturbances in fluid, electrolyte, and acid-base balance occur. In addition, endocrine functions of the kidney such as erythropoietin production and vitamin D activation begin to fail.
- Uremia is a constellation of signs and symptoms observed with advanced CKD and is an indication for dialysis.
- Cardiovascular disease is the greatest modifiable risk factor affecting morbidity and mortality in the CKD population.

INTRODUCTION

The magnitude of chronic kidney disease (CKD) worldwide is growing exponentially. In the United States, about 20 million people (1/10) have early CKD (about 20 million) and another 40 million are at risk due to underlying medical conditions. **Hypertension** and **diabetes mellitus** are the most common conditions leading to CKD. Other factors that predict a higher risk of developing CKD include: age over 60 years, family history of kidney disease (e.g., adult polycystic kidney disease), recurrent urinary tract infections, autoimmune diseases like systemic lupus erythematosus, and exposure to certain drugs (e.g., chronic nonsteroidal anti-inflammatory drug [NSAID] use). In addition, certain racial and ethnic groups have a higher relative incidence of CKD (African American, Latino, Hispanic, American Indian, Alaskan natives). A prior episode of acute renal failure also puts one at higher risk.

CLINICAL PRESENTATION

Overt signs and symptoms of early CKD are few, due to the remarkable capacity of the kidney to adapt to the reduction in functioning nephrons. CKD thus remains an insidious problem until more advanced stages manifest the complications of CKD. Patients may come to clinical attention presenting with consequences of anemia or volume overload. Some present with frank uremic manifestations (e.g., nausea, vomiting, and change in mentation) and others with biochemical abnormalities, including electrolyte imbalances. Therefore, early identification of patients with CKD is imperative. Serum creatinine determination alone is an imperfect indicator of glomerular filtration rate (GFR) and may remain "normal" despite substantial kidney damage. For example, in those with reduced muscle mass (e.g., elderly patients or patients with advanced liver disease), minor elevations in serum creatinine above reported normal laboratory values might represent significant reductions in GFR. Similarly, diet, gender, and race influence the interpretation of serum creatinine values. The use of mathematical calculations to estimate GFR has greatly augmented the detection and recognition of early stages of CKD. Most hospital and commercial laboratories are now automatically reporting serum creatinine with accompanying calculated estimate of GFR using these formulae. These tools are only useful, however, in patients with **stable** kidney function, not with acute renal failure.

Findings on ultrasonography can lend supporting data to the diagnosis of CKD, as well as suggesting the likely etiology. Bilateral, small (<10 cm), echogenic kidneys suggest chronic hypertension. Large kidneys are seen in diabetic nephropathy, especially in early stages when GFR is actually excessive (with ensuing glomerular damage); less common causes of large kidneys in CKD are multiple myeloma, HIV nephropathy, amyloidosis and autosomal-dominant polycystic kidney disease.

Classification: CKD comprises a spectrum from those with mild decrements in GFR or microalbuminuria to those requiring renal replacement therapy (RRT) (i.e., dialysis). The National Kidney Foundation-Kidney Disease Outcomes Quality Initiative (NKF-DOQI) guidelines define the stages of CKD based on level of GFR impairment (stages 2–5) and/or evidence of kidney

Table 33-1 **Stages of CKD***

Stage	Description	GFR (mL/min/1.73 m²)
1	Kidney damage, nl/↑ GFR	≥90
2	Kidney damage, mild ↓ GFR	60–89
3	Moderate ↓ GFR	30–59
4	Severe ↓ GFR	15–29
5	Kidney failure	<15 or RRT

*Abnormalities present for >3 months.

nl = normal

parenchymal damage as manifested by proteinuria, biopsy proven renal disease, or radiographic evidence of renal impairment (Table 33-1).

MANAGEMENT

The care of the CKD patient is complex and necessitates a comprehensive evaluation of four major components:

- Specific therapies for the underlying kidney disease
- The complications that ensue from diminished nephron function
- Strategies to slow down the progression of CKD
- Managing patient comorbidities, particularly cardiovascular disease risk factors

Complications of Chronic Kidney Disease

Complications of CKD generally begin to occur when GFR declines below 60 mL/min (i.e., stage 3) and persist through the progression to/development of end-stage renal disease (ESRD). Therapies to **delay progression** of CKD and address comorbidities should be implemented at all stages of CKD. By stage 4, physicians need to adequately prepare patients for smooth **transition to RRT**.

As progressive loss of functioning nephrons ensues in CKD, the remaining nephrons have a remarkable capacity to adapt by increasing the filtration, reabsorption, and secretion of solutes and water. Thus, in early stages of CKD when GFR is relatively well maintained, total body fluid and electrolyte balance and acid-base balance are relatively well preserved. A progressive decline in renal function, however, is accompanied by more or less predictable abnormalities in sodium balance (volume control), water balance (water excess), blood pressure (BP) control (hypertension), potassium balance, acid-base balance, anemia, and bone mineral metabolism (calcium, phosphorus).

Sodium and water imbalance: Retention of extra sodium (and water) as the kidney is failing is manifested by the development of peripheral **edema** of the lower extremities. Patients may also develop congestive heart failure (CHF) and may present with dyspnea, orthopnea and paroxysmal nocturnal dyspnea. This may be associated with **systemic hypertension** and decreases in urine output. These patients are in positive sodium (Na^+) and water balance, that is, more input than output of solutes and water. In most forms of advanced CKD, despite enhanced solute excretion per remaining nephron, patients may develop volume overload more readily if ingested dietary sodium exceeds the kidney's capacity for excretion.

Dietary sodium restriction is an effective way to target sodium balance; however, many patients also require loop diuretics to facilitate a negative sodium balance by enhancing urinary Na excretion. Furthermore, patients may be more responsive to the effects of their antihypertensive agents if they are in negative sodium balance.

Patients with CKD have both defects in urinary concentration and dilution. With disease progression, the range of urinary concentration and dilution becomes even more limited and results in urine that is typically isotonic to plasma. This may manifest clinically as **hyponatremia** if water intake far exceeds the kidneys' capacity for free water excretion.

Potassium imbalance: The kidney is the main way ingested potassium (K^+) is eliminated from the body, largely by secretion of K^+ in the distal nephron. As renal function declines, attention to serum potassium is important to prevent adverse effects of **hyperkalemia** on nerve and muscle function. Dietary restriction of K^+ becomes particularly important in those patients with CKD who have underlying difficulty handling potassium due to impaired renal secretion of K^+, for example, patients with diabetes mellitus and type IV renal tubular acidosis (RTA). If the patient has hyperkalemia and is also edematous, the use of diuretics can have dual function to assist in control of volume, as well as facilitate renal K excretion. Control of metabolic acidosis may also facilitate control of serum K by resulting in transcellular shifts of potassium from the extracellular to intracellular space, as the acidemia is treated.

Metabolic acidosis: Metabolic acidosis invariably develops with worsening kidney function. Patients may have an elevated anion gap metabolic acidosis, due to retained acids such as sulfates or phosphates, or a nonanion gap, hyperchloremic metabolic acidosis, the latter due to reduced renal ammoniagenesis. As a consequence of reduced capacity of the kidney to produce NH_4^+ (ammonium), the kidney, which normally excretes 1 meq/kg acid load per day, may only be able to excrete 30–40 meq daily with resultant acid retention.

Interestingly, the long-term consequences of metabolic acidosis are those related to bone health, as metabolic acidosis stimulates bone turnover and has been associated with increased bone resorption (thus decreased skeletal calcium). This is a consequence of bone minerals buffering the systemic acidosis. Metabolic acidosis is also associated with muscle wasting and weakness. Oral bicarbonate supplementation is used as an adjunctive therapy to optimize bone health and prevent bone loss.

Metabolic bone disease: Disturbances in calcium and phosphorus homeostasis and abnormal regulation of bone turnover are interrelated processes that contribute to skeletal morbidity in the CKD population. The metabolic bone disease of CKD is known as **renal osteodystrophy,** of which there are several subtypes (secondary hyperparathyroidism, adynamic bone disease, osteomalacia, mixed renal osteodystrophy).

Hyperphosphatemia: Hyperphosphatemia results from impaired ability to excrete excess dietary phosphorus and is an important risk factor for cardiovascular events and sudden cardiac death. This excess risk is independent of serum calcium levels or compliance with treatments and is perhaps linked to calcium deposition in the myocardium and coronary arteries. Control of phosphorus and calcium and restoration of a Ca × P product <55 (i.e., the serum level of Ca multiplied by the serum level of P in mg/dL) optimizes bone health and potentially can decrease cardiovascular morbidity.

Anemia: With the introduction of synthetic erythropoietin to treat **anemia** associated with renal failure in the 1980s, patients have benefited with improved quality of life, quality of sleep, cognitive function, and exercise performance. Correction of anemia has resulted in decreased cardiovascular mortality and in regression of left ventricular hypertrophy (LVH). Anemia management should begin early when recognized in CKD with use of recombinant erythropoietin to maintain Hgb >11 g/dL, with a target of 12–12.5 g/dL. (Iron stores must be repleted for erythropoietin to work.)

Malnutrition: One of the most significant clinical indicators of progressive kidney failure is an apparent decrease in appetite. Nutritional compromise may begin when GFR falls <50 mL/min/1.73 m^2 (i.e., stage 3 CKD). Spontaneous decreases in dietary protein and energy intake can be regarded as an early index of uremia. Attention to nutritional status improves outcomes of patients with CKD and ESRD.

Uremia: Uremia represents a constellation of signs and symptoms observed with progressive CKD, particularly in the advanced stages. Most common are gastrointestinal manifestations (nausea, anorexia, hiccups, weight loss) and cognitive dysfunction (hypersomnolence, impaired concentrating ability). Uremic neuropathies include peripheral neuropathy (characterized by paresthesias and hypalgesia), "restless" leg syndrome, myoclonic jerks, and uremic encephalopathy that can even lead to seizures. Uremic platelet dysfunction can cause bleeding. Pruritus may occur as a manifestation of uremia or as a consequence of hyperphosphatemia. Despite extensive efforts, the "uremic toxin" has yet to be defined.

Strategies to Slow Progression of Chronic Kidney Disease

It is well established that timely introduction of strategies to slow the progression of CKD not only smoothes the transition to RRT, but actually significantly delays the time for need of RRT. Many of these strategies focus on **optimum control of BP** and **control of proteinuria** to <500 mg daily. These strategies should be implemented even with stage 1 or 2 CKD and continue through stage 5 CKD.

BP: The vast majority of patients are hypertensive even in early stages of CKD, with a prevalence of nearly 100% by the time the GFR falls below 10 mL/min. Hypertension often requires the use of three to four medications to achieve control in the CKD population, particularly those with diabetic kidney disease. Evidence overwhelmingly demonstrates that control of BP retards progression of any type of renal disease, but the effect is particularly dramatic in those with high risk of progressive renal disease (e.g., diabetics, established renal disease, and proteinuric renal diseases). BP goals are <130/80 mmHg for patients with CKD, and <125/75 mmHg for those with significant proteinuria (>1 g/day).

Proteinuria: Proteinuria is a marker for progression of renal disease, and routine screening for proteinuria is indicated in patients at risk for CKD. Overt **proteinuria** (>300 mg daily) can therefore be detected on routine dip-stick analysis. If the dipstick is positive, the degree of proteinuria should be quantitated. Screening for **microalbuminuria** can be performed on a random spot urine specimen by measuring a microalbumin:creatinine ratio (30–300 mg/g on two occasions suggests microalbuminuria).

Control of proteinuria delays the progression of CKD to ESRD and reduces cardiovascular risk. The target of proteinuria should be <500 mg/day. Pharmacologic inhibition of the renin-angiotensin-aldosterone system (RAAS), using agents like **angiotensin-converting enzyme (ACE) inhibitors** or **angiotensin II receptor blockers**, slows progression of renal failure in chronic proteinuric nephropathies, that is, both diabetic and nondiabetic pro-teinuric renal disease. When using agents that block the RAAS, particular attention to electrolytes to avoid hyperkalemia should be made. Nondihydropyridine calcium channel blockers may afford some antiprotein-uric benefits as a second- or third-line therapy.

Comorbidities and Impact on Renal Disease

In patients with CKD, it is important to optimize control of comorbid condi-tions, particularly diabetes mellitus, cardiovascular disease, CHF, hyperlipi-demia, and peripheral vascular disease. The psychosocial impact of CKD and patients' coping behaviors also influences patient outcomes.

Renal disease is an increasingly important risk factor for cardiovascular disease. Approximately 40% of patients with CKD die of cardiovascular dis-ease **before** developing ESRD. Once patients do reach ESRD, death from car-diovascular events is considerable and is most prominent in young adults (aged 15–35 years), in whom the annual cardiovascular mortality is several 100-fold that of the general population.

Preparation for Renal Replacement Therapy

The "30-20-10 rule" is a frequent paradigm used to help prepare patients for RRT. Referral to a nephrologist is recommended when patient's GFR falls to ≤30 mL/min or sooner. RRT options should be discussed with the patient at stage 4 CKD, to begin initiating plans for vascular access placement once GFR falls to 20 mL/min. Dialysis is initiated at approximately 10 mL/min. Options for dialysis include peritoneal dialysis (PD) or hemodialysis. If the patient is a suitable candidate, the option of kidney transplantation should be discussed and patient referred for evaluation for either a living related or deceased donor renal transplant. Outcomes with renal transplantation are considerably better than with maintenance hemodialysis. This improvement in survival is most pronounced in the diabetic population.

Hemodialysis involves circulating the patient's blood through a machine that results in flow of blood along one side of a semipermeable membrane with a cleansing solution, or dialysate, along the other. Diffusion and convection allow the dialysate to remove unwanted substances from the blood (e.g., excess potassium) while adding back needed components. Most patients require chronic hemodialysis three times a week, 3–4 hours per session. With **PD**, the capillary bed that lies between the visceral and parietal layers of the peritoneal membrane is the "dialyzer." The dialysate enters and leaves the peritoneal space through an indwelling catheter. It can be performed as continuous ambulatory peritoneal dialysis (CAPD), which requires fluid exchanges four to six times a day using gravity rather than machinery for flow, or as continuous cyclic peritoneal dialysis (CCPD), which does require a cycler machine to perform exchanges at night. There are advantages and disadvantages with both forms of dialysis so the decision must be individualized. However, PD does require a high level of patient sophistication to perform safely.

Vascular access for hemodialysis requires the surgical creation of a connection between the artery and vein of the forearm or upper arm, using native vessels (arteriovenous fistula [AVF]) or a synthetic material like gortex interposed between the artery and vein (arteriovenous graft [AVG]). The vascular access needs time to mature, longer in the case of AVFs and shorter with AVGs, but usually in the order of 8–12 weeks. Infection, thrombosis, and aneurysm formation are more common with grafts, so fistula is preferred when native vessels are of sufficient integrity. Intravascular catheters can also be used but are more prone to infection and thus preferably used only in the acute setting or in the cases of access failure. PD catheters can be placed more in proximity to timing of first dialysis, usually within 1 month of RRT initiation.

Timely placement of access for dialysis will ensure that the patient is properly prepared to start RRT when the time comes. This usually occurs with GFR <10–15 mL/min (closer to 15 in diabetic patients and closer to 10 in nondiabetic patients). The initiation of RRT is based on several medical indications:

1. Symptomatic uremia
   - Nausea, anorexia, weight loss
   - Hypersomnolence, impaired concentrating ability
   - Neuropathy, myoclonic jerks
   - Bleeding diathesis from uremic platelet dysfunction
2. Acute pericarditis, as a manifestation of uremia
3. Fluid overload (pulmonary edema or uncontrollable hypertension)
4. Hyperkalemia unresponsive to medical management
5. Metabolic acidosis unresponsive to medical management
6. Other acute electrolyte abnormalities (hyperuricemia, hypercalcemia)

ACID-BASE DISORDERS

Joel A. Gordon
Lisa M. Antes

KEY POINTS

- The three mechanisms that help maintain a normal pH (7.38–7.42) are buffering, compensation, and correction.
- The serum anion gap is normally 10 ± 2 meq/L and represents the difference between the unmeasured anions and cations.
- Calculation of the anion gap is the key in determining the etiology of a metabolic acidosis.
- A random urine [Cl⁻] is the key in determining the etiology of metabolic alkalosis.
- There are six steps in evaluating any acid-base problem. Following these six steps will help to make acid-base problems easy (relatively speaking) and help to uncover existing triple disturbances. The six steps are:
  1. Do the numbers make sense?
  2. Is this an acidemia or an alkalemia? Even if the pH is normal, one still must check the PCO_2, HCO_3^-, and the anion gap.
  3. What is the primary disturbance (metabolic or respiratory)?
  4. Is the compensation appropriate for the primary disturbance?
  5. What is the anion gap? If it's normal, one may stop here!
  6. If the anion gap is elevated, is the bicarbonate appropriate for the anion gap?

INTRODUCTION

Understanding acid-base problems is essential to the practice of clinical medicine. Correctly evaluating acid-base problems is often challenging for many clinicians, but can be less daunting if approached in a systematic fashion. In addition to reviewing causes of acid-base disorders, this chapter intends to demonstrate a practical approach, walking the reader through sample acid-base problems.

PATHOPHYSIOLOGY

An acid is a compound that donates a hydrogen ion, and a base is a compound that accepts a hydrogen ion. The acid-base status is expressed as the hydrogen ion concentration $[H^+]$ or pH. The normal $[H^+]$ is 40 neq/L (normal range 36–44 neq/L) or 40×10^{-9} eq/L. The normal pH is 7.40 with the normal range being 7.38–7.42. The pH and the hydrogen ion concentration are inversely related. An increase in the hydrogen ion concentration will lower the pH, and a decrease in the hydrogen ion concentration will increase the pH. **Acidemia** is defined as a pH <7.38 and is the result of accumulation of hydrogen ions. **Alkalemia** is defined as a pH >7.42 which is the result of a lowering of the hydrogen ion concentration. **Acidosis** and **alkalosis** refer to the processes by which the acid or alkali accumulate.

The $[H^+]$ is regulated by three mechanisms: (1) **chemical buffers**; (2) the **lungs** regulate the excretion of CO_2; and (3) the **kidneys** regulate the excretion of H^+ ions and the reabsorption and generation of HCO_3^-. The lungs regulate CO_2 through either hyperventilation or hypoventilation. H^+ ions are secreted in the distal tubule and combine with NH_3 and are excreted primarily in the form of NH_4^+. For every 1 meq of H^+ ion combining with NH_3 to form NH_4^+, 1 meq of "new" HCO_3^- is formed and returned to the systemic circulation. An acidosis or alkalosis can be characterized by being primarily a respiratory or a metabolic problem depending on whether the primary disturbance involves a change in PCO_2 or HCO_3^-.

Carbonic acid is a weak acid which is formed by carbon dioxide and water:

$$CO_2 + H_2O \leftrightarrow H_2CO_3 \leftrightarrow HCO_3^- + H^+$$
$$\text{Carbonic acid}$$

H_2CO_3 is an acid because it can donate a hydrogen ion. Thus, an increase in the CO_2 will cause an acidosis, and a decrease will cause an alkalosis. The serum CO_2 is in equilibrium with the PCO_2; since the lungs regulate the PCO_2, the lungs in turn regulate the amount of H_2CO_3. The normal PCO_2 is 40 mmHg with a range of 38–42 mmHg.

Bicarbonate (HCO_3^-) is an alkali because it can accept a hydrogen ion:

$$H_2CO_3 \leftrightarrow H^+ + HCO_3^-$$
$$\text{Carbonic acid} \qquad \text{Bicarbonate}$$

Thus, an increase in the serum bicarbonate will decrease the $[H^+]$ and result in an alkalosis, and a decrease in the serum bicarbonate will increase the [H^+] and result in an acidosis. The bicarbonate will decrease with the addition of acid, an increased excretion of bicarbonate or a decreased excretion of acid from the kidney. The bicarbonate will increase as a result of addition of alkali, a decreased excretion of bicarbonate or an increased excretion of acid from the kidney. The kidneys regulate the serum bicarbonate and help determine the [H^+]. The normal serum bicarbonate is 26 mmol/L with a range of 22–28 mmol/L.

When initially evaluating an acid-base problem, four laboratory values are required: (1) **pH**, (2) **PCO_2**, (3) **HCO_3^-**, and (4) **anion gap**. The pH and PCO_2 values are obtained from an arterial blood gas (ABG), and HCO_3^- is determined from venous or arterial blood. The HCO_3^- is part of many routine serum chemistries. It may be listed as CO_2, and it must not be confused with the PCO_2. On the blood gas slip, there may also be a value listed for HCO_3^-. This is often a **calculated value** and is usually not directly measured. This value is what the serum bicarbonate should be if the measured values, the pH, and PCO_2 are correct from the ABG.

There are three general mechanisms that describe how the body attempts to maintain a normal pH (7.38–7.42). They are buffering, compensation, and correction. **Buffering** is the first line of defense against acid-base disorders. It occurs very rapidly and includes both intracellular and extracellular processes. The HCO_3^- buffer system is the major **extracellular** buffer. **Intracellular** buffers include hemoglobin, phosphates, sulfates, and proteins. **Compensation** is the next mechanism that helps restore pH toward normal. **The first rule is that one cannot overcompensate!** Respiratory compensation in metabolic disorders occurs rapidly. With metabolic acidosis, carotid chemoreceptors stimulate ventilation in response to a falling pH and the change in the cerebrospinal fluid (CSF) pH will maximize hyperventilation. It may take up to 24 hours for this mechanism to be complete. In metabolic alkalosis, hypoventilation is the response to an increase in pH. The ability to compensate for a metabolic alkalosis is limited by the fall in PO_2. Acute metabolic compensation for primary respiratory disorders begins with buffers as discussed above. The renal compensation for a primary respiratory acidosis (increased production and excretion of ammonium) does not begin for 12–24 hours and will take up to 48 hours to be complete. The renal compensation for a primary respiratory alkalosis (decrease in HCO_3^- production and decreased reabsorption of HCO_3^-) will take up to 72 hours to reach equilibrium. Thus, the degree of compensation for an acute respiratory acidosis/alkalosis will be less than that of a chronic respiratory acidosis/alkalosis.

Correction is the final mechanism that helps restore pH toward 7.40. In primary metabolic disorders, further correction occurs when the kidney alters excretion of either H^+ or HCO_3^-, a process that generally takes 3–5 days. In primary respiratory disorders, correction occurs when the lungs alter excretion of CO_2.

Table 34-1 **Simple Acid-Base Disorders**

Acid-Base Disorder	pH	PCO$_2$	HCO$_3^-$
Metabolic acidosis	↓↓	↓↓	↓↓↓
Acute respiratory acidosis	↓↓	↑↑	↑
Chronic respiratory acidosis	↓	↑↑	↑↑
Metabolic alkalosis	↑↑	↑↑	↑↑↑
Acute respiratory alkalosis	↑↑	↓↓	↓
Chronic respiratory alkalosis	↑	↓↓	↓↓

Examples of the changes in pH, PCO$_2$, and HCO$_3^-$ in **simple acid-base disorders** are shown Table 34-1. As one can see, examining the directional changes in pH, PCO$_2$, and HCO$_3^-$ can be useful in quickly assessing the primary acid-base disorder that is present.

APPROACH TO ACID-BASE DISORDERS

Based on the index of suspicion, obtain an ABG to determine the pH and PCO$_2$ and obtain a HCO$_3^-$ from a chemistry panel. Next, follow the six basic steps:

1. Do the numbers make sense?

The following equation is a derivation of the Henderson-Hesselbach equation and does not require log function.

$$[H^+] = 24 \times \frac{PCO_2}{HCO_3^-}$$

Using this equation requires converting pH to [H$^+$]. Between a pH of 7.25 and 7.48, for every 0.01 increase in pH the [H$^+$] decreases 1 neq/L and for every 0.01 decrease in pH the [H$^+$] increases 1 neq/L. Therefore, for a pH of 7.28: 7.40 (normal pH) − 7.28 = 0.12; the [H$^+$] will increase by 1 for every 0.01 decrease in pH, so therefore the [H$^+$] should increase by 12. Normal [H$^+$] is 40, so 40 + 12 = 52 neq/L, the calculated [H$^+$] for a pH of 7.28. For pH variations that are wider (severe acidosis or alkalosis), another way to estimate the [H$^+$] is for every 0.3 change in pH, the [H$^+$] changes by a factor of 2 (since pH is on a log scale); for a pH of 7.40 the [H$^+$] is 40 neq/L, thus at a pH of 7.10 the [H$^+$] is 80 neq/L, at a pH of 6.80 the [H$^+$] would be 160 neq/L, and for a pH of 7.70 the [H$^+$] would be 20 neq/L (it should be noted that a pH of 7.70 would be incompatible with life!).

If the left and right sides of the above equation are not within ~10%, one must assume that either the pH, the PCO_2, or the HCO_3^- are incorrect and one should recollect the ABG and the blood chemistry. One major reason that the numbers may not fit is that the ABG and HCO_3^- are obtained at different times. One should also remember that there often will be a discrepancy in PCO_2 and serum HCO_3^- for specimens collected during a cardiopulmonary resuscitation. A shortcut for the above is to compare the HCO_3^- from the chemistry panel with the HCO_3^- from the ABG (if the HCO_3^- from the blood gas is a calculated value).

2. Is this an acidemia (pH <7.38) or an alkalemia (pH >7.42)? Even if the pH is normal, one must check the PCO_2, HCO_3^-, and the anion gap.

3. What is the primary disturbance (metabolic or respiratory)?
   For acidemia:
   - Respiratory acidosis   pH <7.38, PCO_2 >42
   - Metabolic acidosis   pH <7.38, HCO_3^- <22
   For alkalemia:
   - Respiratory alkalosis   pH >7.42, PCO_2 <38
   - Metabolic alkalosis   pH >7.42, HCO_3^- >28

4. Is the compensation appropriate for the primary disturbance? If the answer is no, then there is a secondary disturbance. The following should be used to calculate the level of expected compensation for each of the primary disturbances:

Example 1: In a patient with a pH of 7.25, PCO_2 of 23, and HCO_3^- of 10 meq/L, the first step is to be sure the numbers fit, and the numbers fit, 55 = $24 \times 23/10$ (55 was derived from $7.40 - 7.25 = 0.15$, so [H$^+$] will change by 15; $40 + 15 = 55$). Step 2: is this an acidemia or alkalemia? It is an acidemia in this case. Step 3 is to determine the primary disturbance. For an acidemia, is the PCO_2 increased or is the HCO_3^- decreased? In this instance, the HCO_3^- is decreased, so is a metabolic acidosis. From Table 34-2, for a HCO_3^- of 10, one would expect the PCO_2 to be $(1.5 \times 10) + 8 \pm 2$ or 23 and the PCO_2 is 23, the expected level.

Table 34-2 **Expected Compensation**

Metabolic acidosis	$PCO_2 = 1.0 - 1.4 \times \Delta HCO_3^-$
Metabolic alkalosis	$\Delta PCO_2 = 0.5 - 1.0 \times \Delta[HCO_3^-]$; PCO_2 not >55 mmHg; no hypoxia
Acute respiratory acidosis	$\Delta[HCO_3^-] = 1$ meq/L↑/10 mmHg ↑ in PCO_2
Chronic respiratory acidosis	$\Delta[HCO_3^-] = 4$ meq/L↑/10 mmHg ↑ in PCO_2
Acute respiratory alkalosis	$\Delta[HCO_3^-] = 2$ meq/L↓/10 mmHg ↓ in PCO_2
Chronic respiratory alkalosis	$\Delta[HCO_3^-] = 5$ meq/L↓/10 mmHg ↓ in PCO_2

Example 2: With a pH of 7.10, PCO_2 of 32, and HCO_3^- 10, follow the same steps as above. The numbers fit, $80 = 24 \times 32/10$. Again, there is an acidemia (step 2) and the primary disturbance is a metabolic acidosis (the HCO_3^- is decreased—step 3). Step 4 is to determine the expected PCO_2 for the level of HCO_3^-. For a HCO_3^- of 10, you would expect the PCO_2 to be $(1.5 \times 10) + 8 \pm 2$ or 23. The PCO_2 is actually 32, so the patient is hypoventilating relative to the expected PCO_2, thus the patient has a secondary respiratory acidosis in addition to the metabolic acidosis.

5. What is the anion gap? If normal one may stop here! If the primary disturbance is a metabolic acidosis, calculating the anion gap is the first step in determining the cause of the metabolic acidosis. Also, one should always calculate the anion gap regardless of the primary disturbance or the pH. In the setting of primary metabolic alkalosis or respiratory acidosis or respiratory alkalosis, the presence of an elevated anion gap provides evidence of a secondary disturbance.

The **anion gap (AG)** is calculated as $AG = Na^+ - (Cl^- + HCO_3^-)$. The normal anion gap is 8–12 mmol/L. An increase in the anion gap results from an increase in an unmeasured anion (phosphate, sulfate, and other organic anions). Causes of anion gaps will be discussed below.

6. If the anion gap is elevated, is the bicarbonate appropriate for the anion gap? If the answer to this question is yes, the cause of the elevated anion gap is a metabolic gap acidosis. If the answer is no, then there is a metabolic anion gap acidosis plus a metabolic alkalosis OR an anion gap metabolic acidosis plus a nongap metabolic acidosis.

For step 6, one needs only the anion gap and the HCO_3^-.

For instance, consider a situation where the HCO_3^- is 13 and the anion gap is 23. The ΔGap represents the increase in gap over normal, in this case $23 - 10$ (normal gap) $= 13$. Normal HCO_3^- is 26; normal bicarb minus the ΔGap will yield the expected HCO_3^-, so $26 - 13 = 13$. Since the measured bicarb equals the expected bicarb, this represents a pure anion gap metabolic acidosis. In contrast, consider the example of the HCO_3^- of 19 with a gap of 25; $25 - 10 = 15$, the ΔGap. Therefore, $26 - 15 = 11$, the expected HCO_3^-. The actual HCO_3^-, however, is 19 mmol/L, 8 mmol/L higher than the expected value of 11 mmol/L. Thus, there must also be a metabolic alkalosis in addition to the anion gap metabolic acidosis. Finally, consider if one has a HCO_3^- of 8 with a gap of 22; $22 - 10 = 12$, the ΔGap. Then $26 - 12 = 14$, the expected HCO_3^-. The actual HCO_3^-, however, is 8 mmol/L, or 6 mmol/L lower than expected. Thus, there may also be a metabolic nongap acidosis in addition to the anion gap metabolic acidosis.

An important exception to this rule is in cases where the primary disturbance is a respiratory acidosis or alkalosis, where the baseline HCO_3^- will not be 26 but will be based on whether the process is acute or chronic (see Table 34-2 for the expected compensation). For example, a patient with chronic respiratory acidosis from chronic obstructive pulmonary disease

(COPD) may have a chronically elevated PCO_2 of 60. Sixty is 20 higher than normal PCO_2 of 40. Therefore, from Table 34-2, one would expect that patient's HCO_3^- to not be a normal 26, but one should expect compensation of 4 meq/L for every 10 increase in PCO_2, or 8 meq/L for a PCO_2 of 60. Therefore, in the above calculations, one expects the baseline HCO_3^- to be 34 (26 + 8).

METABOLIC ACIDOSIS

Metabolic acidosis is defined as a primary acid-base disturbance that lowers the pH to <7.38 as a result of either addition of H^+ ions or the loss of HCO_3^- ions. Metabolic acidosis is further classified on the basis of the anion gap into an **increased anion gap** metabolic acidosis or **normal or nonanion gap** (hyperchloremic) metabolic acidosis. Increases in the anion gap associated with metabolic acidosis are shown in Table 34-3.

Causes of metabolic **nongap** acidosis include inorganic acid ingestion (HCl), inhibition of the carbonic anhydrase enzyme on the brush border in proximal tubule of kidney (acetazolamide), failure to secrete H^+ ions in the distal tubule (chronic kidney disease), type 1, 2, and 4 renal tubular acidosis,

Table 34-3 **Causes of Anion Gap Metabolic Acidosis**

Mnemonic	Disturbance	Key Feature/Clinical Characteristic
S	Salicylate intoxication	Intentional or unintentional intoxication
L	Lactic acidosis	Organ hypoperfusion and production of lactic acid
U	Uremia (renal failure)	Accumulation of the unmeasured anions SO_4^{2-} and PO_4^{2-}
M	Methanol	Renal failure, retinal toxicity, and an elevated osmolar gap
P	Propylene glycol	Vehicle used in many drugs. Metabolite glycolic acid accumulates in renal failure
E	Ethylene glycol	Renal failure, oxalate crystals, and an elevated osmolar gap
D	Diabetic ketoacidosis	Anions are acetoacetate and β-hydroxybutyrate
Plus other ketoacidoses	Alcoholic and starvation ketoacidosis	Anions are acetoacetate and β-hydroxybutyrate

loss of HCO_3^- from diarrhea, ureteroenterostomy, and infusion of large quantities of chloride-containing fluids (termed volume expansion acidosis).

METABOLIC ALKALOSIS

Metabolic alkalosis is defined as a primary disturbance that raises the systemic pH to >7.42 as a result of net gain of HCO_3^- or loss of H^+ ions. Metabolic alkalosis is further classified into two broad categories: **chloride (volume) responsive** or **chloride (volume) resistant**. The pivotal diagnostic test that helps distinguish chloride responsive from chloride-resistant metabolic alkalosis is a **random urine [Cl⁻]**.

Metabolic alkalosis is frequently discussed in terms of the "generation" and the "maintenance" of this disturbance. The "generation" of metabolic alkalosis generally refers to the conditions that lead to the loss of H^+ ions or the addition of HCO_3^- ions, such as vomiting or diuretic administration, respectively. In contrast, the "maintenance" of metabolic alkalosis refers to factors that result in the kidney's inability to excrete HCO_3^- ions and correct the disturbance. These factors include volume depletion and hypokalemia, both commonly seen in metabolic alkalosis.

The common theme that characterizes **chloride responsive metabolic alkalosis** is loss of isotonic or hypotonic fluid with resulting decrease in the effective circulating volume. The urine [Cl⁻] in this case, in the absence of diuretics, is <10 meq/L. Causes of chloride responsive metabolic alkalosis include vomiting, nasogastric suction, diuretics, villous adenoma, and posthypercapnia.

Chloride-resistant metabolic alkalosis is characterized as a hypermineralocorticoid state. The urine [Cl⁻] in this case is >20 meq/L. The chloride-resistant metabolic alkaloses can be further divided on the basis of blood pressure and are often classified as hypertensive (primary hyperaldosteronism [Conn's syndrome], Cushing's syndrome, licorice intoxication, and Liddle's syndrome) or normotensive (Bartter's syndrome and Gitelman's syndrome).

RESPIRATORY ACIDOSIS

Respiratory acidosis is the primary disturbance that lowers the pH to <7.38 from hypoventilation. The PCO_2 increases as a result of failure of the lungs to excrete CO_2 produced via the metabolism of carbohydrates, fats, and proteins. Decreased minute ventilation or ventilation-perfusion (V/Q) mismatches are the two common ways that produce a rise in PCO_2 and a subsequent decline in systemic pH.

Causes of acute respiratory acidosis include neuromuscular abnormalities (brain stem injury, Guillain-Barre syndrome, myasthenia gravis, and narcotic, sedative, or tranquilizer overdose); airway obstruction (foreign body and severe bronchospasm); thoracic-pulmonary disorders (pneumothorax, severe pulmonary edema, severe pneumonia), and iatrogenic ventilator problems (inadequate frequency, inadequate tidal volume, and large dead space). The major causes of chronic respiratory acidosis are thoracic-pulmonary disorders (COPD and kyphoscoliosis) and neuromuscular abnormalities (obesity hypoventilation syndrome, primary hypoventilation, obstructive sleep apnea, and chronic narcotic or sedative ingestion).

RESPIRATORY ALKALOSIS

Respiratory alkalosis is a primary disturbance that raises the pH to >7.42 as a result of a decrease in PCO_2. The PCO_2 falls as a result of respiratory excretion of CO_2 that exceeds its production. This occurs as a result of increased alveolar ventilation. The increase in alveolar ventilation occurs from two general processes: (1) increased neurochemical stimulation of ventilation by peripheral or central neural mechanisms and (2) increased ventilation, either voluntarily with increased conscious effort or via inappropriate settings on mechanical ventilators.

Causes of acute and chronic respiratory alkalosis include central nervous system stimulation of respiration (salicylates, fever, pain, pregnancy, head trauma, and anxiety), peripheral stimulation of respiration (pulmonary embolus, congestive heart failure, high altitude), pulmonary diseases (pneumonia, asthma, and interstitial lung disease), combined causes (sepsis and cirrhosis), and iatrogenic mechanical ventilation problems (increased tidal volume and increased rate).

HYPONATREMIA AND

HYPERNATREMIA

Matthew Fitz
Paul Hering

KEY POINTS

- Hyponatremia reflects a low serum concentration, but actual sodium stores may be decreased, normal, or increased.
- The differential diagnosis depends on the patient's volume status.
- Correction of serum sodium should be targeted for 1–2 meq/L/h.
- Hypernatremia results predominantly from a free water deficit from either inadequate intake or increased loss.
- Neurologic symptoms can develop if serum sodium surpasses 160 mg/dL.

HYPONATREMIA

Introduction

Hyponatremia occurs in 2% of hospitalized patients and is the most commonly encountered electrolyte abnormality. Most cases of hyponatremia are associated with a low serum osmolality. Serum osmolality is principally determined by the serum sodium concentration with minor contributions from urea and glucose. Thus, a normal or high osmolality in the face of hyponatremia implies that another osmotically active substance is present in the blood (Fig. 35-1). Hypotonic hyponatremia is a low concentration of sodium, which reflects a water imbalance in relation to decreased, normal, or increased total body sodium.

Pathophysiology

Evaluation of hyponatremia requires a thorough understanding of the hormonal systems which control sodium and water homeostasis. The serum

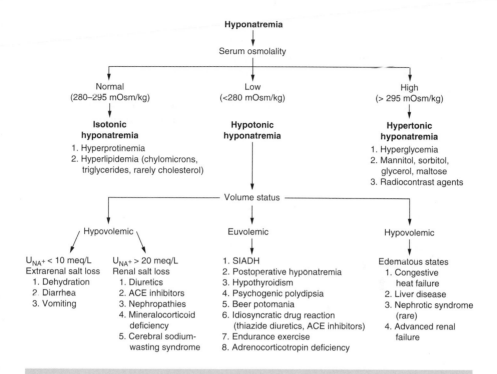

Figure 35-1 **Evaluation of hyponatremia using serum osmolality and extracellular fluid volume status.** (*Source:* Tierney LM et al. *Current Medical Diagnosis and Treatment.* 2006.)

concentration is tightly regulated within the range 275–290 mOsm/kg. Increases in concentration are detected by chemoreceptors in the anterolateral hypothalamus. Initially, an increase in concentration stimulates thirst and subsequent increase will stimulate the release of **arginine vasopressin** (AVP or antidiuretic hormone). AVP stimulates water reabsorption from the collecting ducts in the kidney. A secondary stimulus for AVP release is volume depletion. A decrease in mean arterial pressure stimulates baroreceptors in the carotid sinus which will also stimulate the release of AVP and water reabsorption in the kidney. Several less potent factors are also known to stimulate AVP release including nausea, pain, pregnancy, stress, and multiple medications. **To excrete free water, sufficient volume must be delivered to the kidney, sodium must be reabsorbed in the nephrons, and AVP must be suppressed.** Most causes of hyponatremia reflect impairment in one of these three mechanisms rather than improper sodium balance. The sodium balance reflects the intake of sodium (which is usually adequate) and the ability of the body to excrete that sodium load, predominantly by the kidneys. Sodium freely passes through the glomerulus and most is reabsorbed in the proximal convoluted tubule with the remainder being reabsorbed in the loop of Henle or the distal convoluted tubule. Aldosterone stimulates sodium reabsorption in the distal convoluted tubule in exchange for potassium or hydrogen ion and is the major hormone responsible for controlling body sodium. Any state which impairs aldosterone activity can cause hyponatremia; however, mineralocorticoid deficiency is usually best recognized by the concomitant hyperkalemia. The release of aldosterone is stimulated by either a decreased effective volume in the glomerulus or elevated serum potassium. Because of the interaction of volume and sodium regulation, disorders of sodium homeostasis usually result either in volume expansion or contraction rather than hypo- or hypernatremia.

Hyponatremia that develops acutely and rapidly causes an intracellular osmotic shift of water. Although most organs can tolerate this increase in cellular volume, the brain located in a closed compartment will develop **cerebral edema** and dysfunction with rapid changes. Gradual chronic hyponatremia rarely causes symptoms because of the adaptive responses of body systems. Within hours of developing hyponatremia, solutes begin leaving the brain thus reducing edema. Cerebral dysfunction may also develop if hyponatremia is corrected without allowing for the gradual reversal of these adaptations. Rapid increases in serum tonicity will result in the osmotic shift of water to the extracellular compartment. This loss of intracellular water can cause demyelination (**central pontine myelinolysis**).

Clinical Presentation

Most cases of hyponatremia are **asymptomatic** unless it is severe (Na <120 meq/L) or has occurred rapidly (within hours). Most symptoms are neurologic in origin with patients initially developing headache, nausea, restlessness, and disorientation. More severe hyponatremia can result in seizures, coma, brain herniation, and death from worsening cerebral edema.

Evaluation

Hyponatremia is a manifestation of a diverse number of disease states (Fig. 35-1) and the evaluation is dictated by the patient's history and examination. The most essential step in diagnosis is to assess the patient's volume status as hypervolemia, euvolemia, or hypovolemia. **Hypervolemia** is suggested by a report of weight gain and the finding of elevated jugular venous pressures, edema or ascites. **Hypovolemia** is often suggested by a history of vomiting, diarrhea or diuretic use, and findings of tachycardia, hypotension, or orthostasis.

Several laboratory tests can be useful in determining the etiology of hyponatremia (Table 35-1). The **plasma osmolality** can be confirmed to be low if causes of hypertonic or isotonic hyponatremia are suspected. In patients with hypovolemia, a **urine sodium** can determine if sodium losses

Table 35-1 **Laboratory Findings in Major Categories of Hyponatremia**

	Urine Osm	Urine Na
Hypovolemic		
Renal Na loss	Variable	>20 meq/L
Extrarenal Na loss	High	<10 meq/L
Euvolemic		
SIADH	Usually >300 mOsm/kg	>40 meq/L
Polydipsia	<100 mOsm/kg	>20 meq/L
Hypervolemic		
Congestive heart failure/cirrhosis	High	<10 meq/L
Renal failure	High	>20 meq/L

occurred from renal (>20 meq/L) or extrarenal (<10 meq/L) etiologies. In patients with normal effective circulating volume, the **urine osmolality** should be maximally dilute (<100 mOsm/kg). If the urine osmolality is not maximally dilute, then AVP release is being stimulated from other causes, such as the syndrome of inappropriate antidiuretic hormone secretion (SIADH). Other clues to SIADH include low serum levels of uric acid (<4 mg/dL) and blood urea nitrogen (BUN, <10 mg/dL) due to the mild volume expansion. One important etiology to remember is Addison's disease. Patients with mineralocorticoid deficiency will be volume-depleted with a high serum potassium and a high urine sodium (>20 meq/L).

Patients with SIADH should also be evaluated for the etiology of their condition. Physiologic release of AVP is stimulated by pain, nausea and stress, any of which can result in SIADH. Most pathologic causes of SIADH are from either neurologic or pulmonary conditions. Because AVP is released from the pituitary, virtually any neurologic condition can increase AVP release, including meningitis, stroke, hemorrhage, or trauma. All types of pneumonia are commonly associated with SIADH although the mechanism remains unclear. Last, small cell lung carcinoma is a common source of ectopic AVP production.

Management

Treatment of the patient's hyponatremia is best accomplished by management of the patient's underlying condition; however, a few principles must be taken into consideration. The initial step is to ensure that all patients have an **effective circulating volume** to suppress AVP release. For patients with hypovolemia, crystalloid should be administered, and patients with hypervolemia generally require diuresis to improve cardiac output. Subsequent management is dictated by the symptoms of the patient. Any patient with neurologic symptoms should be aggressively managed to **correct the serum sodium to 125 meq/L** (the level generally considered safe to not cause neurologic dysfunction). In patients with hypervolemia or euvolemia, this may require the administration of hypertonic (3%) saline to prevent volume expansion. Patients who are asymptomatic can be managed more conservatively with a gradual correction of their sodium. For example, asymptomatic patients with SIADH will generally respond to fluid restriction alone to correct their serum sodium. Another option for patients with SIADH is to administer both saline and furosemide. Furosemide reduces the efficacy of AVP by decreasing the amount of free water in the nephron which can be reabsorbed.

Management of hyponatremia should avoid rapid correction of sodium and its complications. **Central pontine myelinolysis** manifests with quadriplegia, pseudobulbar palsy, seizures, coma, and even death. This is a rare complication but occurs more commonly in patients with hepatic failure, hypokalemia and/or malnutrition. To ensure a slow progressive correction of sodium, the target rate of correction is 1–2 meq/L/h. The effect of 1 L of crystalloid can be estimated using the following formula:

$$\text{Change in serum Na} = \frac{\text{crystalloid Na} - \text{patient Na}}{\text{total body water} + 1}$$

The sodium content of normal saline is 154 meq/L and the content of hypertonic saline (3%) is 513 meq/L. The total body water is estimated by multiplying the patient's weight (kg) by 0.6.

HYPERNATREMIA

Introduction

Hypernatremia is another common electrolyte disorder in hospitalized patients. Hypernatremia reflects a rise in serum concentration of sodium and an invariable rise in serum osmolality; however, total body sodium can be either depleted, normal, or increased depending on the underlying etiology (Table 35-2). Although most cases occur from either inadequate intake or increased loss of water, an important iatrogenic cause is the unintentional administration of excessive sodium.

Pathophysiology

For a review of the mechanisms of water and sodium balance, see "Hyponatremia," above. **Hypernatremia is usually prevented by an intact thirst mechanism and the action of AVP.** Patients who are unable to drink (intubated or with altered mental status) and those with impaired thirst (elderly or hypothalamic dysfunction) are at the highest risk. Contributing to this risk are conditions which result in significant losses of water. The

Table 35-2 **Causes of Hypernatremia**

Hypovolemia (Unreplaced Water Loss)	Euvolemic (Diabetes Insipidus)	Hypervolemic (Hypertonic Sodium Gain)
Impaired thirst	Central	Primary hyperaldosteronism
Renal losses	Tumors	Cushing's syndrome
Osmotic diuresis	Meningitis	Iatrogenic
Postobstructive diuresis	Encephalitis	Hypertonic saline
Polyuric ATN	Head trauma	Sodium bicarbonate
Gastrointestinal losses	Nephrogenic	Hypertonic enemas
Vomiting	Hypercalcemia	
Infectious diarrhea	Hypokalemia	
Osmotic diarrhea	Medullary cystic	
Nasogastric suction	disease	
Dermal losses	Lithium	
Burns		
Excessive diaphoresis		

most common would be **gastrointestinal losses**, especially associated with infectious gastroenteritis or osmotic diarrhea (sorbitol and lactulose). **Renal losses** can occur as well and are usually related to osmotic diuresis (hyperglycemia or mannitol), postobstructive diuresis, polyuria associated with acute tubular necrosis (ATN) or diabetes insipidus. **Diabetes insipidus** occurs either from a lack of AVP secretion from the pituitary (central) or from collecting duct resistance to AVP stimulation (nephrogenic).

Acute rapid increases in sodium result in brain shrinkage which causes vascular rupture (intracerebral or subarachnoid hemorrhage) and neurologic dysfunction. Within hours of these changes, electrolytes begin to accumulate in the brain to prevent the osmotic loss of water. Slower adaptations will occur over the next several days with the intracellular accumulation of organic substances to prevent intracellular water loss. Similar to hyponatremia, rapid correction of hypernatremia can result in severe neurologic consequences. Because of the accumulation of osmotically active substances within the brain, sudden decreases in extracellular sodium will cause an intracellular water shift and cerebral edema.

Clinical Presentation

Neurologic symptoms from hypernatremia only occur if the serum sodium is severely elevated (>160 meq/L) or the change has occurred rapidly (within hours). The major manifestations are muscle weakness, confusion, and irritability which can progress to seizures and coma.

Evaluation

Similar to hyponatremia, the underlying cause of hypernatremia can be deduced from the patient's volume status (Table 35-2). Measurement of urine volume and serum osmolality is often helpful in cases where the underlying cause is unclear. **The body's natural response to hypernatremia should be minimal volume (<500 mL/day) of maximally concentrated urine (>800 mOsm/kg).** If the urine is appropriate, urine sodium concentration can differentiate between excessive sodium administration (>100 meq/L) and primary water loss (<25 meq/L). If the urine is not of minimal volume and maximally concentrated, the patient either has an osmotic diuresis (should be hypovolemic) or diabetes insipidus (should be euvolemic). The etiology of diabetes insipidus can be determined by the administration of desmopressin (synthetic AVP), which will result in a 50% increase in urine osmolality with central causes and no change with nephrogenic causes.

Management

The initial therapeutic goals are to prevent further water loss and to correct the underlying water deficit. Patients with hemodynamic compromise should be treated initially with isotonic fluids to correct volume depletion. Once patients are hemodynamically stable, the serum sodium should be gradually corrected (<0.5 meq/L/h) in patients with unknown duration of their hypernatremia, and more rapidly (1 meq/L/h) if the change is documented to be acute. The preferred route of administration is always via the gastrointestinal tract to minimize transcellular shifts. If intravenous administration is necessary, hypotonic fluids, such as D_5W (0 meq/L of Na), 1/4NS (38 meq/L of Na), or 1/2NS (77 meq/L of Na) are required. The change in serum sodium can be estimated by using the same formula mentioned in the hyponatremia section. When selecting fluids, the volume of crystalloid should always be minimized to prevent cerebral edema from excessive fluid administration.

Central diabetes insipidus is safely managed with either oral or intranasal desmopressin titrated to normal serum sodium. Targeting the underlying cause of nephrogenic diabetes insipidus will usually result in resolution of hypernatremia, although lithium-induced injury may be irreversible. Acute management requires the combination of a low sodium diet and thiazide diuretics. Amiloride can be used as an adjunct and is particularly useful in cases associated with lithium.

HYPERKALEMIA

Matthew Fitz

KEY POINTS

- Hyperkalemia is common in the inpatient setting and can be life threatening.
- Because the primary toxicity from hyperkalemia is cardiac, an ECG is necessary in managing patients with various degrees of hyperkalemia.
- Treatment for hyperkalemia consists of both short- and long-term management.

INTRODUCTION

It is estimated that approximately 10% of all inpatients will have hyperkalemia, defined as potassium level **>5 meq/L**. Even small elevations beyond normal level can be dangerous. Of particular note, the acuity of change in elevation of potassium is often more important than the actual number. Hyperkalemia can be life threatening due to fatal arrhythmias; therefore, diagnosis and subsequent treatment must be expedient.

PATHOPHYSIOLOGY

Hyperkalemia occurs from either **release of K$^+$ from cells** or **decreased renal clearance**; increased intake of K$^+$ is rarely the etiology due to renal adaptation. One of the most common causes of reported hyperkalemia is **pseudohyperkalemia**, that is, an artificial elevation usually as a result of phlebotomy-related hemolysis or clot formation. Potassium, predominantly an intracellular cation, shifts out of cells to balance **acidosis** or **hypertonicity** (e.g., hyperglycemia), therefore, does not actually represent total body potassium excess. **Hypoaldosteronism** causes hyperkalemia because of impaired Na$^+$ absorption in the proximal convoluted tubule and may be primary, secondary, or due to aldosterone resistance. Patients with diabetes, mild renal

Table 36-1 **Mechanisms of Hyperkalemia**

Cellular release or shift	Pseudohyperkalemia, intravascular hemolysis, cell death (tumor lysis syndrome, compartment syndrome, snakebite), rhabdomyolysis, metabolic acidosis, hypertonicity
Renal failure	Oliguric renal failure from any cause, especially hypovolemia
Hypoaldosteronism:	Impaired Na$^+$ reabsorption
A. Primary hypoaldosteronism	Adrenal insufficiency (Addison's disease)
B. Secondary hypoaldosteronism	Hyporeninemia from chronic kidney disease or drugs: NSAIDs—inhibit renin and vasodilatory prostaglandins ACE inhibitors—impair aldosterone release Heparin—inhibits adrenal synthesis of aldosterone
C. Aldosterone resistance	Tubulointerstitial disease, K$^+$-sparing diuretics, trimethoprim

Abbreviations: NSAIDs, nonsteroidal anti-inflammatory drugs; ACE, angiotensin-converting enzyme.

insufficiency, or chronic tubulointerstitial disease are predisposed to developing hyporeninemic hypoaldosteronism (Table 36-1).

Hyperkalemia partially depolarizes cell membrane resting potential which if prolonged, impairs membrane excitability causing weakness. The most serious complication, **cardiac toxicity**, first manifests on the electrocardiogram as **peaked T waves**, then loss of P waves, and progresses to PR and QRS

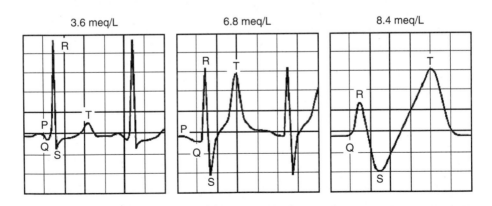

Figure 36-1 **Progression of hyperkalemia from peaked T waves to widening of the QRS complex to sine wave pattern.** (*Source:* Reproduced with permission from Morgan GE Jr, Mikhail MS, Murray MJ. Clinical Anesthesiology, 4th ed. New York: McGraw-Hill, 2006, Figure 28-6.)

prolongation which may eventually incorporate the T wave and an ominous **sine wave** pattern (Fig. 36-1). Of note, cardiac toxicity does not correlate well with plasma K^+ concentration.

MANAGEMENT

Management of hyperkalemia depends on the degree of potassium concentration (rarely fatal unless >7.5 meq/L), presence of profound weakness, or ECG changes. If the patient is asymptomatic, pseudohyperkalemia should be suspected and another specimen collected. The history may uncover medications associated with hyperkalemia. The physical examination should evaluate the volume status of the patient. An ECG should be obtained to detect any of the above abnormalities detected. If confirmed, and in addition to correcting the precipitant mechanism, treatment of hyperkalemia is often a two-step process:

1. Short-term measures may be necessary to stabilize the cardiac membrane. Calcium, insulin + glucose, or sodium bicarbonate (Table 36-2) can be instituted rapidly but **do not deplete potassium**.

Table 36-2 **Treatment of Hyperkalemia**

Treatment	Onset of Action	Duration	Mechanism
Short-term measures			
Calcium gluconate or calcium chloride	Seconds to minutes	30 min	Membrane stabilization
Insulin + glucose	Minutes to hours	Hours	Transcellular shift of potassium into the cells
Sodium bicarbonate	Minutes	1–2 h	
β2-Agonist	Minutes to hours	Hours	
Long-term measures			
Sodium polystyrene sulfonate (Kayexalate)	Variable	Permanent	Binds potassium in gut (can be given oral or per rectum)
Furosemide (Lasix)	Variable	Permanent	Inhibits potassium reabsorption
Dialysis	Variable	Permanent	Potassium removal in the dialysate bath

2. All cases of true hyperkalemia will require more definitive treatment which effectively removes potassium from the body. If potassium is not lowered adequately, short-term measures may have to be repeated.

If the etiology of hyperkalemia is not readily apparent from the history, physical, or tests of renal function, hypoaldosteronism should be considered. Primary adrenal insufficiency can be differentiated from hyporeninemic hypoaldosteronism by examining the renin-aldosterone axis. The transtubular potassium gradient: [urine K/(urine osm/serum osm)]/serum K should be <10 in hypoaldosteronism and increase after the administration of mineralocorticoid. Plasma renin activity will be high in primary hypoaldosteronism and low in secondary hypoaldosteronism.

BASICS OF FLUID

MANAGEMENT

Lisa M. Antes
Joel A. Gordon

KEY POINTS

- Total body water is approximately 60% of total body weight and is distributed into two major body fluid compartments: 1/3 in the ECF compartment and 2/3 in the ICF compartment.
- Electrolytes are compartmentalized into either predominantly the ECF or ICF. Na^+ is the predominant cation in the ECF and K^+ is the predominant cation in the ICF.
- Because isotonic saline (0.9% NaCl, or NS) contains no solute-free water, it is an excellent way to expand the ECF space.
- Maintenance fluid and electrolyte balance per 24 hours requires 1.5–2.0 L of water, 100–150 g of carbohydrates, 60–100 meq K^+, and 100–150 meq Na^+. D5 1/2 NS with 30 meq/L KCl infused at 75 mL/h is an excellent way to meet these requirements.
- Disease states such as congestive heart failure or renal failure will require modification of fluid management to address altered fluid and electrolyte dynamics.

INTRODUCTION

Physiology of Body Fluids and Body Fluid Compartments

From the time of conception to the time of death, fluids are central to the proper functioning of cells, tissues, and organs, and thus to our everyday existence. Water is the most ubiquitous component of the human body, composing 60% by body weight. Water distributes between the two main body

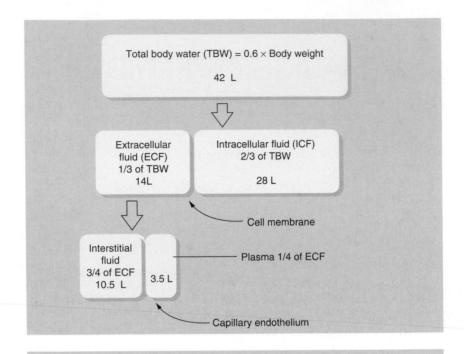

Figure 37-1 **Body fluid compartments in a 70-kg individual.** (*Source:* Adapted from Koeppen BM, Stanton BA. *Renal Physiology,* 3rd ed. St. Louis, MO: Mosby, 2001.)

fluid compartments, 1/3 in the extracellular fluid (ECF) and 2/3 in the intracellular fluid (ICF). The ECF has two main compartments, the vascular space and the interstitial space, each respectively comprising 1/4 and 3/4 of the ECF space. Water moves freely across the cell membrane (between the ICF and ECF) and the capillary membranes (between the vascular space and interstitial space) into and out of all body fluid compartments (Fig. 37-1).

Electrolytes in the body, however, compartmentalize into preferentially the ICF or ECF. This differential residence establishes transmembrane electrochemical gradients, which are important for the normal physiologic function of cells. Na^+ is the main cation in the ECF and K^+ is the main cation in the ICF. The main anion in the ECF is chloride (Cl^-). The main anions in the ICF are phosphates, organic ions, and negatively charged proteins (nonalbumin).

Plasma Osmolality and Plasma Tonicity

Cell volume is regulated by the **osmolality** of the ECF. Plasma osmolality is determined by the following equation:

$$P_{osm} = 2Na + glucose/18 + BUN/2.8\ (+\ unmeasured\ osmoles).$$

Thus, under normal circumstances one can readily see that the plasma osmolality is roughly twice the serum Na concentration. In cases of severe hyperglycemia or renal failure, however, glucose and urea nitrogen (respectively) contribute more substantially to the plasma osmolality. Other substances, aside from Na, urea, and glucose, may also contribute to the plasma osmolality. Such substances include alcohols like ethanol, methanol, ethylene glycol, and isopropyl alcohol.

Water moves across the cell membrane from areas of low osmolality to areas of high osmolality in an attempt to equalize osmolality on both sides of the membrane. The driving force for this is called "osmotic pressure." Osmotic pressure is created only by solutes that are confined to the ECF space, that is, are not permeable across cell membranes. Such substances are called **effective osmoles** and contribute to the **tonicity** of the ECF by creating a driving force for the movement of water from inside the cell to outside the cell. Effective osmoles include NaCl, glucose, and KCl. Although K is an effective osmole, it is not normally included in the calculation of plasma osmolality due to its predominant intracellular location.

Plasma tonicity under normal circumstances is determined by the following equation:

$$P_{tonicity} = 2Na + (glucose/18)$$

Note that urea nitrogen contributes to the plasma osmolality but does not contribute to the tonicity of the ECF because it is freely permeable across most cell membranes, and thus creates no driving force for water movement.

The concept of hyperosmolality and hypertonicity can be illustrated in two common clinical conditions: severe hyperglycemia and advanced renal failure. Because **glucose** is an **effective osmole** it exerts osmotic pressure in the ECF, and as a consequence water moves from the ICF to the ECF in an effort to normalize plasma osmolality. Severe hyperglycemia thus results in **intracellular** dehydration due to **hyperosmolality** of the ECF. In renal failure, urea is elevated; however, because urea is **freely permeable** across cell membranes (it is an ineffective osmole), no intracellular dehydration occurs despite ECF hyperosmolality. (Cerebral dehydration will occur, however, as urea is not freely permeable across the cerebrospinal fluid [CSF].)

Intravenous Fluids

When patients are hospitalized it is common that intravenous fluids (IVFs) are administered, either as a maintenance fluid (to accommodate normal daily fluid and electrolyte requirements) or tailored to address specific fluid, electrolyte, or acid-base disturbances.

Normal saline (0.9% NaCl, or abbreviated NS) contains 154 meq/L Na$^+$ and has a calculated osmolality of 308 mOsm/L. It is an **effective osmole** and contributes to the **tonicity** of the ECF, since the Na$^+$ and Cl$^-$ each contribute independent osmotic effects. Normal plasma osmolality is 280–290 mOsm/kg H_2O, yet NS at 308 mOsm/L is termed **isotonic** (i.e., equivalent to plasma osmolality). The discrepancy is partly due to the fact that the activity of 0.154 molar NaCl is actually slightly <0.154, and partially due to the fact that the volume of water in 1 mL of plasma is only about 0.95 mL (the rest is mostly the volume of dissolved proteins). Thus, plasma with a Na^+ concentration of 140 meq/L, actually has a Na concentration in plasma water of 147 meq/L. **Normal saline contains no free water**.

Fluids with total ion composition less than the "equivalent" of NS are **hypotonic**. Examples of such fluids include D_5W, 1/2 NS (0.45% NS), and 1/4 NS (0.2% NS). Administration of hypotonic fluids dilutes ALL body fluid compartments, as the free water component is freely diffusible across all cell membranes. Solutions that are greater than the osmolality of NS are **hypertonic**. An example of a hypertonic solution is 3% saline, which contains 513 meq/L Na (Table 37-1).

Interestingly, a solution of D_5W (5%, or 50 g/L, dextrose) is actually **isotonic to plasma as it is infused**; however, because glucose is normally metabolized to carbon dioxide and water it behaves clinically as though it were free water without solute. Distilled water infused directly into the vein would result in hemolysis and thus can *never* be infused directly into the circulation.

How do fluids administered intravenously distribute into the ICF and/or ECF? This is dependent on several factors, including the water content of the solution, the electrolyte content of solution, and the content of osmotically active substances in the solution. It is helpful to look at how normal saline (0.9% NaCl) and D_5W (5% dextrose in water), two different and opposing solutions, distribute in the body after intravenous infusion. **Normal saline is confined to the ECF space** (vascular plus interstitial) and thus is an ideal solution to expand ECF volume in cases of volume depletion. **D_5W readily moves across all body fluid compartments as free water**, preferentially

Table 37-1 **Composition of Common Electrolyte Solutions**

	Osm (mOsm/L)	Glucose (g/L)	Na (meq/L)	Cl (meq/L)
D5W	252	50		
D$_{10}$W	505	100		
1/4 NS	77		38	38
1/2 NS	154		77	77
NS	308		154	154
3% NS	1026		513	513
Ringer's lactate*	273		130	108

*Ringer's lactate also contains 4 meq/L Ca, 3 meq/L K, and 28 meq/L HCO_3.

moving into the intracellular space (2/3), with only 1/12 (1/3 [distribution into ECF] × 1/4 [i.e., the fraction in the vascular space]) of the fluid staying in the intravascular space. Thus, it is a poor volume expander but ideal for treating cellular dehydration.

It is convenient to think of IVFs in terms of the **"free" water content** and the electrolyte content (the **ionic composition**) of the solution. **Osmotically active substances** (i.e., effective osmoles) like potassium will **contribute to the tonicity** of the solution and must be taken into account when analyzing the free water content of the solution. One liter of 1/2 NS, for example, conceptually contains 500 mL of solute-free water and 500 mL of isotonic saline. D_5W + 30 meq KCl/L contains less free water than D_5W alone because K is an osmotically active substance. Any fluid with **more osmotically active substances will have less free water content**.

The rate of infusion of the solution is as important. **Potentially fatal errors can result if incorrect fluid orders are administered** (see Chap. 35). **Central pontine myelinolysis** can result if hyponatremia is corrected too rapidly with a hypertonic solution (e.g., 3% NS). **Intracerebral edema** can result if hypotonic fluid is rapidly administered to a patient who has a serum Na of 120 meq/L (i.e., is hypo-osmolar).

Depending on what underlying electrolyte disturbance is being treated, solutions can be chosen that are isotonic or hypotonic, and in rare circumstances hypertonic. The following clinical examples illustrate how to integrate treatment of the primary fluid disturbance with which body fluid compartment is being targeted:

- If a patient is intravascular volume-depleted due to excessive diuretic use and is orthostatic on examination, this implies ECF sodium deficit. **Isotonic saline** is an excellent choice to expand the ECF volume and restore blood pressure (BP).
- If a patient presents with hypernatremia but has normal BP, this implies water deficit. A **hypotonic solution** is an excellent choice to provide free water. Due to the differential distribution of water between the ICF and ECF, this type of fluid would serve its purpose in predominantly rehydrating the ICF compartment.

Pure water losses can be replenished enterally (orally) or parenterally (intravenously). If the patient has a functioning gastrointestinal (GI) tract, water can be given **enterally**, either orally or via nasogastric (NG) tube or Dobhoff tube. In some patients, for instance with ileus and resultant inability to properly absorb fluid from the GI tract, water may need to be replenished intravenously in the form of a dextrose-containing solution.

Parenteral Additives

Parenteral additives, consisting of a variety of different cations and anions, are frequent constituents of IVFs. Examples of parenteral additives include potassium chloride, sodium bicarbonate, calcium chloride, potassium phosphate, and magnesium sulfate. When considering which additives would be appropriate, one must consider the goals of treatment:

- Provide a patient with maintenance fluid and electrolytes which cannot be provided enterally.
- Address specific electrolyte or fluid imbalances (losses or excesses).

Parenteral additives should be added to **hypotonic** fluids, as a parenteral additive in NS will result in a hypertonic solution, which in most circumstances is not indicated. For example, the correct way to administer 40 meq KCl/L in a sodium chloride-containing solution would be as D5 1/2 NS + 40 meq KCl/L (77 meq Na + 77 meq Cl + 40 meq K + 40 meq Cl = total osmolality of 234 mOsm/L) and **NOT** as NS + 40 meq KCl/L (154 meq Na + 154 meq Cl + 40 meq K + 40 meq Cl = total osmolality of 388 mOsm/L). It is important to remember that certain parenteral additives are not compatible in solution. For example, calcium and bicarbonate cannot be combined in the same IV bag because of resultant precipitation of calcium, and must therefore be administered separately. This is why Ringer's lactate solution actually contains lactate, which is then metabolized by the body to bicarbonate.

Maintenance Daily Fluid and Electrolyte Requirements

WATER

Daily, each one of us has certain obligate fluid losses which must be replenished through appropriate intake to stay in electrolyte and water balance. Insensible water losses can occur as a result of skin (evaporative), respiratory, or stool losses. Similarly, urinary output will result in a certain degree of obligate losses of solute and water. Counterbalancing these losses, cellular metabolism produces a certain quantity of water daily. As a result, humans living in temperate climates require on average 1.5–2 L of water daily to remain in balance.

- Insensible water losses: 500–1000 mL/day (negative)
  - Skin (500 mL), respiratory tract (400 mL), stool (150 mL)
- Urine output: 1000–1500 mL/day (negative)
- Water production: 300 mL/day (positive)
  - Endogenous metabolism (oxidation of H^+ in protein, carbohydrate, and fat)
  - 15 mL H_2O generated for every 100 kcal energy produced

GLUCOSE AND ELECTROLYTES

Daily carbohydrate intake of 100–150 g/day is necessary to minimize protein catabolism and prevent ketosis. The average dietary intake of potassium (K^+) is 60–100 meq K^+. The minimum required intake of K^+ in hospitalized patients (with normal renal function) is at least 40 meq daily. There is considerable interindividual variation in dietary intake of sodium (Na^+). Because Na conservation and excretion is quite efficient under normal circumstances, sodium intake can be safely varied over a wide range without adverse consequences. In certain disease states, however, like congestive heart failure or renal failure, the excretion of sodium may be impaired and Na restriction coupled with a diuretic to achieve a natriuresis may be necessary to prevent volume or sodium overload.

Maintenance IVF for a hospitalized patient without congestive heart failure, renal failure, or liver dysfunction is not difficult and in a 70-kg person might be administered as:

$$D5\ 1/2\ NS + 20\text{–}30\ meq\ KCl/L \times 2\ L$$

This solution per 2 L would provide 154 meq Na^+ (77 meq/L × 2 L), 40–60 meq of K^+, and 100 g dextrose (50 g/L × 2 L). The total cations in solution per liter are thus 97 meq (77 meq Na and 20 meq K). Using 154 meq/L as the "standard" isotonic solution (i.e., NS), then the nonionic, or free water, portion of this solution is 37% (i.e., 97 meq ions in solution/154 meq/L is equal to 63% ionic solution, with the remaining 37% solute-free water).

ELECTROLYTE CONTENT OF BODY FLUIDS

Electrolyte and water losses occur on a daily basis, as mentioned previously, through insensible losses. If these losses occur in excess and cannot be adequately replenished, however, significant imbalances of electrolytes and water can result. The source of excess fluid losses assists in determining the type of intravenous replacement fluid chosen, as the ionic composition, and thus free water content, of different body fluids differs.

As Table 37-2 illustrates, even *within* the GI tract, the ion content of secretions differs. Gastric secretions contain mostly hydrochloric acid (HCl) and

Table 37-2 **Ion Composition of Specific Body Fluids**

	Na (meq/L)	K (meq/L)	Cl (meq/L)	HCO₃ (meq/L)
Plasma	135–145	3.5–5.0	98–106	24–26
Gastric	100	10	120	0*
Duodenum	60	15	60	15
Jejunum	140	6	100	30
Ileum	140	8	60	70
Rectum	40	90	15	30
Sweat	8–50	6–10	15–40	0

*Contains 10–120 meq H^+/L.

no bicarbonate. Patients on continuous NG tube suction are at risk for developing metabolic alkalosis, due to loss of H^+ and Cl^- in the gastric aspirate. Note that the final stool output, designated as rectum, is significantly higher in potassium content, reflecting potassium secretion between the ileum and rectum. In general, Na losses in intestinal tract secretions approximately equal the sum of HCO_3^- and Cl^- losses. A patient with viral enteritis with large stool outputs will be at risk for developing hyperchloremic metabolic acidosis (loss of HCO_3) and hypokalemia (loss of K^+). Hypovolemia may also occur (Na^+ losses).

Systematic Approach to Water and Electrolyte Imbalances

1. Assess which body fluid compartment is affected
   a. ICF
   b. ECF
   c. Both
2. Assess where losses or excesses are occurring from
   a. Sensible and insensible fluid losses
   b. Surgical drains or GI losses (aliquot body fluids to determine electrolyte content)
   c. Quantity (volume) and quality (electrolyte content) of totality of oral and intravenous intakes (composition/volume) relative to outputs
3. Assess the magnitude of the deficits or excesses
   a. Quantify volume and content of fluids
   b. Review serial laboratory data
   c. Mathematical equations to quantify magnitude of fluid excesses
4. Assess the rate of continuing loss or gain of fluid or electrolytes
   a. Monitor inputs and outputs
   b. Review serial laboratory data
   c. Assess cardiac, renal, and liver function
5. Assess volume status of patient on physical examination

It is helpful to maintain flow sheets of daily body weights as well as intakes (IV and PO) and outputs (urine, stool, respiratory, skin). In addition, monitoring response to therapy and **frequent reassessment** is vital to ensure the proper rate of correction and steady resolution of the disturbance, without overcorrection. Physical examination to assess orthostatic BP and pulse, skin turgor, and jugular venous distention is central when assessing a patient's volume status. Similarly, serial monitoring of serum $[Na^+]$ is necessary when correcting hypo- or hypernatremia, as disastrous consequences can result from overzealous or imprudent repletion. In certain instances, it is helpful to analyze the specific body fluid from which fluid/electrolyte losses are occurring to determine the concentrations of solutes in the losses. This is extremely helpful in certain instances of diarrhea, ostomy drainages, or drainage from intra-abdominal surgical sites, and helps guide therapy.

Certainly knowing from which source electrolyte and fluid losses are occurring is pivotal in selecting the proper **ionic composition** of IVFs. Equally important is assessing the volume status of the patient to facilitate prescribing fluids of the proper **tonicity**. Solutions can be made isotonic using combinations of electrolytes. In a patient who is hypotensive and has a severe hypokalemic metabolic acidosis as a consequence of secretory diarrhea, for instance, a solution can be tailored made to provide Na, K, and bicarbonate in an isotonic solution. Such a fluid prescription might be written as D_5W + 3 ampules $NaHCO_3$/L + 20 meq KCl/L, that would give an osmolality of 304 mOsm/L (132 meq Na/L + 20 meq K/L = 152 meq/L or 304 mOsm/L considering the osmotic contribution of the anions HCO_3^- and Cl^-), that is, of similar tonicity to isotonic saline. This solution would contain no free water, but would be an excellent volume and address specific acid-base and electrolyte abnormalities. Certain ions, as mentioned previously, are not compatible in solution and thus must be administered separately.

ENDOCRINE

DIABETIC KETOACIDOSIS

AND HYPEROSMOLAR

HYPERGLYCEMIC STATE

Dan Henry

KEY POINTS

- HHS is usually seen in elderly type 2 diabetics, while DKA occurs mainly in type 1 diabetics.
- Profound insulin deficiency results in ketoacidosis; the primary treatment for DKA is insulin.
- In HHS, hyperglycemia (often >1000 mg/dL) is typically much greater than in DKA but without ketoacidosis because these patients are insulin resistant rather than insulinopenic.
- Significant fluid deficit is present in both diseases, but the deficit is usually greater in HHS due to decreased intake of fluids and more profound osmotic diuresis.
- The mortality rate of HHS is 10 times that of DKA, mainly because it occurs in older and frailer patients.

INTRODUCTION

Diabetic ketoacidosis (DKA) and hyperosmolar hyperglycemic state (HHS) are the two most serious acute metabolic complications of diabetes. While DKA is almost always seen in type 1 diabetes mellitus (DM) and HHS is usually seen in the elderly with "mild" type 2 DM, they share many similarities in their causes and treatments. Both involve hyperglycemia, but only DKA is accompanied by an anion gap (AG) acidosis from ketoacids. Though the hyperglycemia in HHS is much more dramatic, it does not lead

295

to the development of acidosis. Rather hyperosmolality and dehydration are the major features in this condition. Mortality is also 10 times higher in HHS than DKA likely due to the more elderly population with all the associated comorbidities.

PATHOPHYSIOLOGY

Diabetic ketoacidosis is caused by inadequate insulin either from not taking enough (e.g., missing doses) or a stressor (e.g., infection, acute myocardial infarction [MI] causing increased requirements). Stressors increase catecholamines, cortisol, and glucagon, which all work to increase glucose levels. Decreased insulin results in a decrease in the insulin/glucagon ratio, which in turn increases gluconeogenesis and decreases peripheral glucose uptake. Eventually, glucose levels rise to a point that overwhelms the kidneys' maximum tubular resorption of glucose causing glucosuria and an osmotic diuresis. This osmotic diuresis leads to dehydration, total body sodium, potassium, and phosphate depletion, and usually mild renal failure.

Meanwhile as serum glucose levels rise, ketoacids form through hormonally mediated lipolysis that causes increased amounts of fatty acids to be delivered to the liver and converted to β-hydroxybutyrate and acetoacetate. These ketoacids cause a metabolic acidosis that the body tries to buffer with bicarbonate stores, leading to the characteristic low bicarbonate and AG acidosis. Some of the ketoacids are excreted in the urine with either sodium or potassium contributing to further volume depletion.

Patients also develop a compensatory respiratory alkalosis but in the absence of therapy, cannot maintain a neutral pH. As the pH decreases, potassium shifts out of cells to drive protons intracellular leading to the increased plasma potassium despite the total body potassium depletion. The other significant shift occurs as the hyperosmolality from the hyperglycemia drives water out of the cells leading to a degree of hyponatremia in addition to the decrease in total body sodium. A simple correction factor for this phenomenon is to add 1.6 meq to the Na for each rise in glucose of 100 mg/dL.

The pathophysiology of **HHS** is less well understood. Patients may have a partial or relative insulin deficiency, in the sense that insulin-sensitive tissues become less responsive to insulin ("insulin-resistance"). The insulin concentration is adequate to prevent lipolysis and subsequent ketogenesis, but is not enough to facilitate glucose entry into muscle, fat, and liver. Hyperglycemia ensues, which in turn causes an osmotic diuresis and volume depletion. Severe volume depletion and hyperglycemia are the primary mechanisms for the hyperosmolality in HHS (osmolality = $2Na + [glucose/18] + [BUN/2.8]$). This alters the patient's mental status, further diminishing the patient's oral intake and worsening the dehydration. Additionally, the marked hyperglycemia promotes a vicious cycle of exacerbating the dehydration and worsening the hypernatremia, hyperkalemia, hyperglycemia, and causing acute renal failure.

CLINICAL PRESENTATION

Patients with DKA and HHS typically present after a precipitating event. The most common event in DKA is poor adherence to insulin therapy. Other precipitating factors for DKA and HHS include:

- Infections
- MI
- Pregnancy (DKA)
- Intoxication from alcohol and/or other drugs of abuse (mainly DKA)
- Pancreatitis
- Steroid therapy
- Strokes (mainly HHS)
- Gastroenteritis with insufficient intake of water (more in HHS)

Therefore, the history should include questions about fever, cough, chest pain, vomiting, diarrhea, abdominal pain, last menstrual period, neurologic symptoms, and recent changes in medications, oral intake, and physical activity. Symptoms more specific for uncontrolled diabetes include polyuria polydipsia, polyphagia, and weight loss. Patients with DKA may also complain of dyspnea since there is a need to increase baseline alveolar ventilation to compensate for metabolic acidosis.

Patients with HHS are usually elderly and many have a baseline decreased mental status due to dementia or a previous stroke(s). The decreased intake of fluids with profound dehydration is a major factor in their symptoms, which include dry mouth, thirst, and presyncope. However, impaired mental status is the major symptom, which frequently limits the ability to take a thorough history from the patient. Therefore, family members and/or nursing home staff should be contacted.

In **DKA**, the blood pressure is usually normal, but can be low depending on the degree of dehydration. Patients often are tachycardic. Respirations are deep, and depending on severity of acidosis, may be increased (Kussmaul-Kien respirations). Often there is a "fruity" breath due to ketones. The remainder of the examination is usually normal unless there is superimposed disease. Signs of a precipitating infection should be actively sought (e.g., dullness and crackles on lung examination suggesting pneumonia).

In **HHS**, patients exhibit more severe evidence of volume depletion, including hypotension, tachycardia, dry mucous membranes, and poor skin turgor.

Neurologic examination often reveals decreased mental status, even coma. As in DKA the rest of the examination depends on whether there is superimposed disease.

Table 38-1 **Features of DKA and HHS**

Lab	DKA	HHS
Glucose (mg/dL)	300–800	>1000
Plasma sodium	Decreased	Normal or increased
Plasma potassium	Normal or increased	Normal or increased
Total body potassium	Significantly decreased	Decreased
Plasma HCO_3	<15 meq/L	Slightly decreased
Fluid deficit (L)	3–6	Up to 8–10
Mental status at presentation	Usually normal	Often significantly decreased

EVALUATION

Routine chemistries (Na, K, Cl, HCO_3, blood urea nitrogen [BUN], creatine [Cr], and glucose) are critical and allow calculation of the AG [Na – (Cl + HCO_3)]. Serum ketones, phosphate, urinalysis, arterial blood gas (ABG), and complete blood count (CBC) are usually ordered. ECG is needed to look for signs of ischemia or MI. Other tests to consider in the appropriate setting include cardiac enzymes, triglycerides, lipase, hCG, and chest x-ray. Table 38-1 contrasts key differences in the clinical presentations of DKA and HHS.

MANAGEMENT

Management always involves treating any precipitating event for the DKA or HHS. Correction of dehydration and insulin are mainstays in the treatment of both conditions.

Patients with **DKA** do require volume replacement but correcting the AG with **insulin is the critical aspect** of successful therapy. Patients have a significant decrease in total body potassium (despite the initial hyperkalemia from osmolar and acid-related fluid shifts) which will require correction. It is common for the glucose to normalize before the AG is completely corrected. Therefore, glucose is a typical addition to the later part of treatment, even though it may seem counterintuitive. Whenever there are major electrolyte and fluid abnormalities, electrolytes should be monitored frequently to avoid causing cerebral edema (usually seen in younger patients, felt to be from too rapidly lowering glucose) and other metabolic complications. The following treatment guidelines can be applied to most patients:

1. Fluid replacement
   - NS 500–1000 mL/h × 4 hours
   - 1/2 NS 250–500 mL/h × 4 hours
   - Switch to D5 or D10 1/2 NS when serum glucose <250 mg/dL
2. Insulin
   - Regular insulin 10 units IV push
   - Regular insulin 0.1 unit/kg/h continuous IV infusion
   - If glucose does not drop 10% every hour or the AG is not improving, double the rate
   - Reduce the rate once glucose <250 mg/dL or if glucose is lowering more than 100–125 mg/dL/h
   - Continue to decrease until the AG resolves
2. Potassium—KCl is added to the IV fluids as soon as the serum potassium falls to 5–5.5 meq/L, assuming urine output is achieved. Usually, 20–40 meq in each liter of fluid is sufficient to maintain K of 4–5 meq/L.
3. Phosphate—Phosphate levels will decrease rapidly with insulin therapy. However, in general, there is no need to replace phosphate unless the patient is not eating. Exceptions would be severe hypophosphatemia (a level <1 mg/dL), to avoid cardiac and skeletal muscle weakness, and the potential for respiratory depression.
4. Bicarbonate—It is unnecessary to replace this as insulin will reverse the cases of the acidosis. Some clinicians give $NaHCO_3$ initially only if the pH <6.9.

In order to keep up with the electrolyte changes and drip adjustments, glucose should be checked every 1–2 hours and electrolytes with AG calculation every 2–4 hours during the first 24 hours. Most DKA can be reversed in 24 hours. Once the AG had corrected, if the patient can eat, then he/she can be converted to long-acting insulin subcutaneously. The initial dose of subcutaneous insulin should be given 1–2 hours before discontinuing the insulin drip, to insure continuous levels of circulating insulin.

Since patients with **HHS** are markedly dehydrated, treatment focuses on initial fluid resuscitation with NS 1–3 L. However, once the patient is hemodynamically stable, the free water deficit must be calculated and carefully repleted over several days (see Chap. 34). Fluid alone will help correct the hyperglycemia but insulin is required at lower doses than with DKA.

INPATIENT GLYCEMIC CONTROL

Christopher S. Newell

KEY POINTS

- Tight glucose control can improve outcomes for hospitalized patients.
- Glycemic targets for hospitalized patients should be <110 mg/dL for preprandial glucose and <180 mg/dL for random blood glucose.
- Insulin is the best option to achieve tight glucose control.
- Insulin administration is conceptualized as basal dosing, prandial dosing, and correction factor dosing.
- Monitor fingerstick blood glucoses frequently to avoid hypoglycemia.

INTRODUCTION

Diabetes mellitus (DM) and stress-induced hyperglycemia represent very common comorbid conditions in the hospitalized patient. Regardless of what medical condition brings your patient to the hospital, recent studies show that **elevated blood glucoses have substantial effects on both morbidity and mortality**. For example, among diabetics and nondiabetics admitted with an acute myocardial infarction hyperglycemia is associated with greater in-hospital mortality and a higher incidence of congestive heart failure (CHF). Similarly, patients admitted with an acute stroke have a greater mortality and a higher risk of poor functional recovery if they have hyperglycemia during their hospitalization. Further, studies have shown that using insulin to control hyperglycemia will improve outcomes. In the ICU, patients who are aggressively managed to keep blood sugars <110 have lower rates of sepsis and renal failure as well as overall reduction in mortality. Given this background, aggressive control of hyperglycemia has become a standard of care for every hospitalized patient.

PATHOPHYSIOLOGY

Why control of hyperglycemia has such a substantial impact on outcomes continues to be debated. Hyperglycemia is known to impair many basic physiologic processes. One of the most recognized areas is on immune function. Hyperglycemia is known to impair phagocytosis T-cell function and the binding of antigen by immunoglobulin. This is known to delay wound healing and resolution of infections, but may also put patients at risk for developing infections. In addition, hyperglycemia will increase certain cytokines, such as C-reactive protein (CRP) and tumor necrosis factor (TNF), which will have proinflammatory effects. Hyperglycemia also has significant effects on the vasculature, primarily by impairing vasodilation and reducing blood flow to organs and damaged tissue. Last, hyperglycemia increases platelet activation and reduces fibrinolysis, which may also play a role in expanding the size of the infarct. These mechanisms may explain why patients with an acute myocardial infarction and hyperglycemia have been noted to have reduced collateral blood flow and larger infarct size.

Insulin administration may also have beneficial effects independent of lowering blood glucose. Insulin inhibits lipolysis, thereby decreasing the production of free fatty acids which have been linked to cardiac arrhythmias. Insulin positively affects the endothelium by stimulating nitric oxide production which has a vasodilatory effect. Insulin may also have anti-inflammatory properties. Insulin may protect the brain, kidney, and lung from ischemia, and may actually improve the fibrinolysis at the time of acute coronary events. Finally, insulin is an anabolic hormone which promotes wound healing and deposition of lean body tissue during times of catabolism.

MANAGEMENT

Diabetics, regardless if they are type 1 or type 2, and patients with stress-induced hyperglycemia should all have aggressive glucose management. The goals of management are to maintain blood glucoses **<110 for preprandial** measures and **<180 for any blood glucose**, because levels higher than these have been associated with worse outcomes.

In order to achieve this tight of blood glucose control, patients should generally be managed with insulin. Oral medications are not considered effective for aggressive glucose management in the hospital. Hospitalized patients frequently miss meals or are made NPO (nothing by mouth) which often precludes oral medications. In addition, individuals with acute illness tend to have greater elevations in blood sugar due to stress and require frequent adjustments of their regimen to control blood sugar. Finally, oral medications have been associated with adverse events in the inpatient setting. **Sulfonylureas** have a variable duration of action between individuals and predispose to hypoglycemia, particularly if the patient is not eating. **Metformin** is associated with lactic acidosis, so should be avoided in patients with CHF, hypoperfusion, renal disease, old age, or pulmonary disease, because all increase the risk. **Thiazolidinediones** have been known to increase intravascular volume, which may needlessly complicate the management of CHF, liver disease, renal disease, or acute myocardial infarctions. Given these concerns, one should consider discontinuing oral diabetes medications while the patient is hospitalized.

Most hospitalized patients should be managed with either the continuous infusion of intravenous insulin or subcutaneous insulin preparations. The preferred method of insulin administration in the critical care setting or patients who are NPO is IV infusion, because it allows more frequent and tighter dosing adjustments. However, in the lower acuity setting, subcutaneous administration of insulin is efficacious and cost-effective. Standardized protocols have been developed and offer a more rational, individualized approach to blood glucose control. In general, standardized protocols address three principal components of insulin therapy:

1. **Basal** insulin reflects what the body typically produces during the fasting state. This must be provided to any patient with insulin deficiency. Such patients include those with type 1 diabetes, pancreatectomy or a history of diabetic ketoacidosis (DKA). Most patients with wide fluctuations in their glucose levels, insulin use for over 5 years, or diabetes for >10 years will also be insulin deficient as well. A rough estimate of basal insulin production for patients already on insulin is approximately **40–50% of total daily insulin** requirements. Basal insulin should be provided with a long-acting insulin analogue, such as glargine insulin or NPH insulin.
2. **Prandial** insulin is used for any patient who is eating a diet and should be dosed to account for the meal they are about to eat. Prandial insulin usually consists of 50% of the total insulin dose and should be a short-acting insulin, such as regular, aspart, or lispro insulin.
3. **Correction factor** insulin is supplemental insulin required to tightly control blood glucoses. Correction factor is given before meals to correct for existing premeal hyperglycemia (generally defined as a glucose >150 mg/dL). Correction factor is an important component for hospitalized patients, because concomitant illness typically requires greater insulin doses than usual. This should also be a short-acting insulin.
   a. Type 1 DM: Use the patient's calculated correction factor or assume that 1 unit of insulin will lower glucose by 50 mg/dL.
   b. Type 2 DM: Assume that 1 unit of insulin will lower glucose by 30 mg/dL.
   c. Calculation for correction factor = **1700/total daily insulin dose** (e.g., if a patient takes 53 total units of insulin per day, 1700/53 = 32, so 1 unit of insulin should lower their glucose by 32 mg/dL).

Why Not Sliding Scale Insulin?

With sliding scale insulin dosage regimens, a set amount of insulin is administered per results gathered from fingerstick blood glucose monitoring. First, and perhaps most importantly, when a patient is just managed with sliding scale insulin, no basal insulin is provided, which most patients need to achieve adequate control. This is a **reactive approach** usually to an event which occurred several hours ago and led to the hyperglycemia. As a result, patients usually have **alternating bouts of hypoglycemia and hyperglycemia**. Second, sliding scale is often administered without regard to meals or previously administered insulin doses. Thus, it is not uncommon to have "**insulin stacking**," when sliding scale is administered despite the fact that previously administered insulin has not reached its peak effect yet. This can lead to hypoglycemic episodes when all of the insulin doses reach their effect. Last, sliding scale is usually written as a standard algorithm and does not take into account the individual patient's sensitivity to insulin.

Glucose Monitoring and Hypoglycemia

An intensive insulin regimen requires frequent testing of blood sugar to both maintain tight control and to monitor for hypoglycemia. Anytime tight glucose control is achieved, the patient has a higher risk of hypoglycemia. **Fingerstick glucose should be monitored prior to meals and prior to bedtime at a minimum**. Consideration should also be given to monitoring glucose 2–3 hours after a meal to ensure that prandial insulin is sufficient and in the middle of the night to ensure nighttime hypoglycemia is not occurring.

Hypoglycemia is the major "side effect" of intensive insulin regimens. In addition, patients with DM type 1 may have impaired counterregulatory hormonal responses such as the release of glucagons and epinephrine which will further increase the risk of hypoglycemia. Patients may become symptomatic with a blood glucose level of 80 mg/dL. They may become obtunded when blood glucose levels dip to <50 mg/dL. Classic signs and symptoms that you may observe if your patient is becoming hypoglycemic include: sweating, tremor, hunger, anxiety, difficulty concentrating, uncoordination, weakness, lethargy, blurred vision, and confusion.

Any episode of symptomatic hypoglycemia or glucose <60 mg/dL should be promptly treated. Glucose administration is usually preferred, particularly if the patient is awake and alert and able to eat. Such patients should be given 15 g of simple carbohydrates such as found in 4 oz of fruit juice or soda, 8 oz of nonfat milk, or 3–4 glucose tablets. Alternatively, glucose can be administered intravenously by giving 25 g (25 mL) of a 50% dextrose solution. If glucose cannot be administered, glucagon can be given as a subcutaneous or intramuscular injection of 0.5–1.0 mg. Fingerstick glucose should be monitored every 15 minutes until it rises above 80 mg/dL.

CHAPTER 40

HYPERCALCEMIA

Steven Durning
John Poremba

KEY POINTS

- Symptoms in hypercalcemia are due to both the rate and the degree of calcium elevation.
- Primary hyperparathyroidism is the most common cause of asymptomatic hypercalcemia.
- Malignancy is the most common cause of symptomatic hypercalcemia in the inpatient setting.
- The etiology for hypercalcemia can be ascertained by a careful history and physical, and a limited laboratory evaluation.
- The first step in the laboratory workup of hypercalcemia is determining if the hypercalcemia is PTH or non-PTH-mediated.
- Symptomatic hypercalcemia can be managed with volume repletion, loop diuretics to enhance renal calcium excretion ± bisphosphonate therapy.

INTRODUCTION

Calcium has two major biologic functions—calcium salts provide strength to the skeleton, and ionized calcium plays a key role in membrane stability, blood clotting, and neuromuscular function. As the biologically active form, free or ionized calcium levels are normally tightly regulated. Serum calcium levels represent the net balance of calcium influx from the diet, storage, and release of calcium from bone, and loss of calcium through the kidneys. Hypercalcemia results when the calcium influx from bone and the gastrointestinal tract overwhelms the capacity of the kidneys to excrete calcium. Hypercalcemia can be a manifestation of a serious illness such as an underlying malignancy or it can be detected coincidentally in an asymptomatic patient.

PATHOPHYSIOLOGY

Total body calcium is regulated by a variety of hormones, but principally by parathyroid hormone (PTH) and vitamin D. The dominant hormonal control of serum calcium is **PTH** which is produced in response to calcium-sensing receptors on the parathyroid glands (Fig. 40-1). A small decrease in serum ionized calcium stimulates PTH release. Likewise, small increases in serum ionized calcium suppress PTH release. High phosphate levels also stimulate PTH secretion as PTH lowers serum phosphate by reducing renal tubular phosphate reabsorption. PTH increases serum calcium through several mechanisms:

1. Stimulates bone resorption with release of calcium
2. Stimulates renal 1-α hydroxylase which converts calcidiol to calcitriol
3. Increases renal tubular absorption of calcium

Vitamin D (calciferols) are a group of steroids that raise serum calcium levels by promoting intestinal absorption of calcium and phosphate, and by stimulating bone resorption (Fig. 40-1). Vitamin D can be obtained from dietary sources, or produced de novo in sun-exposed skin. Vitamin D must be sequentially converted to calcidiol (25-hydroxy vitamin D) in the liver, then calcitriol (1,25-dihydroxy vitamin D) by renal 1-α hydroxylase. Calcitriol is the bioactive form of vitamin D and is regulated by PTH.

Calcitonin only plays a minor role in calcium regulation by opposing the action of PTH. It promotes uptake of calcium into bone and promotes renal calcium excretion.

As PTH is the dominant hormone for calcium regulation, a general classification is to divide the disorders into those caused by PTH and those independent of PTH (Table 40-1). The majority of patients with **PTH-dependent hypercalcemia** will have **primary hyperparathyroidism**, the most common form of hypercalcemia in outpatient practice. Primary hyperparathyroidism is usually the result of a single parathyroid adenoma (85%) or multigland hyperplasia (15%), but rarely may be caused from parathyroid carcinoma. The overproduction of PTH results in hypercalcemia and hypophosphatemia. **Lithium** therapy can cause excessive PTH release and is a reversible cause of primary hyperparathyroidism. **Familial hypocalciuric hypercalcemia or FHH** is a hereditary disorder resulting from a mutation of the calcium-sensing receptor on the parathyroid gland and kidney, leading to mild hypercalcemia through elevated PTH release and diminished renal calcium clearance. Last, in advanced renal failure, **tertiary hyperparathyroidism** can develop as a result of long-standing PTH hypersecretion from low calcitriol levels (due to renal failure and/or chronic hyperphosphatemia).

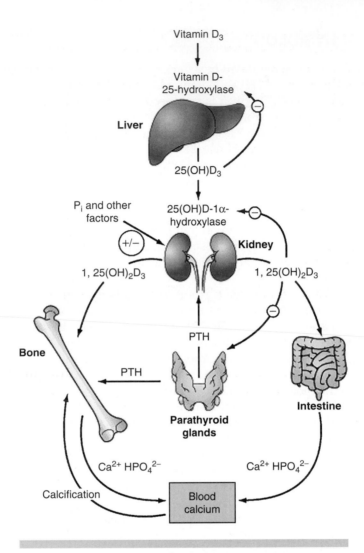

Figure 40-1 **Calcium hormonal control: schematic representation of the hormonal control loop for vitamin D metabolism and function. A reduction in the serum calcium below approximately 2.2 mmol/L (8.8 mg/dL) prompts a proportional increase in the secretion of PTH and so mobilizes additional calcium from the bone. PTH promotes the synthesis of 1,25(OH)$_2$D in the kidney, which, in turn, stimulates the mobilization of calcium from bone and intestine and regulates the synthesis of PTH by negative feedback.** (*Source:* Reproduced with permission from Kasper DL, Braunwald E, Fauci AS, et al. *Harrison's Principles of Internal Medicine,* 16th ed. New York: McGraw-Hill, 2005, Figure 331-5.)

Table 40-1 **Differential Diagnosis of Hypercalcemia by Mechanism of Action**

PTH Dependent	PTH Independent
Primary hyperparathyroidism	Malignancy
Solitary adenoma	PTHrp
Multiple endocrine neoplasia	Cytokine-mediated (multiple myeloma)
Parathyroid carcinoma	Direct invasion of bone
Tertiary hyperparathyroidism	Vitamin D intoxication
Benign familial hypercalcemia (FHH)	Granulomatous disease
Ectopic PTH (neuroendocrine tumors)	Thyrotoxicosis
	Adrenal insufficiency
	Prolonged immobilization
	Rhabdomyolysis
	Paget's disease
	Pheochromocytoma

This leads to chronic parathyroid hyperplasia with dysregulation and autonomous secretion of PTH.

Note that secondary hyperparathyroidism is a compensatory process, usually from vitamin D deficiency or renal failure, and does not cause hypercalcemia.

PTH-Independent Hypercalcemia

Malignancy can lead to hypercalcemia through a variety of mechanisms. Some tumor cells, including **squamous cell carcinoma** of the lung, can produce a bioactive PTH fragment (similar actions), termed PTH-related protein or PTHrp. Malignancy can also lead to hypercalcemia through extensive local bone invasion with release of calcium salts or production of osteolytic cytokines by tumor cells (multiple myeloma). **Excessive intestinal absorption of calcium and phosphate** can lead to hypercalcemia. Causes of hypercalcemia by this mechanism include **vitamin D intoxication** (excess of 20,000 IU/day) and occasionally **vitamin A intoxication**. **Milk-alkali syndrome** (ingestion of large amounts of calcium-containing antacids) can also lead to hypercalcemia through excessive intestinal calcium absorption. **Granulomatous diseases** (i.e., sarcoidosis, tuberculosis, berylliosis, and fungal diseases) can also be associated with hypercalcemia. Macrophages can express 1-α hydroxylase (similar to the kidney), resulting in unregulated calcitriol production and hypercalcemia.

CLINICAL PRESENTATION

The clinical setting of the patient will often not only clarify the diagnosis, but also direct therapy. For example, most patients with primary hyperparathyroidism are either asymptomatic or with minimal symptoms are detected because of mild elevations of calcium on screening. On the other hand, most patients with hypercalcemia from malignancy have clinically obvious symptoms related to their underlying cancer. Only rarely is hypercalcemia the first manifestation of cancer.

Symptoms of hypercalcemia itself can vary substantially, because symptoms are related to not only the degree of calcium elevation but also the rapidity in the rise. As calcium plays an important role in neuromuscular function, typical symptoms and signs in hypercalcemia include **fatigue, weakness, neurocognitive impairment,** and **depressed mental status**. Neurocognitive impairment is usually the first symptom, but may only be apparent on careful questioning or neuropsychological testing. Mental status may progress to coma, but is a late finding associated with severe elevations in serum calcium. Gastrointestinal symptoms may also occur from alteration of smooth muscle activity, including anorexia, nausea, vomiting, abdominal pain and **constipation. Polyuria** is common in symptomatic hypercalcemia as the renal response to vasopressin is impaired, resulting in a reversible form of nephrogenic diabetes insipidus. Significant intravascular **volume depletion** is also common in hypercalcemia. Volume depletion occurs as a result of reduced oral intake due to nausea, anorexia, and vomiting and increased urinary losses form the diabetes insipidus.

The physical examination may reveal distress, tachycardia, hypotension, orthostasis, diaphoresis, lymphadenopathy, palpable parathyroid gland (parathyroid carcinoma), thyroid goiter (thyrotoxicosis), Horner's syndrome, breast masses, crackles, wheezes, lobar consolidation, abdominal mass or tenderness, costovertebral angle tenderness, hyperreflexia, or diminished mental state, strength, and sensation.

An ECG can also aid in recognizing hypercalcemia; hypercalcemia is one of the clinically relevant causes of a **shortened** QT interval. A chest x-ray should be considered if a malignant etiology is suspected, because of the prevalence of lung cancer.

EVALUATION

Despite the numerous causes for hypercalcemia, the mechanism for hypercalcemia can usually be ascertained after a complete history and physical examination, and a limited series of laboratory tests. The first step is to verify that the calcium is high. Most serum assays measure total calcium, both free and protein bound, and normal values vary slightly between labs. About

half of circulating calcium is bound to serum proteins, predominantly albumin, and is not active. The remaining free or unbound calcium is responsible
for the cellular action of calcium. When elevations in serum proteins such as
albumin are present, the total serum calcium levels may be elevated, but the
free serum calcium level is normal. Ionized calcium level can be measured
directly, but measurement is often unavailable or unreliable. The following
formula should be used to correct total serum calcium levels for albumin concentrations >4 g/dL:

$$\text{Corrected calcium} = \text{total calcium} - 0.8 \,(\text{albumin} - 4)$$

The next step is to determine if the PTH level is appropriate or inappropriate (non-PTH-mediated or PTH-mediated hypercalcemia, respectively) for
the serum calcium level. When measured, serum PTH should always be
ordered with a serum calcium and albumin measurement, because PTH elevations can be compensatory rather than pathologic. Likewise, a "normal"
PTH value in the setting of hypercalcemia is inappropriate as PTH should be
suppressed. **In the setting of elevated serum calcium, a PTH which is normal
or high reflects a PTH-dependent mechanism, whereas a PTH <10 ng/mL
reflects a PTH-independent mechanism**. Other essential labs to understand
the patient's calcium regulation include the phosphorous, 25-OH vitamin D,
1,25-OH vitamin D, and 24-hour urinary calcium excretion. Note that in PTH-
mediated diseases, the serum calcium and phosphorous tend to move in
opposite directions, while in PTH-independent processes, the serum calcium
and phosphorous tend to move in the same direction.

For PTH-dependent hypercalcemia, these labs will often provide the
diagnosis (Table 40-2). Patients with renal failure should be suspected of
having tertiary hyperparathyroidism. If a hypercalcemia is marked and a
palpable neck mass is evident, parathyroid carcinoma should be suspected.
Similarly, in the setting of PTH-independent hypercalcemia, a careful history
and physical in addition to the basic labs will generally guide the evaluation
(Table 40-3).

Table 40-2 **Essential Lab Tests in Common Causes of PTH-Dependent
Hypercalcemia**

	PTH	Phosphorous	Urine Calcium	1,25-OH Vitamin D
Primary hyperparathyroidism	High/normal	Low	High	High
FHH	High	Normal	Very low	Low

Table 40-3 **Lab Results in the Common Causes of PTH-Independent Hypercalcemia**

	Phosphorous	25-OH Vitamin D	1,25-OH Vitamin D
Malignancy (PTHrp)	Low or normal	Low or normal	Normal to high
Malignancy (bony metastasis)	Variable	Low or normal	Low or normal
Granulomatous disease	High	Normal	High
Vitamin D intoxication	High	High	Normal
Milk-alkali syndrome	High	Normal	Low or normal

MANAGEMENT

Primary hyperparathyroidism is the most common cause of hyperparathyroidism in the outpatient setting. The essential question for primary hyperparathyroidism is if treatment is necessary. Asymptomatic patients generally require no further therapy, but should be followed closely for complications. Symptomatic patients require surgical resection of the adenoma, which is curative in 95% of patients with primary hyperparathyroidism. Other indications for surgery include: age <50, total serum calcium >1 mg/dL over the upper limit of normal, marked hypercalciuria (>400 mg/24 h), osteoporosis, and impaired renal function (creatinine clearance reduced by 30%). Medical options are typically directed at preventing bone loss, using bisphosphonates or raloxifene.

Symptomatic hypercalcemia, particularly associated with malignancy is typically managed in the hospital. Initial management must be directed at identification and treatment of the underlying cause of hypercalcemia. For the hypercalcemia, the first step is to replace any fluid losses with **normal saline**. Intravascular expansion and increased sodium delivery to the kidney will both result in an increase in urinary calcium excretion. Once the patient is volume resuscitated, loop diuretics such as furosemide can be administered, because they block tubular reabsorption of calcium, further increasing urinary calcium excretion. As inhibitors of bone resorption, **bisphosphonates** are effective in reducing serum calcium. Intravenous pamidronate is the most widely used agent and can return serum calcium to normal within 1–2 days and its effects can last several weeks.

INFECTIOUS

DISEASES

INPATIENT HIV-RELATED

CONDITIONS

Terri Postma

KEY POINTS

- The differential diagnosis of presenting symptoms is different for PLWH than the general population.
- The CD4+ T-cell count can be used as a guide for susceptibility to certain opportunistic infections.
- Managing a PLWH in the hospital often requires multiple disciplines and a higher level of suspicion for serious pathology.

INTRODUCTION

There are approximately 1,000,000 persons living with HIV (PLWH) in the United States. Since the first descriptions and relatively primitive treatment in the 1980s, the medical community's knowledge about HIV/AIDS has expanded significantly and highly effective treatments for both HIV and opportunistic infections have been developed. In spite of this, the diagnosis and treatment of HIV/AIDS and its associated diseases remains a challenge. One of the significant challenges is due to the fact that patients with compromised immune function are susceptible to almost any pathogen and many malignancies which can present in any system of the body. This chapter will focus on some of the more severely involved systems and etiologies of illness in PLWH.

PATHOPHYSIOLOGY

After inoculation, HIV attaches, invades, and eventually destroys CD4 (helper) T cells which are integral to many aspects of immune function (see

Chap. 35 in *First Exposure to Internal Medicine: Ambulatory Medicine*). Therefore, loss of CD4 cells over time produces severe compromise of all branches of the immune response in those infected with the virus. For example, patients with HIV are particularly prone to infection by encapsulated microbes such as *Haemophilus influenzae* and *Streptococcus pneumoniae*, perhaps secondary to depressed B cell or neutrophil function. If untreated, after a median of 10 years, the CD4 count reaches a critical value at which the patient is at risk for opportunistic infections (see Table 41-1). Progression from HIV to AIDS is defined as occurring when the CD4 count falls below 200 cells/µL or with the development of an "AIDS defining condition," usually an opportunistic infection or malignancy (Table 41-2).

Table 41-1 **Infections Associated With CD4+ T-Cell Counts**

CD4+ Count (Cells/µL)	Pathogen/Manifestation
<500	*S. pneumoniae, H. influenzae*
	Mycobacterium tuberculosis (pulmonary TB)
	HSV (orolabial, genital, perirectal lesions)
	Candida albicans (thrush, vaginitis)
	HHV-8 (KS)
	EBV (oral hairy leukoplakia), VZV (shingles)
<200	*Pneumocystis jiroveci* pneumonia (PCP)
	Toxoplasma gondii (pneumonia)
	M. tuberculosis (miliary/extrapulmonary TB)
	HIV encephalopathy
	Cryptosporidium (diarrhea), *Salmonella* (diarrhea)
<100	EBV (primary CNS lymphoma)
	T. gondii (encephalitis)
	Cryptococcus neoformans (meningitis)
	Microsporidia (diarrhea)
	Histoplasma capsulatum (disseminated)
	C. albicans (esophagitis)
	Progressive multifocal encephalopathy (PML, JC virus)
	Rhodococcus equi (pneumonia)
<50	MAC (disseminated)
	CMV (disseminated, retinitis, diarrhea, encephalitis, esophagitis, pneumonitis)

Abbreviations: HHV-8, human herpesvirus 8; EBV, Epstein-Barr virus; VZV, varicella zoster virus.

Table 41-2 Disease Management in Hospitalized PLWH

Disease (Differential)	Clinical Characteristics	Evaluation	Treatment
Pneumonia CAP, PCP, TB, MAC, *Histoplasma, Aspergillus, Cryptococcus,* toxoplasmosis, lymphoma, KS, interstitial pneumonitis	Fever, cough, night sweats, weight loss, or pleuritic chest pain	CXR in PCP may be normal or faint bilateral infiltrates. Suspect PCP when CD4 <200 and not on prophylaxis. Consider isolation until TB is ruled out—PPD may not be reliable in fulminant disease. KS is associated with bilateral lower lobe infiltrates and effusions. Bronchoalveolar lavage may be necessary for neoplasm or pneumonitis	CAP—appropriate antibiotics PCP-TMP/SMX, dapsone, or inhaled pentamidine; consider steroids if PaO_2 <70 mmHg TB—per usual; avoid rifampin if on HAART Neoplasia—radiation or chemotherapy
Esophagitis *Candida,* CMV, HSV, KS, lymphoma	Odynophagia, dysphagia, or retrosternal chest pain	Often treated empirically. Barium esophagram may be helpful. Upper endoscopy with biopsy is required to make an accurate diagnosis	Hydration and nutrition. Antifungals or antivirals. In severe cases, steroids to reduce inflammation
Diarrhea Community enterics, TB, CMV, *Clostridium difficile,* Cryptosporidia, Microsporidia, Isospora, HIV enteropathy, HAART	Fever, anorexia, fatigue, abdominal pain. Note recent travel and drinking water source. Suspect CMV colitis if CD4 <50	Stool for culture, ova/parasite × 3, *C. difficile* toxin, AFB, fecal leukocytes. Colonoscopy and/or upper endoscopy with biopsy if no pathogen is identified. If unrevealing, consider HIV enteropathy	Hydration and nutrition Antibiotics as indicated

(Continued)

315

Table 41-2 **Disease Management in Hospitalized PLWH** *(Continued)*

Disease (Differential)	Clinical Characteristics	Evaluation	Treatment
General neurologic Encephalopathy Metabolic, infectious, HIV dementia, PML **Seizures** Toxoplasma, PML, lymphoma, electrolyte imbalance	Acute confusion, delirium, or seizures; progressive decline General—metabolic Focal—lymphoma or toxoplasmosis	At minimum, CT and unless contraindicated, LP must be performed on any HIV patient that presents with neurologic complaints. Abnormalities on imaging may include lesions with surrounding edema ("ring-enhancing" lesions) suggestive of abscess (usually toxoplasma), a solitary lesion may suggest lymphoma, periventricular contrast enhancement may suggest CMV or VZV, widespread white matter abnormalities may suggest PML or HIV encephalitis, atrophy, and enlarged ventricles (ex vacuo) suggestive of HIV dementia. The CSF should be examined for opening pressure, Gram stain and culture, cell count, protein and glucose, AFB stains and cultures, cryptococcal antigen, VDRL, cytology, and other studies depending on clinical suspicion	
Toxoplasmosis PML, CNS lymphoma, *Cryptococcus*, TB, fungal	Fever, headache, focal neurologic deficits, seizures	MRI or double-contrast CT scan reveals ring-enhancing lesions. Brain biopsy is definitive but reserved pending empiric treatment failure	Often empiric. Sulfadiazine and pyrimethamine with leucovorin; alternatives clindamycin, atovaquone

Cryptococcal meningitis *Histoplasma*, CMV, HSV, VZV, EBV, *Listeria*, *Treponema pallidum*, lymphoma	Subacute meningoencephalitis symptoms. Kernig's and Brudzinski's signs	CSF may be normal or modest pleocytosis and elevated protein. Send for cryptococcal antigen and India ink examination. Consider VDRL, AFB, cytology	Amphotericin and flucytosine IV followed by long-term oral fluconazole
Primary CNS lymphoma Systemic lymphoma, toxoplasmosis	Focal seizures, mass lesions, extranodal disease	MRI or CT shows limited number of lesions—often ring-enhancing—in any location	Palliative radiation; median survival <1 year
Systemic lymphoma Disseminated infection, KS	Adenopathy, abdominal pain, dysphagia, dyspnea	Lymph node or bone marrow biopsy	Combination chemotherapy
Disseminated infection TB, MAC, CMV, *Candida*, *Histoplasma*, *Bartonella*, HIV wasting	Rash, fever, cough, night sweats, weight loss, joint pain, adenopathy, organomegaly	CXR, blood cultures, PPD, CT of chest or abdomen, bronchoscopy for biopsy or culture, skin biopsy and culture, bone marrow biopsy and culture	Appropriate antimicrobials

Abbreviations: CXR, chest x-ray; TMP/SMX, trimethoprim-sulfamethoxazole; AFB, acid fast bacilli; CT, computed tomography; LP, lumbar puncture; CSF, cerebrospinal fluid; VDRL, Venereal Disease Research Laboratory.

CLINICAL PRESENTATION

In PLWH, common diseases are still common and any differential should include all the etiologies one would consider for a patient not infected with HIV. That being said, the HIV patient population is susceptible to a spectrum of illness that changes as the CD4+ count declines, with most occurring once CD4+ count falls below 500 cells/μL.

In addition to duration of HIV disease, medications, opportunistic infections, and most recent CD4 cell counts and viral load, a comprehensive history and physical is essential. Constitutional symptoms such as fever and weight loss might herald tuberculosis (TB), Mycobacterium-avian complex (MAC), Bartonella, or lymphoma. Lymphadenopathy could indicate lymphoma, toxoplasmosis, or even immune reconstitution. Headache or other focal neurologic complaints may indicate toxoplasmosis, cryptococcal meningitis, or central nervous system (CNS) lymphoma. Vision changes should prompt investigation for cytomegalovirus (CMV) retinitis or herpes simplex virus (HSV) keratitis. Oral complaints and especially odynophagia could be related to candidiasis, aphthous ulcers, HSV, or CMV. Dyspnea and cough are common and one must consider community-acquired pneumonia (CAP), of course, but also pneumocystic pneumonia (PCP), Rhodococcus, TB, MAC, and fungal infections. Diarrhea is common with highly active antiretroviral therapy (HAART) but infectious etiologies to be considered are Cryptosporidia, Microsporidia, and Isospora as well as enteric pathogens that may be more virulent in PLWH such as *Salmonella*, *Campylobacter*, and *Shigella*. Dermatologic problems such as zoster, HSV, and Molluscum are common; fortunately Kaposi's sarcoma (KS) is rare. PLWH seem particularly susceptible to drug eruptions, including Stevens-Johnson syndrome.

Laboratory evaluation often reveals anemia, lymphopenia, and thrombocytopenia frequently due to medications or direct result of HIV. PLWH being treated with zidovudine typically have an elevated mean corpuscular volume. The CD4 T-cell count can be transiently suppressed during any acute illness.

MANAGEMENT

Management of an HIV patient admitted to the hospital will depend on the symptoms and diagnosis and will require a team approach to management and care. Because information related to HIV management is both enormous and ever-expanding, a key team member will be the infectious disease consultant. Since resistance to antiretrovirals is an ever-present problem in the treatment of HIV/AIDS, care should be taken to **continue the patient's home regimen** when they are admitted. However, should the patient not have regular monitoring as an outpatient, special attention to plans for follow-up care at time of discharge is critical.

FEVER IN THE
HOSPITALIZED PATIENT

Christine Yasuko Todd

KEY POINTS

- Fever within the first 3 days of hospitalization generally reflects a community-acquired process; after 3 days of admission, consider nosocomial or iatrogenic processes.
- UTIs, line infections, *C. difficile*-associated colitis and pneumonia are common causes of fever in hospitalized patients.

INTRODUCTION

Fever is a common reason for admission to the hospital, and a common development in patients during the course of their hospitalization. Patients who develop fever within 3 days of their hospitalization are usually harboring a pathogen they acquired in the community. Fevers occurring after 3 days of hospitalization are typically nosocomial or iatrogenic and are the focus of this chapter.

PATHOPHYSIOLOGY

Fever is caused by a cascade of events triggered by pyrogenic cytokines (e.g., interleukin [IL]-1, IL-6, and tumor necrosis factor [TNF]) that induce the synthesis of prostaglandin E2 (PGE2). In addition to causing the shivering, vasoconstriction, and elevation of the temperature set point, PGE2 also causes the myalgias and arthralgias classically associated with fever. Exogenous pyrogens from microorganisms (e.g., lipopolysaccharide endotoxin) are the most common cause of fever. However, there are noninfectious triggers of this cytokine-mediated pathway as well, such as drug reactions.

CLINICAL PRESENTATION

Fever is not difficult to diagnose. By definition it is an oral temperature in the morning >37.2°C (98.9°F) or in the evening >37.7°C (99.9°F). Tympanic temperatures should correspond to oral temperatures, while in general, rectal temperatures are 1°F higher and axillary 1°F lower than oral temperatures. As people age, they tend to mount less of a febrile response so even modest temperature elevations can be clinically significant. Patients on immunosuppression will also have the fever response blunted or even blocked.

EVALUATION

The evaluation of the febrile hospitalized patient begins with repeating a detailed, unbiased history, physical examination, and a thorough chart review. When patients are hospitalized and settled into a prescribed course of therapy, it is easy to become overly focused in history taking and physical examination. The following questions will help guide a more comprehensive fever evaluation in the hospitalized patient:

1. Is the fever the result of a partially treated infection (e.g., patient with lung abscess but being treated for "pneumonia")?
2. Is the fever the result of an incorrectly treated infection (e.g., the organism is resistant to the antibiotic)?
3. Does the patient have any new, localizing symptoms (e.g., cough or diarrhea)?
4. Does the patient have a special risk for fever (e.g., is the patient neutropenic or postoperative)?
5. Does the patient have a catheter or pressure ulcer?
6. Could the patient have developed a common, noninfectious nosocomial complication (e.g., pulmonary embolism [PE], myocardial infarction [MI], pancreatitis, or drug reaction)?

These questions generally can be answered by repeating or reviewing the diagnostic studies that were performed on admission. Pay special attention to results or findings that may have been overlooked or underemphasized on admission.

Immunocompetent patients typically develop an inflammatory response to a new infection which leads to localizing symptoms (e.g., cough, pain, dysuria) and signs (e.g., pulmonary crackles, abdominal tenderness, skin erythema). Evaluation is targeted to the localizing symptom (chest x-ray [CXR], urinalysis [UA]). In contrast, **immunocompromised patients** may **not** develop localizing symptoms, due to lack of an inflammatory response. In these cases, initial evaluation and management focuses on **the most common**

hospital acquired infections—urinary tract infection (UTI), pneumonia, and line-associated infections. Unless the source of infection is obvious, patients who develop a fever in the hospital are "pan-cultured"—two sets of blood cultures, a UA with culture and sensitivity (C&S), and sometimes a sputum culture are obtained. A CXR is commonly ordered in these settings as well but **it is critical to obtain blood cultures and urine prior to initiating antibiotics**. Areas frequently overlooked in the evaluation of a febrile, hospitalized patient are catheters and complete skin examinations despite the frequency of catheter-related and pressure ulcer-related infections.

MANAGEMENT

It is very tempting to give the patient a course of broad-spectrum antibiotics before a clear diagnosis is made. However, one must resist this temptation as it can cloud an already complicated picture and cause further iatrogenesis (e.g., by inducing *Clostridium difficile* colitis). **Empiric antibiotics are indicated when patients are toxic appearing, septic, or neutropenic**. For patients who are clinically stable, there is time to pursue a diagnosis that will allow targeted therapy. Hospitalized patients are closely monitored and antibiotics can be started in a matter of minutes should their clinical situation change. Loss of valuable microbiological data through the hasty institution of therapy, however, can never be regained.

Vascular access in the form of IVs or central lines puts patients at risk for fever as they easily can become colonized with skin flora. Therefore, all old and new IV sites should be inspected for signs of thrombophlebitis. If present, the IV should be removed. All central lines, particularly those more than a week old, are suspect in febrile patients. A set of blood cultures must be obtained through the line as well as through a peripheral vein. This technique helps determine whether the patient has a line infection only or if the positive line cultures are due to systemic bacteremia from another source. Whenever possible the line should be pulled, the access site relocated, and the tip sent for culture. However, there are instances when the infection can be treated successfully through the line though this is reserved for patients with difficult access. If both line and peripheral cultures are positive, look for other sources of the bacteremia. If a febrile patient with a central venous catheter appears toxic, the line is pulled immediately once cultures and alternate access are obtained. Line infections are usually due to gram-positive organisms.

A search for pressure ulcers should happen at the same time as an inspection of IV sites in the febrile, hospitalized patient. These ulcers are very common (see Chap. 45), and if there is surrounding cellulitis or purulent discharge then debridement and antibiotic treatment is indicated. Cultures of the ulcer are rarely helpful as these infections are commonly polymicrobial, but the presence of methicillin-resistant *Staphylococcus aureus* (MRSA) should lead to the addition of vancomycin.

Special consideration is given to patients with **neutropenic fever**. There is clear evidence that neutropenic patients have improved survival when treated empirically with antibiotics covering gram-positive and gram-negative organisms, especially *Pseudomonas* (see Chap. 53). Patients with a history of MRSA infection or who are at high risk of MRSA colonization should receive vancomycin therapy as well. Though every attempt should be made to collect cultures prior to the administration of antibiotics, antibiotics should never be delayed, as neutropenic fever is a medical emergency with a 70% mortality rate if antibiotics are delayed.

Postoperative fever is common and usually noninfectious for the first few days after surgery. For example, **atelectasis** is thought to be a common cause of low-grade fever in the initial postoperative period. Noninfectious acute problems such as PE, fat embolism, pancreatitis, and MI should be considered as well. Other common causes of fever in the first postoperative week include **UTI, ventilator-associated pneumonia, aspiration pneumonia**, and in patients with nasogastric tubes, **sinusitis**. Most of these are iatrogenic and reinforce the principle of eliminating invasive catheters and other devices as rapidly as possible. Later in the postoperative period, **surgical site infections** become much more common, as do treatment-related fevers from *C. difficile* **colitis or line infections**. Specific types of procedures carry special risks that must be considered, such as bacterial meningitis after neurosurgical or head and neck procedures.

Noninfectious etiologies for fever in hospitalized patients are typically considered when cultures are negative and the fever fails to respond to broad-spectrum antibiotics. However, astute clinicians will consider these possibilities earlier in the appropriate clinical setting, particularly when the patient does not appear toxic. Drug fever is caused commonly by penicillins, cephalosporins, and sulfa drugs, but any drug can be implicated, even if the patient has been previously exposed to them without problems. Accompanying rash, eosinophilia or temporal relationship of fever to drug administration are helpful in suspecting the diagnosis, but are not necessarily present in all cases. Other noninfectious causes to consider include MI and Dressler's syndrome (consider ECG/cardiac enzymes and CXR on patients with multiple cardiac risk factors who develop fever); PE/deep vein thrombosis (DVT); fat embolus (occurs primarily in the setting of long bone fractures); collagen-vascular diseases such as lupus or rheumatoid arthritis; pancreatitis (due to the massive inflammation that accompanies this disease); stroke (through reset of the hypothalamic thermostat); transfusion reactions; hyperthyroidism; and Addisonian crisis.

FEVER OF UNKNOWN ORIGIN

Raymond Y. Wong

KEY POINTS

- The classic definition of FUO was established over 40 years ago.
- Patients who are hospitalized, have neutropenia, or are HIV positive may require a different approach to FUO.
- Most diagnoses made in FUO are infections, malignancies, or collagen-vascular diseases.
- Even in undiagnosed cases (up to 25–30% of all FUO) the prognosis is excellent.
- The history and physical examination remain the most useful diagnostic "tests."

INTRODUCTION

The majority of fevers experienced by patients are either self-limited or relatively easy to diagnose. A fever of unknown origin (FUO) is one of the few which elude diagnosis and for decades has been a challenge for clinicians. The first formal definition of FUO was established over 40 years ago: **fever higher than 38.3°C** on several occasions, **duration of fever for at least 3 weeks**, and an uncertain diagnosis after 1 week of study in the hospital. More recently, the acceptable period of evaluation has changed to include **no diagnosis after three clinic visits or 3 days in the hospital**. In addition to this classic definition of FUO, additional classes of patients have been described which may have specific evaluations and treatments and are discussed elsewhere:

1. Nosocomial FUO: Patient who develops a fever after admission to the hospital who remains undiagnosed after 3 days of investigation (see Chap. 42).

2. Immunodeficient or neutropenic FUO: Patients with an absolute neutrophil count of <500 cell/mL and fever who remain undiagnosed after 3 days of evaluation (see Chap. 53).
3. HIV-associated FUO: HIV-positive patient with fever for 4 weeks as an outpatient or 3 days as an inpatient who remains undiagnosed after 3 days of evaluation (see Chap. 41).

PATHOPHYSIOLOGY

The definition of FUO was established with fever duration of 3 weeks to exclude typical viral causes as an etiology. The eventual diagnosis of FUO generally falls into one of four categories: infections, malignancies, collagen-vascular disease, or miscellaneous causes. However, even after extensive evaluation, many patients remain undiagnosed. The general causes in reported series will vary depending on the geographic area, age of patient, and other factors. For example, infections predominate in children and young adults, whereas infections and malignancy account for most cases in older adults. In general, most patients with FUO have common diseases with unusual presentations and not rare diseases.

Infections are the most common cause ranging from 25 to 50% of cases. Even though 3 weeks of fever should exclude most viral etiologies, some still occur, most commonly viral hepatitis, Epstein-Barr virus, and cytomegalovirus. Other important infections to consider are:

- Tuberculosis, especially extrapulmonary tuberculosis, is a great mimicker of disease and presents in many diverse populations. Tuberculosis is the most common infection identified in most reported series of FUO patients.
- Endocarditis is the second most commonly identified infection.
- Abscesses, particularly intra-abdominal abscesses, are often difficult to diagnose by history and physical.

The typical **malignancies** causing FUO are lymphomas, especially **non-Hodgkin's**, but may also include **leukemia**, **renal carcinoma**, and **liver cancer**. As opposed to these malignancies which are commonly associated with fever, multiple myeloma, and chronic lymphocytic leukemia (CLL) rarely cause fever and patients with these malignancies should be evaluated for infection.

The predominant **collagen-vascular diseases** which cause FUO vary with age. In older patients temporal arteritis and polymyalgia rheumatica need to be considered, as these conditions are common in elderly patients. The frequency of FUO caused by collagen-vascular disorders in elderly patients may approach or exceed that of infectious causes. In younger patients, juvenile rheumatoid arthritis (Still's disease) is the most common rheumatologic disease causing prolonged fevers.

Miscellaneous causes for FUO range from drug fever, pulmonary embolism, endocrine disorders to factitious fever. Patients with factitious fevers are often young women with backgrounds in the health-related fields. A list exceeding 150 causes of FUO in the United States appears in one standard textbook of internal medicine.

EVALUATION

The first step in the evaluation is to verify the presence of fever. This may require independent or unbiased confirmation if a factitious fever is suspected. Up to one-third of patients actually do not have fever or have fever of factitious origin. The pattern of fever may also provide useful information. Examples include the Pel-Ebstein fever seen in Hodgkin's disease (bouts of several days of continuous fever followed by days without fever), reversal of the normal diurnal pattern in disseminated tuberculosis (fever pattern higher in the morning than late afternoons or evenings), the lack of rise in pulse seen with fevers in typhoid fever, or the tertian (paroxysms separated by an intervening normal day) and quartan (fevers occur with two intervening normal days) patterns in malaria.

An accurate and complete history and physical, which should be repeated with each evaluation, is essential to directing the workup. Asking about recent travel experience, pet or other animal exposures, elements in the work environment, family history, or exposures to patients with similar symptoms is critical. Review of previous medical conditions (especially treated cancers) may provide possible clues to relapses of these conditions. Every medication that a patient is taking needs to be reviewed and considered as a possible culprit. **All unnecessary medications should be discontinued**. Most drug fevers will resolve within 72 hours of stopping the medication. If a patient has a fever with flu-like symptoms that persists, West Nile virus infection is a consideration depending on the regional risk and time of year. A thorough physical examination can provide significant clues. Examples would be suspecting sinusitis in a patient with sinus tenderness. A nodular or weakly pulsatile temporal artery might suggest temporal arteritis. A new heart murmur would obviously bring endocarditis into consideration. Enlarged lymph nodes or splenomegaly might suggest the possibility of lymphoma. **Careful repetition of the physical examination** may uncover earlier missed findings.

The recommended approach to the workup utilizes the idea of "potentially diagnostic clues that are key findings of history, key symptoms, or localizing signs." This should direct the workup toward evaluation of the presenting condition.

Table 43-1 **Evaluation of FUO**

Routine Studies	Advanced Testing
Complete blood count (CBC) with differential	Antinuclear antibodies
Routine blood chemistries (including liver function)	Rheumatoid factor
	HIV antibody
Urinalysis and urine culture	Cytomegalovirus antibodies
Blood cultures	Epstein-Barr virus antibodies
Chest x-ray	Hepatitis serologies
PPD (if risk factors present)	CT of the abdomen
ESR	Echocardiogram

Noninvasive laboratory testing may result in a diagnosis in approximately a quarter of cases. The most helpful tests are outlined in Table 43-1. A few cases of endocarditis (<5%) are culture negative as some species of microorganisms are difficult to isolate. In cases where endocarditis is likely but no growth appears after 5–7 days, the microbiology lab should be instructed to continue incubation for 14 days in order to detect HACEK (*Haemophilus parainfluenza* and *Haemophilus aphrophilus*; *Actinobacillus actinomycetemcomitans*; *Cardiobacterium hominis*; *Eikenella corrodens*; *Kingella kingae*) organisms, slow-growing gram-negative bacilli (see Chap. 48). In the FUO workup, the erythrocyte sedimentation rate (ESR) may be measured. Although mild to moderate elevations are typical and nonspecific, a marked elevation of the ESR is suggestive of vasculitis, particularly polyarteritis nodosa or giant cell arteritis. A screen for tuberculosis utilizing intermediate-strength purified protein derivative (PPD) skin testing should be considered in patients with risk factors. Unfortunately, negative results may occur in patients with miliary tuberculosis, other granulomatous disorders, Hodgkin's disease, or AIDS. The PPD skin test is negative in >50% of patients ultimately diagnosed with tuberculosis as the cause of the FUO.

Imaging studies such as computed tomography (CT) of the abdomen and/or pelvis are routinely utilized in patients with FUO. Nuclear studies with tagged leukocytes have a role in cases where infection or neoplasm is suspected; however, these scans commonly produce both false positive and false negative results. Many patients will require some form of invasive procedure, biopsy, or even laparotomy. In a patient with a prolonged fever and negative noninvasive workup, one should **consider biopsies of liver or bone marrow**. The yield for biopsies is obviously higher if the procedure is suggested by abnormalities of previous testing. However, even "blind" liver biopsies in the absence of liver disease have been found to be diagnostic in a small number of cases. In elderly patients, biopsy of the temporal artery can occasionally yield a diagnosis in the absence of localizing symptoms.

MANAGEMENT

Therapy should be delayed in cases of classic FUO pending the establishment of a specific diagnosis to treat. Empiric therapy is rarely curative and will likely just further delay a diagnosis. Exceptions may be made for the occasional patient for whom all approaches have been unfruitful or for the patient who is gravely ill. This differs from patients with neutropenic FUO or nosocomial FUO where the prevalence of serious bacterial infections is high and the risk of delay bodes poorly for patients. In these situations, broad-spectrum antibiotics should be administered and targeted at the most likely organisms and make adjustments according to the microbiology results and patient response. This approach is often utilized in nosocomial FUOs as most are caused by infections. Risk factors include surgical procedures, placement of intravascular catheters, instrumentation of the respiratory and urinary tracts, as well as the consequences of immobilization.

The prognosis of FUO is related to both the cause of the fever and the underlying condition of the patient. The worst outcomes occur in elderly patients and those with neoplastic disorders. Obviously, delays in diagnosis may affect outcomes in conditions such as intra-abdominal infections, miliary tuberculosis, disseminated fungal infections, and recurrent pulmonary emboli as examples. Interestingly, patients who are not diagnosed despite an extensive workup generally have a favorable outcome and tend to resolve their fevers. The 5-year mortality for undiagnosed FUO is <5%.

CELLULITIS

Andrew J. Koon

KEY POINTS

- Cellulitis is a clinical diagnosis based on spreading involvement of the skin and subcutaneous tissues with erythema, swelling, and local tenderness, accompanied by fever.
- Skin flora such as streptococci (groups A, G, and B) and *Staph aureus* are the most common etiologic agents; however, in certain situations (bites, associated with diabetic ulcers) other bacteria should be suspected.
- Necrotizing fasciitis requires early and urgent surgical debridement in addition to antibiotics.

INTRODUCTION

Cellulitis is a common medical problem in both the inpatient and outpatient settings. This diffuse spreading infection of the dermis and subcutaneous tissues may affect any region of the body; the most common site is the lower leg. It commonly occurs in association with other disorders of the skin such as abscesses, folliculitis, and dermatitis.

PATHOPHYSIOLOGY

The skin is the body's largest natural barrier to infection. Yet, there are risk factors for disrupting the barrier leading to cellulitis. Dermatitis, folliculitis, and other underlying skin conditions disrupt this barrier and may allow for the proliferation of normal skin flora. Organisms may also be introduced through the skin by other means such as trauma. The most common portal of entry in otherwise healthy persons is from fissuring of the toe webs. The inflammatory response to these pathogens results in erythema, swelling, and pain at the site of infection. Venous or lymphatic drainage problems can further increase the risk of cellulitis.

Table 44-1 **Settings and Pathogens in Cellulitis**

Etiology	Organism
Cat bite	*Pasteurella multocida*
Dog bite	*Capnocytophaga canimorsus* (DF-2)
Human bite	*Eikenella corrodens*
Salt water exposure/eating raw seafood	*Vibrio* species
Fresh water exposure	*Aeromonas hydrophila*
Nail puncture wound	*Pseudomonas aeruginosa*
Whirlpool	*P. aeruginosa*
Hospitalized patient	MRSA
Fish and meat handlers	*Erysipelothrix rhusiopathiae*

CLINICAL PRESENTATION

Historic events are extremely helpful in determining the underlying etiology and in guiding therapy. Although Group A Streptococcal (GAS) and *Staphylococcus aureus* are the most common organisms identified in cellulitis, Table 44-1 outlines pathogens that should be considered in the appropriate context.

Fever may be present and is the body's systemic response to infection. **Erythema, tenderness,** and **swelling** are apparent in the region involved. **Lymphangitis** and **lymphadenopathy** are commonly noted in the regions surrounding the infection.

Fluctuance over a region of erythema may indicate an underlying abscess which may need drainage. **Crepitus of the skin** or **sensory anesthesia** may indicate subcutaneous air and gas forming organisms such as *Clostridium* species. These findings are worrisome for necrotizing infections which involve the fascia and subcutaneous tissues. When these findings are present, immediate surgical intervention is warranted.

EVALUATION

A complete blood count (CBC) will reveal a leukocytosis. Blood cultures are often unnecessary in the absence of systemic symptoms such as fever due to the infrequent isolation of pathogens. Swabs of affected skin regions or aspirations of leading skin edges are typically **not** performed. However, if there is the presence of an underlying abscess, a specimen may be sent for organism identification. In the hospital setting, medical patients often get frequent, even daily, laboratory tests for their multiple medical conditions.

Findings suggestive of early necrotizing infections are those which suggest tissue breakdown, such as acidosis, hyperkalemia, rising leukocytes, altered coagulation profile, increased creatinine kinase (muscle origin), or rising creatinine.

Cellulitis is a clinical diagnosis and typically involves fever with associated erythema and edema of the skin. When borders of this inflammation are diffuse, this is classified as **acute cellulitis**. However, when the erythema has discrete raised borders, indicating involvement of the dermis and lymphatics, this is classified as **erysipelas**. Erysipelas is associated with *Streptococcus pyogenes* and the skin is often described as having a peau d'orange appearance, classically occurring on the cheek. **Necrotizing fasciitis** involves the subcutaneous tissues and superficial fascia. It classically presents with associated sensory anesthesia in the regions of involvement due to disruption of penetrating nerve fibers, resulting in pain out of proportion to local skin findings in early stages (when ideally diagnosed). Late stages exhibit skin discoloration, from red-purple to a dusky blue, progressing to necrosis and formation of hemorrhagic bullae (Fig. 44-1).

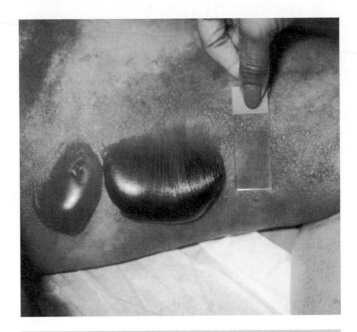

Figure 44-1 **Necrotizing fasciitis. Large cutaneous bullae are seen on the leg of this patient with necrotizing fasciitis. Note the dark purple fluid in the bullae.** *(Courtesy of Lawrence B. Stack, MD.)* (*Source:* Reproduced with permission from Knoop KJ, Stack LB, Storrow AB. *Atlas of Emergency Medicine*, 2nd ed. New York: McGraw-Hill, 2002, Figure 12-17.)

MANAGEMENT

Most cases of cellulitis can be treated in the outpatient setting with oral antibiotics. However, if the patient is clinically unstable, unable to take oral medications, or is immunocompromised, parenteral therapy is typically indicated. Historic information will guide antibiotic selection and clinical response will determine overall duration of therapy. Typically, clinicians will empirically use beta-lactam antibiotics which cover staphylococcal and streptococcal organisms for 1–2 weeks of therapy. Examples include first-generation cephalosporins (IV cefazolin, oral cephalexin) or antistaph penicillins (IV nafcillin, oral dicloxacillin). If the patient has a penicillin allergy, macrolides, clindamycin, or vancomycin may be used. Alternative antibiotic regimens may be considered if historic risk factors for a particular organism are present. For example, animal bites, infected diabetic foot ulcers, and trauma usually require broad-spectrum antibiotics such as ampicillin-sulbactam (or orally, amoxicillin-clavulanate) that cover anaerobes and gram-negative organisms as well. Methicillin-resistant *Staphylococcus aureus* (MRSA) has been emerging as a more frequent cause of cellulitis, certainly in the hospital setting, but also in the community. If a patient is severely ill, or not improving on usual antibiotic therapy, one should have a low threshold to switching to trimethoprim-sulfamethoxazole, vancomycin, or linezolid.

Surgical debridement is typically reserved for those patients with underlying systemic conditions such as an abscess or foreign body. Other necrotizing conditions of the subcutaneous tissues and fascia (**necrotizing fasciitis**) require urgent surgical intervention in addition to parenteral antibiotic therapy.

For all patients, treatment of preexisting skin conditions, removal of foreign bodies, drainage of an underlying abscess, and maximizing venous/lymphatic drainage (such as elevation of the affected leg) are important steps in treating cellulitis. Risk factor identification and modification may prevent recurrences.

PRESSURE ULCERS

Caridad A. Hernandez

KEY POINTS

- Pressure ulcers are a common, but often preventable complication of hospitalization.
- Patients with pressure ulcers have increased in-hospital morbidity and mortality.
- Prevention strategies should include early identification and correction of risk factors before ulcers occur.
- Mechanical pressure reduction and frequent repositioning are the mainstays of both prevention and treatment.

INTRODUCTION

Pressure ulcers are local areas of necrosis caused by the compression of soft tissues between a bony prominence and an external surface. Pressure ulcers are a significant problem present in ~10% of hospitalized patients (up to 30% at some institutions), and **most initially develop in the acute hospital setting**. Although pressure ulcers are most commonly associated with the elderly and immobilization, many risk factors can lead to their development (Table 45-1). Patients with pressure ulcers are susceptible to infectious complications such as cellulitis, osteomyelitis, and sepsis. Furthermore, patients who develop these complications have an increased risk of in-hospital mortality.

PATHOPHYSIOLOGY

The development of pressure ulcers requires two factors—unrelieved **external pressure** and **time**. Anytime external pressure exceeds the capillary filling pressure (~32 mmHg), microcirculation is disrupted, and oxygen delivery

Table 45-1 **Risk Factors for the Development of Pressure Ulcers**

	Intrinsic Factor	**Extrinsic Factor**
Immobility	Neurologic disease	Activity restrictions
	Spinal cord injury	Sedative administration
	Cerebrovascular accident	Poor pain control
	Dementia	
	Decreased pain sensation	
Shear forces	Loss of subcutaneous fat	Bed transfers
		Incline position in bed
Moisture	Incontinence	Fistula drainage
	Perspiration	Wound drainage
Friction	Patient agitation	Bedding
	Contractures	Bed pans
	Spasticity	
Wound healing	Advanced age	Malnutrition
	Poor local blood supply	Steroid administration
	Diabetes	

is compromised. Thus, pressure ulcers develop over bony prominences, particularly the sacrum, ischial tuberosity, greater trochanter, and calcaneus, because higher pressure can be attained by the compression of soft tissue between bone and the external surface. The amount and duration of pressure determines how much tissue damage occurs. For example, a continuous pressure of 60 mmHg **for as little as 2 hours** will cause muscle damage. In normal individuals, this prolonged pressure causes pain and the person will reposition before tissue damage occurs. However, in individuals who are immobile or who do not have normal pain sensation, repositioning will not occur.

Although skin breakdown is the first sign of a pressure ulcer, muscle and subcutaneous tissue are more susceptible to pressure-induced injury. The additional factors of friction, moisture, and shear forces contribute to skin injury. **Shear force** is generated when a force tangential to the skin (e.g., patient resting on an incline) causes a lateral shift of dermal and epidermal tissues. This further reduces the microcirculation, making the skin more susceptible to pressure-induced injury. **Friction** and **moisture** both cause skin breakdown, which further contribute to ulcer formation. Once an ulcer is formed, wound healing is dependent on relief of pressure, adequate nutrition, and sufficient blood flow to the affected area.

CLINICAL PRESENTATION

Identifying patients at risk for pressure ulcers is critical. Although immobility is the primary cause, other contributing factors should be identified (Table 45-1). A thorough skin examination is essential to diagnosing a pressure ulcer particularly early in its course. The untrained eye may easily miss the early signs. Since muscle and soft tissues are more susceptible than skin to ischemic injury, the only early evidence of a pressure ulcer may be skin erythema or a small ulceration accompanied by a much greater area of involvement subcutaneously. Early ulcers may be difficult to detect in darkly pigmented skin and ulcers covered by dry eschars must first be debrided so that the lesion may be properly accessed. Pressure ulcers are typically classified into stages based on severity:

- **Stage 1**: Nonblanchable erythema of intact skin, which heralds skin ulceration. In persons with darker skin, skin discoloration, warmth, edema, induration, or hardness may also be indicators.
- **Stage 2**: Partial thickness skin loss involving epidermis, dermis, or both.
- **Stage 3**: Full thickness skin loss involving damage or necrosis of subcutaneous tissue that may extend down to, but not through, underlying fascia. The ulcer presents clinically as a deep crater with or without undermining adjacent tissue.
- **Stage 4**: Full thickness skin loss with extensive destruction, tissue necrosis, or damage to muscle, bone, or supporting structures (tendon or joint capsule).

All wounds should also be evaluated for secondary infection—superficial infection, cellulitis, osteomyelitis, or bacteremia. Careful examination of the ulcer and surrounding tissues will usually reveal local infections; however, poor wound healing can be the only manifestation. Any patient with systemic signs (fever, elevated WBCs) should be evaluated for osteomyelitis and bacteremia. Every patient should also have a screening sensory examination to identify those with the additional risk factor of sensory neuropathy.

MANAGEMENT

For either prevention or management of pressure ulcers, risk factors must be initially addressed. The most essential step in management is to relieve or eliminate the causative pressure. This can be achieved by a combination of turning or **repositioning schedules** and the use of either static (pads, cushions, and foam mattress overlays) or dynamic (low air loss and air-fluidized beds) **pressure-relieving surfaces**. Patients should also undergo a thorough nutritional assessment to ensure **adequate nutrition** and wound healing.

Any urinary or fecal **incontinence** must also be addressed to ensure that the skin is not in prolonged contact with moisture.

For patients with existing pressure ulcers, aggressive wound care is necessary with the goals of preserving intact skin and preventing deeper tissue injury. An ideal dressing maintains a moist wound environment (necessary for dermal repair), keeps surrounding tissues dry, promotes granulation tissue, and prevents bacterial contamination (Table 45-2). Wound debridement is necessary as the presence of necrotic tissue will promote bacterial growth and slow wound healing. Most dressings provide either mechanical debridement or autolytic debridement (allow normal body enzymes to digest necrotic tissue) which are adequate for most patients. Vacuum-assisted closure (VAC) is an emerging technique which applies negative pressure to remove exudates in chronic, open, wounds. Patients with thick eschar or extensive necrotic tissue generally require surgical debridement.

If a wound infection is present, antibiotics active against *Staphylococcus* and *Streptococcus* should be administered. Superficial infections can generally be treated with topical antibiotics (silver sulfadiazine, bacitracin). Topical antiseptics such as hydrogen peroxide and iodine solutions are avoided because they delay wound healing. A 2-week trial of topical antibiotic therapy should be considered for nonhealing ulcers. Systemic antibiotics may be indicated if the pressure ulcer is complicated by cellulitis, osteomyelitis, or sepsis.

Table 45-2 **Dressings for Pressure Ulcers**

Dressings	Indication	Consideration
Wet-to-damp	Deep ulcers	Provides mechanical debridement, but may remove healthy granulation tissue if it dries
Hydrocolloid	Ulcers with minimal exudate	Occlusive dressing promotes autolytic debridement. Avoid if infection is present
Hydrogel	Ulcers with minimal exudate	Occlusive dressing promotes autolytic debridement and wound rehydration
Alginate	Deep ulcers with copious drainage (large cavity)	Combines with wound exudates to form a hydrophilic gel which promotes autolytic debridement and wound rehydration
VAC	Chronic, open, exudative	Effective for removing exudates

Pressure ulcers require close and regular follow-up to assure appropriate healing. While the rate of healing may vary, most stage 1 ulcers will heal within 1 week whereas stage 4 ulcers can take 6 months to 1 year. Despite adequate healing, patients who have had a pressure ulcer have recurrence rates as high as 90%. Even though the epithelial and dermal layers can be fully restored, the muscle layer never returns to normal.

MENINGITIS

Edward Cutolo

KEY POINTS

- The classic triad of meningitis is fever, nuchal rigidity, and mental status changes.
- Meningitis should be considered a medical emergency.
- Treatment should not be delayed for diagnostic studies (including lumbar puncture).
- A CT scan of the head is not needed prior to lumbar puncture unless the patient is at risk for mass lesions in the brain.

INTRODUCTION

Meningitis is defined as an **inflammation of the meninges**, which include the three membranes (dura mater, pia mater, and arachnoid) that surround the brain and spinal cord. Meningitis is often separated into categories based on the time course with acute designating symptoms which have developed over hours to days and chronic over weeks. Acute meningitis may be caused by a variety of infectious and noninfectious agents (Table 46-1). **Aseptic meningitis** is defined as occurring in patients with signs and symptoms of meningeal irritation but with negative bacteriologic cultures. Aseptic meningitis is usually caused by viral pathogens and the majority are self-limited illnesses that resolve without specific therapy. This chapter will focus on acute bacterial and viral meningitis.

PATHOPHYSIOLOGY

The predominant organisms causing acute bacterial meningitis are listed in Table 46-2. The majority of cases are caused by *Streptococcus pneumoniae*, *Neisseria meningitidis*, or *Haemophilus influenzae*, which commonly colonize

Table 46-1 **Causes of Acute Meningitis**

Viral	Bacterial	Spirochetes	Fungal	Other
Enterovirus	S. pneumoniae	Treponema	Cryptococcus	NSAIDs
HSV-2	N. meningitidis	pallidum	Histoplasmosis	TMP/SMX
HIV	H. influenzae	Borrelia	Coccidioides	Cipro-
Arbovirus	L. monocytogenes	burgdorferi		floxacin
West Nile	Group B			PCN
St. Louis	streptococcus			SLE
	Mycobacterium			
	tuberculosis			

Abbreviations: NSAIDs, nonsteroidal anti-inflammatory drugs; TMP/SMX, trimethoprim-sulfamethoxazole; SLE, systemic lupus erythematosus.

the **nasopharyngeal mucosa**. The primary mode of entry for these organisms is to invade across the epithelium and enter the bloodstream. All have polysaccharide capsules which protect against complement-mediated cell lysis and allow them to achieve a sustained high-level **bacteremia**. Bacteria then cross the blood-brain barrier and invade the meninges and subarachnoid space. Once into the central nervous system (CNS), bacterial components stimulate an inflammatory response which results in further **meningeal inflammation** and continued bacterial inoculation of the cerebrospinal fluid (CSF). Activation of neutrophils in the CSF causes increased vascular permeability and **increased intracranial pressure**. Products from both neutrophils and bacteria as well as the increase in intracranial pressure all contribute to neuronal cell death.

Table 46-2 **Major Causes of Acute Bacterial Meningitis in Different Age Groups**

2–18 Years of Age	18–60 Years of Age	>60 Years of Age
60% N. meningitidis	60% S. pneumoniae	70% S. pneumoniae
25% S. pneumoniae	20% N. meningitidis	20% L. monocytogenes
10% H. influenzae	10% H. influenzae	3–4% N. meningitidis
3–4% Group B streptococcus	6% L. monocytogenes	3–4% H. influenzae
1–2% L. monocytogenes	4% Group B streptococcus	3–4% Group B streptococcus

Bacteremic spread is the most common route of infection and mucosal colonization is the most common source. However, any nidus of bacteremia can lead to meningitis, so other sources should be considered, particularly spread from the heart (endocarditis) or urinary tract. Another mechanism involves direct invasion of the organisms from a contiguous site such as the sinuses, mastoid, contiguous soft tissue (trauma), or from medical devices such as shunts.

Certain host factors also play significant roles in the susceptibility to meningitis, mostly immunodeficiency states. Patients with asplenia, complement deficiencies, HIV, and patients on chronic immunosuppressive therapy (particularly corticosteroids) are all at higher risk to develop meningitis.

Enteroviruses are the most common cause of aseptic meningitis, but arboviruses (West Nile virus, St. Louis encephalitis virus), HIV, and herpes must also be considered. As opposed to herpes encephalitis which is caused by HSV-1 and can cause substantial morbidity and mortality, herpes meningitis is associated with a primary HSV-2 genital infection and is typically self-limited. HIV meningitis occurs with the initial viremia associated with acute infection. Similar to bacterial meningitis, most viruses initially infect mucosal surfaces, evade local defenses, and enter the bloodstream. During viremia, entry into the CNS occurs through direct invasion of cerebral capillary endothelial cells. Once in the CSF, initially a neutrophilic and then a lymphocytic inflammatory response is stimulated.

CLINICAL PRESENTATION

Most patients with acute bacterial meningitis have an associated febrile upper respiratory illness, which is most commonly nonspecific, but may include pneumonia, otitis, or mastoiditis. Common symptoms include fever, headache, vomiting, myalgias, and stiff neck. The illness can progress rapidly, with patients developing mental status changes ranging from confusion to coma within a few hours. Physical examination findings of nuchal rigidity are demonstrated by the inability or difficulty in flexing the neck touching the chin to the chest. Lateral neck movement touching the chin to the shoulders is less reliable. Two classic signs of meningeal inflammation, Brudzinski sign (involuntary flexion of the hip and knees when the neck is flexed) and Kernig sign (reluctance to completely extend the knee when the hip is flexed to a 90° angle) are limited by their low sensitivity. The classic triad of bacterial meningitis includes **fever, nuchal rigidity**, and **altered mental status**, but occurs in less than half of all patients. However, virtually all patients with meningitis (>99%) will have at least one of the symptoms. A classic sign that occurs in meningococcal meningitis and less frequently with pneumococcal meningitis is a palpable purpuric rash known as **purpura fulminans**.

Patients may present with a variety of neurologic findings depending on the duration and severity of their infection. Approximately 25% of patients will develop focal neurologic signs including hemiparesis, aphasia, gaze palsies, and visual field defects. Focal or generalized seizures may develop in another 20% of patients and can occur both early and late in the disease. Signs of increased intracranial pressure may include focal neurologic deficits, seizures, and cranial nerve palsies, especially cranial nerve III. Papilledema is uncommon in bacterial meningitis and its presence should make the clinician consider other diagnoses (brain abscess). Elevated blood pressure and brady-cardia may also suggest increased intracranial pressure and is known as the **Cushing's reflex**.

Patients with viral meningitis typically have a more nonspecific presen-tation with low-grade fever, fatigue, headache, nausea, photophobia, and stiff neck. Patients with enterovirus meningitis usually present during the summer and fall months although they can occur throughout the year. Patients commonly have symptoms of enterovirus infection, such as a mac-ulopapular rash, diarrhea, pharyngitis, or conjunctivitis. Herpes meningitis is typically associated with a primary HSV-2 genital infection and patients more frequently develop self-limited neurologic signs (e.g., urinary reten-tion, paresthesias, and motor weakness). Patients with HIV meningitis pre-sent with the classic acute HIV infection: fever, lymphadenopathy, sore throat, diarrhea, headache, nausea/vomiting, and weight loss. Last, West Nile virus meningitis should be suspected in any patient presenting with acute flaccid paralysis from a susceptible area.

EVALUATION

Suspected bacterial meningitis is a medical emergency. Effective manage-ment includes early recognition, appropriate diagnostic evaluation, and immediate therapy. Delay in the initiation of treatment due to diagnostic studies is associated with an increased risk of adverse outcomes.

The diagnosis of meningitis is ultimately made by the evaluation of the CSF from a **lumbar puncture** (see Chap. 3). Essential studies include opening pressure, cell count and differential, glucose, protein, Gram stain, and culture. The CSF findings in different causes of meningitis are listed in Table 46-3. Although acute bacterial meningitis is characterized by a high leukocyte count, a low CSF leukocyte count cannot exclude a bacterial etiology. In fact, cell counts as low as 10–20 cells/μL have been described in meningococcal meningitis. Bacterial meningitis should have a predominance of neutrophils (>80%); however, all causes of meningitis will have a neutrophil predomi-nance early in the course as monocytes usually do not appear prior to 24 hours. CSF glucose is <40 mg/dL in 50% of bacterial meningitis and is caused by inflammatory cells consuming glucose for energy. CSF protein is elevated in most cases of bacterial meningitis.

Table 46-3 **CSF Findings in Various Causes of Meningitis**

CSF	Bacterial	Viral	Tuberculosis	Cryptococcal
Opening pressure (mmH$_2$O)	200–500	<250	180–300	>200
Leukocyte count (cells/µL)	1000–5000	50–1000	50–300	20–500
Predominant cell type	Neutrophilic	Mononuclear	Mononuclear	Mononuclear
Glucose (mg/dL)	<40	>45	<45	<40
Protein	100–500	<200	50–300	>45

Identification of organisms on Gram stain is possible in 60–80% of patients with bacterial meningitis and can be used to immediately guide therapy.

- *S. pneumoniae*: gram-positive diplococci (lancet shaped)
- *H. influenzae*: gram-negative cocobacilli (rods)
- *N. meningitidis*: gram-negative diplococci (kidney bean shaped)
- *Listeria monocytogenes*: gram-positive rod

CSF culture is positive in up to 80% of patients who have not received prior antibiotic therapy, but may take up to 48 hours to grow. Latex agglutination tests have been developed to aid in the rapid diagnosis of bacterial meningitis with results usually available in <15 minutes. However, these tests should be interpreted with caution as they are neither sensitive nor specific. **Blood cultures** should be obtained in all patients although not all patients have persistent bacteremias after developing meningitis. Blood cultures are generally found to be positive in 80% of cases from *H. influenzae*, 50% from *S. pneumoniae*, and 30–40% from *N. meningitidis*.

Both enterovirus and HSV-2 can be diagnosed using polymerase chain reaction (PCR) of the CSF. In addition, CSF viral cultures are positive in approximately 80% of HSV meningitis. For suspected HIV meningitis, serum HIV antibodies and HIV RNA should be tested.

Computed tomography (CT) scan of the head is not indicated in the initial evaluation of the majority of patients presenting with suspected meningitis. Although practitioners commonly worry about an occult mass lesion which could lead to brain herniation if a lumber puncture is performed, this is a rare occurrence. A CT scan of the head should be ordered in patients who are at risk for mass lesions:

- Immunocompromised (HIV infection, immunosuppressive therapy)
- History of CNS disease (mass lesion, stroke, or focal infection)
- New-onset seizure (within 1 week of presentation)
- Papilledema
- Abnormal level of consciousness
- Focal neurologic deficit

MANAGEMENT

Bacterial meningitis is a medical emergency. A rapid but thorough evaluation is essential so appropriate antibiotic therapy is not delayed. A standard antibiotic regimen for suspected bacterial meningitis includes **ceftriaxone or cefotaxime** and **vancomycin**. The cephalosporins have excellent CSF penetration and coverage of the predominant organisms. With the increasing prevalence of penicillin (PCN)-resistant *S. pneumoniae*, vancomycin should be added to any empiric regimen. If the patient is elderly, or is on immunosuppressive therapy, then the addition of **ampicillin** is suggested to cover *L. monocytogenes*. Even if viral meningitis is suspected, many practitioners will empirically start antibiotics because of the poor sensitivity of initial CSF values. If cultures remain negative for 48 hours and the patient has clinically improved, antibiotics can generally be stopped and the patient observed. Directed therapy should be established as soon as the organism is identified:

- *S. pneumoniae* → cefotaxime or ceftriaxone for 14 days
- *S. pneumoniae* (PCN resistant) → cefotaxime or ceftriaxone + vancomycin for 14 days
- *N. meningitidis* → PCN G or ampicillin for 7 days
- *L. monocytogenes* → PCN G or ampicillin for 21 days
- *H. influenzae* → cefotaxime or ceftriaxone for 7 days
- Group B streptococcus → PCN G or ampicillin for 14–21 days

Prior to antibiotic therapy, bacterial meningitis was universally fatal. Although our current therapies have substantially improved outcomes, significant morbidity and mortality still occur. The mortality rates for *S. pneumoniae* and *L. monocytogenes* meningitis remain high (>20%), whereas for *N. meningitidis* mortality rate is low (3–5%). Approximately 25% of individuals will develop a neurologic deficit during the course and 10% will have a permanent neurologic deficit (sensorineural hearing loss, paresis, impaired cognition, or cranial nerve palsies). Neurologic outcomes are significantly worse from infection from *S. pneumoniae* compared to all other causes. Because of the essential role inflammation plays in the pathogenesis of bacterial meningitis, the addition of steroids has been suggested to reduce this mortality and morbidity. Steroids decrease the inflammatory response and may moderate the increases in intracranial pressure and neurotoxicity. **Dexamethasone** (0.15 mg/kg q 6 h for 2–4 days) starting with the first dose of antibiotics has been shown to improve outcomes in patients with meningitis from *S. pneumoniae*. Thus, dexamethasone should be given to any patient with known or suspected pneumococcal meningitis and appears to be most effective in patients with altered mental status (Glasgow coma score ≤11).

Aseptic meningitis is usually treated supportively with no specific therapy other than IV fluids and analgesia. Patients with HIV meningitis should be started on antiretroviral therapy. Although herpes meningitis is a self-limited disease and acyclovir has not been shown to alter the course, most patients with herpes meningitis are started on acyclovir, which will also treat their primary HSV genital infection.

PYELONEPHRITIS

Deborah A. Humphrey

KEY POINTS

- Pyelonephritis is a clinical diagnosis based on the presence of fever, flank pain, and pyuria.
- Most cases are caused by *E. coli* or other gram-negative enterics.
- Early diagnosis and treatment are essential to preventing life-threatening complications.

INTRODUCTION

Acute pyelonephritis is typically a bacterial infection of the kidney and renal pelvis. In the United States, approximately 200,000 adults are admitted to the hospital for this renal infection. It is a clinical diagnosis based on characteristic symptoms, physical findings, and supporting laboratory data. Important definitions in the discussion of pyelonephritis include:

- **Uncomplicated pyelonephritis** is limited to the nonimmunocompromised and nonpregnant patient.
- **Complicated pyelonephritis** is defined by the presence of any of the following conditions: immunocompromised state, pregnancy, male gender, presence of a urinary catheter, and urologic anatomic abnormality such as obstruction (e.g., renal calculi), vesicoureteral reflux, and neurogenic bladder.

PATHOPHYSIOLOGY

Pyelonephritis is an upper urinary tract infection (UTI) involving the kidney and renal pelvis. It can be subdivided into complicated and uncomplicated depending on underlying urologic or medical conditions that predispose the kidney to infection. Almost all cases of acute pyelonephritis arise from an **ascending route of infection**. Most UTIs occur from colonization of the urine by fecal bacteria that grow aerobically. Bacteria enter the urethra, colonize the bladder, then travel through the ureters to the renal pelvis and invade the renal parenchyma.

Anaerobic bacteria that colonize the urine indicate a communication between the urinary tract and the intestinal tract. This can occur via fistula formation after a reconstructive surgery or with abscess formation. Fungi in the urine can occur in patients with bladder catheters or immunocompromised patients.

Risk Factors for UTI and Subsequent Pyelonephritis

- **Female sex**: The urethra in a woman is short and will allow bacteria to enter the bladder.
- **Sexual intercourse**: Sexual intercourse will result in an increase in the number of bacteria in the periurethral area as well as the distal urethra thereby increasing the risk of bacteriuria. Postcoital voiding will decrease this risk.
- **History of UTIs**: Recurrent UTIs may be due to poor hygiene, anatomic abnormality, vesicoureteral reflux, or an undiagnosed metabolic disorder such as diabetes.
- **Spermicide-diaphragm contraception**: There is a documented increase in number of UTIs with use of this type of contraception. This may be due to the mechanical obstruction of the outflow of urine by the diaphragm.
- **Postmenopausal state**: Atrophic vaginal mucosa will alter vaginal flora thereby increasing the chance of colonization of the urine with bacteria.
- **Bladder catheters**: Most patients who have had a bladder catheter for >1 week will develop bacteriuria or funguria. Essentially, all patients with a chronic catheter will develop bacteriuria and need treatment only if they become symptomatic.
- **Pregnancy**: Risk of UTI in pregnancy is higher due to multiple factors such progesterone-mediated decrease in ureteral peristalsis and direct uterine pressure.

The microorganisms responsible for uncomplicated pyelonephritis are similar to those causing an uncomplicated cystitis. Nearly **80% will be** *Escherichia coli*. The remaining organisms include other gram negatives such as *Klebsiella* and *Proteus* sp. Other organisms include the gram-positive *Staphylococcus saprophyticus* (10–15% of pyelonephritis in young women), *Enterococcus* species (common in older men with urologic problems), and on occasion group B streptococci or other streptococci.

The usual culprit of complicated pyelonephritis is also *E. coli*, however, it is typically a less virulent strain. Other Enterobacteriaceae, particularly

Klebsiella, *Proteus*, and *Enterobacter*, are identified as the causative agent in most of the remaining cases and are more frequently encountered in urologic manipulation or obstruction. *Proteus* and *Klebsiella* also contribute to the formation of and reinfection from renal calculi. *Pseudomonas* plays an important role in recurrent infections and complicated pyelonephritis, particularly when a urinary catheter is present. Gram positives such as *Staphylococcus aureus* and *Enterococcus* are occasionally isolated as causative organisms and are more common in complicated pyelonephritis. The presence of *S. aureus* in the urine should raise the suspicion of hematogenous spread to the kidney.

CLINICAL PRESENTATION

The presenting symptoms of an acute pyelonephritis vary widely depending on the characteristics of the host and offending organism. A classic history for pyelonephritis would include several days of increasing **flank pain** associated with **fever and chills**, malaise, and generalized weakness. Patients will often have nausea and vomiting. The patient may or may not have suprapubic tenderness, dysuria, and frequency. Patients with bacteremia will have symptoms consistent with gram-negative sepsis (e.g., tachycardia, hypotension, mental status changes, and oliguria).

The patient typically appears ill and in mild to moderate generalized distress from pain. There is usually fever, tachycardia, tachypnea, and possibly, hypotension. The mucous membranes will likely be dry. Mild to moderate abdominal and suprapubic tenderness may be present as well as the classic tenderness to palpation or percussion over the costovertebral angles.

EVALUATION

- **Urinalysis: Pyuria** (>10 leukocytes/mL urine) and RBCs are usually present. Leukocyte casts are sometimes found in the urine sediment and nearly pathognomonic for pyelonephritis. If hematuria persists after the acute infection, stone, tumor, or tuberculosis should be suspected.
- **Urine culture:** Typically, urine culture is positive although 20% will have <10^5 colony forming unit (CFU)/mL.
- **Gram stain:** Significant bacteriuria is the presence of **>100,000 bacteria/mL of urine**; counts <100,000 bacteria/mL may represent contamination. Bacterial rods or chains of cocci are common and most cases reveal gram-negative rods or bacilli.
- **Complete blood count:** Leukocyte count is typically elevated with a predominance of polymorphonuclear cells (PMNs). Band forms may be seen.

- **Electrolytes and renal function:** There may be evidence of prerenal azotemia if the patient has had prolonged emesis but are typically normal at least in the acute phase.
- **Blood cultures:** All patients suspected of having pyelonephritis should have two sets of blood cultures as 20% of patients will have positive blood cultures.

Imaging studies are not used to establish the diagnosis of pyelonephritis, but are indicated when complications are suspected (see "Management," below). Ultrasound may reveal enlarged kidneys due to inflammation and is useful to assess collecting system obstruction.

MANAGEMENT

If the patient is not pregnant or immunocompromised as well as hemodynamically stable and able to tolerate oral hydration and antibiotics, outpatient management is preferred (see Chap. 39 in the *First Exposure to Internal Medicine: Ambulatory Medicine*). Inpatient management of pyelonephritis involves aggressive fluid resuscitation with normal saline and intravenous antibiotics immediately after the urine and blood cultures are drawn. The choice of antibiotic is somewhat empiric as the results of cultures will not be available for several days (Table 47-1). All patients should receive an antibiotic with activity against the common gram-negative bacilli. Gram-positive organisms and drug-resistant gram-negative organisms should be anticipated in those patients with complicated UTIs or those who have recent

Table 47-1 **Antibiotic Regimens for Pyelonephritis**

	General	Antibiotic	Duration
Uncomplicated pyelonephritis	If require hospitalization (see above)	Gentamicin ± ampicillin, parenteral quinolone, ceftriaxone, or aztreonam	14 days
Complicated pyelonephritis	Identify and/or remove any possible reversible predisposing factor (e.g., catheter)	As above, may require: piperacillin/tazobactam, ticarcillin/clavulanate, or imipenem-cilastatin	14–21 days
Pregnancy	Ceftriaxone or cefazolin. Critical illness or resistant organisms: add gentamicin or aztreonam		

antimicrobial therapy. There have been very few large treatment trials for acute pyelonephritis and so much of the advice on antimicrobial choice is based on anecdotal experience, extrapolation from animal models, or pharmacokinetic studies.

After defervescence, begin an oral fluoroquinolone, cephalosporin, or trimethoprim-sulfamethoxazole. Other issues to consider before conversion to oral antimicrobials are:

- The patient is no longer severely ill or unstable.
- The patient is able to tolerate fluids by mouth.
- The patient's gut is functioning properly.
- There is an appropriate oral agent available based on the culture and sensitivity results that is not otherwise contraindicated by patient allergies, drug-drug interactions, or potential for fetal toxicity.

The majority of patients with pyelonephritis will have significant clinical improvement within the initial 48 hours of treatment. It is common for patients to continue to spike fevers for several days after initiation of appropriate antimicrobial therapy. However, patients who fail to show signs of improvement within this time frame require re-evaluation with imaging with computed tomography (CT) scan for urgent surgical complications. A **renal abscess** is a collection of purulent material within the renal parenchyma, whereas a **perinephric abscess** is a collection in the soft tissues surrounding the kidneys. Perinephric abscesses are particularly concerning, because they carry up to a 50% mortality rate. Both require immediate drainage. **Papillary necrosis** can occur with infection of the renal pyramids, usually in patients with vascular disease, diabetes, or alcoholism. Sloughing of the papilla is often bilateral and may be heralded by flank pain, hematuria, and sudden deterioration in renal function. **Emphysematous pyelonephritis** is an acute necrotizing parenchymal and perirenal infection due to gas-forming pathogens. *E. coli* is the most common organism. It is more common in diabetic and female patients. The overall mortality rate is about 40%. Diagnosis is established by the finding of gas within the renal parenchyma on plain x-ray of the abdomen. **Septic shock** (commonly referred to as **urosepsis**) is a life-threatening complication (mortality rate >30%) resulting from disseminated bacteria into the bloodstream (see Chap. 49).

INFECTIVE
ENDOCARDITIS

Craig J. Hoesley
Ritu A. Kumar

KEY POINTS

- IE is infection of the heart's endocardial surface.
- IE should be suspected in patients with unexplained febrile illness especially in those with valvular heart disease.
- The Duke criteria include blood culture results and echocardiographic findings as major criteria for diagnosing IE.
- TEE is preferred to TTE for detecting vegetations.
- CHF is the major indication for surgical management of IE.

INTRODUCTION

The term infective endocarditis (IE) denotes bacterial infection of the heart's endocardial surface. The heart valves are affected more commonly in this disorder, but the septum or mural endocardium can also be involved. The incidence of IE is difficult to determine, but is approximately 3.6 per 100,000 population per year. IE can be characterized using various classifications including the duration of symptoms (e.g., acute or subacute), the microbial etiology, the anatomic involvement (e.g., right-sided, left-sided, or the specific valve or valves impacted), or even the type of valve (e.g., native or prosthetic).

The microorganisms implicated in native valve endocarditis are most commonly streptococci (**viridans streptococci** being the most prevalent), staphylococci (particularly *Staphylococcus aureus*), and **enterococci**. The incidence of *S. aureus* endocarditis has been increasing over the last several decades and is now the most common etiology. Approximately one-quarter of community-acquired *S. aureus* bacteremia will result in endocarditis, so patients with multiple positive blood cultures should be evaluated for endocarditis. Viridans streptococci, found in the oropharyngeal flora, remain the most common streptococci to cause endocarditis. *Streptococcus bovis* is common in the elderly and is frequently associated with colonic adenocarcinoma. The microbial etiology of prosthetic valve endocarditis may be considered in two time frames: early (<2 months postvalve replacement surgery) and late (≥2 months postvalve replacement surgery). In the "early" period, coagulase-negative staphylococci are a common etiology. In the "late" period, the causative microorganisms are similar to those implicated in native valve endocarditis. Gram-negative bacteria and yeast are uncommon, but difficult to treat, causes of native or prosthetic valve IE. Injection drug users are at high risk for IE, particularly involving the tricuspid valve; *S. aureus* is the most common etiology, but this is a scenario where gram-negative pathogens and yeast may be noted. Although now uncommon, the HACEK group of bacteria are classically associated with endocarditis (*Haemophilus* species [*aphrophilus, parainfluenzae, and paraphrophilus*], *Actinobacillus actinomycetemcomitans, Cardiobacterium hominis, Eikenella corrodens*, and *Kingella kingae*).

PATHOPHYSIOLOGY

The normal endocardial surface of the heart is resistant to infection by all but the most virulent of organisms (*S. aureus*). Most endocarditis begins with damage to the endocardial surface which may lead to direct bacterial invasion or more commonly to the formation of a thrombus. Sites of **endocardial injury** are adhered to by **platelets and fibrin**, which form a sterile vegetation, also known as nonbacterial thrombotic endocarditis. This platelet-fibrin material is a favorable site for bacterial attachment and colonization, so any concomitant **bacteremia** will rapidly result in colonization of the vegetation. The presence of bacteria encourages further platelet and fibrin deposition which provide further sites for bacterial colonization. This circular process continues until a macroscopic vegetation forms housing dense pockets of bacteria. Organisms deep in vegetations are not metabolically active and are relatively resistant to most antimicrobial agents, whereas those close to the surface are continually dividing and being shed into the bloodstream. Once bacteria enter the bloodstream, they can be cleared by the reticuloendothelial system, be deposited in other areas of damaged endocardium, or form septic emboli.

Vegetations have a tendency to occur in areas with the greatest turbulent blood flow (in relation to the greatest endocardial damage). For most valvular diseases, this will be on the valvular side corresponding to the direction of abnormal blood flow. For example, patients with mitral regurgitation develop vegetations on the atrial surface of the mitral valve or on the atrial wall where the regurgitant jet strikes, whereas patients with aortic insufficiency develop vegetations on the ventricular surface of the aortic valve or the chordae tendineae of the mitral valve (the site typically struck by the regurgitant jet). The degree of mechanical stress exerted on the valve also affects the location of IE; thus, the incidence of valvular lesions from most to least common is mitral, aortic, tricuspid, and pulmonic valves.

Bacterial proliferation in the endocardium stimulates both humoral and cell-mediated immunity. Cytokine production results in the systemic manifestations of endocarditis (fever, fatigue, malaise). The constant release of bacteria (antigen) into the bloodstream stimulates a wide proliferation of antibodies including rheumatoid factor (IgM antibody to IgG). Thus, all patients develop circulating immune complexes which can deposit in various tissues resulting in chronic glomerulonephritis, Osler nodes, and Roth spots.

CLINICAL MANIFESTATIONS

No typical presentation exists for IE and clinicians should have a high index of suspicion for the disease. Most patients have risk factors, either cardiac abnormalities (underlying **structural heart disease** or **prosthetic valve**) or **bacteremia** (indwelling intravascular catheters or intravenous drug abuse). The most common complaints are nonspecific systemic symptoms—fever, chills, malaise, weight loss, and myalgias. Patients with suspected endocarditis should also be asked about symptoms related to the complications of endocarditis (Table 48-1). Congestive heart failure (CHF) is a common complication of acute valvular insufficiency and the most common cause of death related to endocarditis. The most common neurologic complication is stroke. Right-sided IE can mimic pneumonia, so respiratory symptoms such as cough and dyspnea may predominate.

The physical examination should include a careful cardiac examination for signs of new regurgitant murmurs or CHF. A careful skin and eye examination is essential to detect several classical stigmata of endocarditis. Petechiae are the most common skin manifestation, but are not specific for IE. They may be present on the skin, usually on the extremities, or on mucous membranes such as the palate or conjunctivae. Splinter hemorrhages are nonblanching, linear reddish-brown lesions found under the nail bed. They are also not specific to IE as they are common in the elderly and with occupation-associated trauma. Several findings are more specific for IE, but occur in <25% of patients. **Janeway lesions** are macular, blanching, painless, erythematous lesions on the palms and soles (Fig. 48-2). By contrast, **Osler nodes** are painful, violaceous nodules found in the pulp of fingers and toes and are seen more often in subacute than acute cases of IE (Fig. 48-1). **Roth spots** are retinal hemorrhages with a pale white of yellow center usually located around the optic disc. Patients with IE may also demonstrate

Table 48-1 **Complications of Endocarditis**

Local invasion	Valve ring abscess (particularly with prosthetic valves)
	Heart block (if abscess affects the conduction system)
	Valvular insufficiency (commonly leading to CHF)
	Myocardial abscess
Embolic	Stroke
	Cutaneous infarction
	Pulmonary emboli (right-sided endocarditis)
	Renal infarction
	Splenic infarction
Metastatic abscess	Septic arthritis
	Vertebral osteomyelitis
	Osteomyelitis
	Epidural abscess
	Renal abscess
Immune complex	Glomerulonephritis
	Arthritis

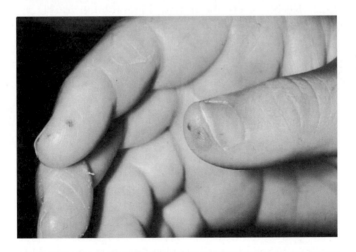

Figure 48-1 **Osler nodes.** *(Courtesy of the Armed Forces Institute of Pathology, Bethesda, MD.) (Source:* Reproduced with permission from Knoop KJ, Stack LB, Storrow AB. *Atlas of Emergency Medicine,* 2nd ed. New York: McGraw-Hill, 2002, Figure 13-9.)

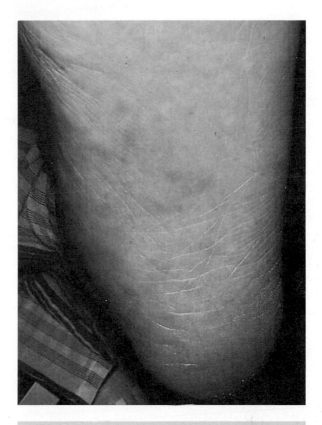

Figure 48-2 **Janeway lesions.** *(Courtesy of the Department of Dermatology, Wilford Hall USAF Medical Center and Brooke Army Medical Center, San Antonio, TX.)* (*Source:* Reproduced with permission from Knoop KJ, Stack LB, Storrow AB. *Atlas of Emergency Medicine*, 2nd ed. New York: McGraw-Hill, 2002, Figure 13-8.)

a wide variety of findings consistent with embolic phenomenon, including focal neurologic deficits, abdominal pain (due to mesenteric ischemia or splenomegaly), and signs consistent with renal insufficiency or pulmonary involvement.

EVALUATION

A definitive diagnosis of endocarditis can be made by the culture of organisms directly from the valve or endocardial surface. As this is rarely recommended, the diagnosis of endocarditis is usually based on the patient's clinical presentation.

The diagnosis can be made with the presence of persistent bacteremia in the absence of another source and a predisposing cardiac abnormality. One of the most widely used clinical criteria is the **Duke criteria** (Table 48-2). Classification as **definite** IE requires two major criteria, one major and three minor criteria, or five minor criteria. Classification as **possible** IE requires one major criterion and 1 minor criterion or 3 minor criteria.

The most essential step in diagnosis is obtaining at least **three sets of blood cultures**. Blood cultures should always be obtained prior to beginning antibiotic therapy, because the bacteremia is usually low grade and can be masked by antibiotics. In most patients, one of the first two blood cultures will be positive; however, patients who have received prior antibiotics may require multiple blood cultures to detect an organism. Patients who clinically have endocarditis but who are culture-negative may have endocarditis secondary to fastidious bacteria. These organisms account for <5% of all confirmed IE cases. Diagnosis of these microorganisms often requires special

Table 48-2 **The Modified Duke Criteria for the Diagnosis of IE**

Major	1.	Positive blood culture
		a. Typical microorganisms: viridans streptococci, *S. bovis*, HACEK group, community-acquired *S. aureus*, or community-acquired Enterococci
		b. Persistently positive blood culture
		Blood cultures drawn more than 12 h apart
		All of 3, or majority of 4 or more separate blood cultures, with first and last drawn at least 1 h apart
		c. Single positive blood culture for *C. burnetii* or antiphase 1 IgG antibody titer >1:800
	2.	Evidence of endocardial involvement
		a. Positive echocardiogram for IE
		Oscillating intracardiac mass
		Abscess
		New partial dehiscence of prosthetic valve
		b. New valvular regurgitation
Minor	1.	Predisposing heart condition or intravenous drug abusers (IVDA)
	2.	Fever ≥38°C
	3.	Vascular phenomenon: arterial emboli, septic pulmonary infarcts, mycotic aneurysm, intracranial hemorrhage, or Janeway lesions
	4.	Immunologic phenomenon: glomerulonephritis, Osler nodes, Roth spots, or rheumatoid factor
	5.	Positive blood culture but not meeting major criterion above, or serologic evidence of active infection with organism consistent with IE

techniques, most commonly prolonged incubation (3–4 weeks) of blood cultures for the HACEK organisms or specialized culture media and serology for *Coxiella burnetii* and *Bartonella* species.

Echocardiogram should be used to evaluate patients with a moderate to high suspicion of endocarditis, such as persistent bacteremia without a known source, peripheral stigmata consistent with endocarditis, or a high clinical suspicion despite negative cultures. Debate still exists regarding whether a transthoracic (TTE) or transesophageal (TEE) echocardiogram should be obtained first. Both tests have a high specificity, but the sensitivity for transthoracic is ~50% compared to ~90% for transesophageal. This must be balanced with the simplicity of a transthoracic approach compared to the relative invasiveness of a transesophageal procedure. Patients without cardiac risk factors can be initially evaluated with a TTE. By detecting the presence of vegetations on an endocardial or valvular surface, the TTE may confirm the diagnosis of endocarditis. Although a negative study (no vegetations) does not preclude the diagnosis, the finding of normal valves (both morphology and function) substantially reduces the probability of IE. Patients with a high clinical suspicion of endocarditis, prosthetic heart valves, congenital heart disease, prior endocarditis, or new cardiac findings (murmur, CHF) should generally be evaluated first with TEE. In addition, TEE is particularly useful in detecting the presence of a perivalvular abscess and in the assessment of embolic risk. Some studies have also suggested that TEE should be performed in the evaluation of all patients with *S. aureus* bacteremia.

The remainder of the workup is used to provide supportive evidence for endocarditis or to evaluate for complications (Table 48-1). A complete blood count with differential should be obtained as most patients with subacute endocarditis have anemia of chronic disease. The white blood cell count is a poor indicator of endocarditis, but is typically elevated with acute *S. aureus* endocarditis. A urinalysis and renal function will provide evidence of glomerulonephritis or septic emboli. Realize that most individuals with endocarditis will have microscopic hematuria or mild proteinuria, so these findings alone do not suggest glomerulonephritis. A chest x-ray should be obtained to evaluate for septic emboli, CHF, or signs of right-sided endocarditis (pleural effusions, consolidation, atelectasis). Many clinicians will order an erythrocyte sedimentation rate and C-reactive protein. They are general markers of inflammation and not specific for endocarditis, but are typically elevated. Approximately half of all patients will also have a positive rheumatoid factor, which will disappear with successful treatment.

MANAGEMENT

Medical management of patients with IE includes prolonged administration of intravenous antibiotics (Table 48-3). In general, antibiotics with bactericidal properties (e.g., penicillins and cephalosporins) are preferred in the

Table 48-3 **Recommended Antibiotic Therapy for IE**

	Treatment of Native Valve	**Treatment of Prosthetic Valve**
Streptococci	Penicillin plus low-dose gentamicin for 2 weeks or penicillin for 4 weeks	Penicillin for 6 weeks, plus low-dose gentamicin for first 2 weeks
MSSA	Nafcillin for 4–6 weeks plus low-dose gentamicin for first 3–5 days	Nafcillin with rifampin for 6 weeks plus low-dose gentamicin for first 2 weeks
MRSA	Vancomycin for 4–6 weeks plus low-dose gentamicin for first 3–5 days	Vancomycin with rifampin for 6 weeks plus low-dose gentamicin for first 2 weeks
Enterococci	Penicillin plus low-dose gentamicin for 4–6 weeks	Penicillin plus low-dose gentamicin for 4–6 weeks
HACEK	Ceftriaxone for 4 weeks	Ceftriaxone for 6 weeks

Abbreviations: MSSA, methicillin-susceptible *Staphylococcus aureus*; MRSA, methicillin-resistant *Staphylococcus aureus*.

treatment of IE. Frequently, the addition of an aminoglycoside (e.g., gentamicin) is also recommended in an effort to provide a synergistic effect. Clinicians should document clearance of bacteria from the blood by surveying blood cultures on appropriate antibiotic therapy.

Despite antimicrobial therapy, valve replacement surgery may be necessary in some IE patients. Surgical indications include: CHF, perivalvular extension of infection (abscess), persistently positive blood cultures despite appropriate antibiotic therapy, and IE caused by microorganisms known to be difficult to treat (fungi). CHF is the most common reason for surgery, because it has a high risk of death that exceeds the risks of immediate surgery. Large vegetations increase the risk of emboli and are often not effectively treated with antimicrobial therapy. Therefore, patients who experience two major embolic events or one major embolic event in the presence of a large mobile vegetation should also be considered for surgery.

PREVENTION

As bacteremia is necessary to develop IE, certain individuals with predisposing heart conditions should receive antibiotic prophylaxis prior to certain medical procedures with a high incidence of transient bacteremia. Persons who are considered at high risk for IE include individuals with prosthetic valves, a prior episode of IE, congenital heart disease, and surgically constructed

Table 48-4 **Antimicrobial Prophylaxis for IE**

Dental, Oral, Respiratory, and Esophageal Procedures	
Oral (1 h prior)	Amoxicillin 2 g
	Clindamycin 600 mg (if penicillin allergic)
	Cephalexin 2 g
	Azithromycin 500 mg
	Clarithromycin 500 mg
Intravenous (30 min prior)	Ampicillin 2 g
	Clindamycin 600 mg
	Cefazolin 1 g

Genitourinary or Gastrointestinal Procedures	
High risk	Ampicillin 2 g IV/IM + gentamicin 1.5 mg/kg IM/IV
	Vancomycin 1 g IV + gentamicin 1.5 mg/kg
Moderate risk	Amoxicillin 2 g PO
	Ampicillin 2 g IM/IV
	Vancomycin 1 g IV

systemic-pulmonary shunts. Individuals at moderate risk include those with congenital heart disease (except for isolated atrial septal defect), acquired valvular disease, hypertrophic cardiomyopathy, and mitral valve prolapse with regurgitation. Patients with mitral valve prolapse without regurgitation are not considered to be at risk for IE. Procedures where prophylaxis is recommended include those dental, respiratory, gastrointestinal, and genitourinary procedures during which the mucosa is traumatized or penetrated. Oral and dental procedures, such as tooth extractions, periodontal surgery, and dental prophylaxis (i.e., cleaning of teeth and removal of tartar) are associated with the highest risk with an incidence of transient bacteremia approaching 50%. The risk of bacteremia is significantly lower for invasive respiratory, genitourinary, and gastrointestinal procedures such as rigid bronchoscopy, cystoscopy, prostatectomy, endoscopy with biopsy, or endoscopic retrograde cholangiopancreatography. Antibiotic prophylaxis options are discussed in Table 48-4.

SEPSIS AND SYSTEMIC INFLAMMATORY RESPONSE SYNDROME

Andrew Bernard
Paul Kearney

KEY POINTS

- The patient's uncontrolled inflammatory response is more often the cause of morbidity than the event triggering SIRS (infection, pancreatitis, and so forth).
- SIRS + infection = sepsis.
- Source control is the primary goal.
- Maintaining tissue oxygenation is an important goal of therapy, accomplished by vigorous fluid resuscitation, vasopressors, red blood cell transfusions, and sometimes inotropic agents.
- Mortality is determined by underlying illness, site and type of insult, organ failure, severity and duration of SIRS, and response to therapy.

INTRODUCTION

Systemic inflammatory response syndrome (SIRS) describes a complex physiologic response to activation of the innate immune system, regardless of cause. Sepsis is defined as SIRS plus infection. Some degree of SIRS affects 40–80% of patients in the ICU while one-fourth of those patients go on to develop sepsis. Diagnostic criteria for SIRS have been established and evidence-based guidelines for the treatment of sepsis have been published, making identification and treatment of SIRS and sepsis more straightforward for the clinician than ever before. Despite these refinements, mortality rates remain high, approximately 60% for septic shock.

PATHOPHYSIOLOGY

Inflammation is intended to be a local or contained response to injury or infection. The local inflammatory response (adherence, chemotaxis, phago-cytosis, bacterial killing) is highly regulated at many levels, but especially by the **production of cytokines** by macrophages. SIRS occurs from excessive and unrestrained triggering of the normal but usually locally contained inflammatory response, incited by infection or other initiating insults. Details of this complex dysregulation are beyond the scope of this text. The basic concept is that the inciting event (infection, pancreatitis, and so forth) is less the cause of morbidity than the patient's uncontrolled inflammatory response. In general, the toxic stimulus activates macrophages, which produce cytokines (such as tumor necrosis factor [TNF] and interleukin [IL]-1). Activation of neutrophils then occurs, resulting in adhesion onto endothelial cells, aggregation and microthrombus formation, and the further production of cytokines which cause alteration of the microvascular wall. The end result is **microvascular injury**, impaired tissue oxygenation and **ischemia**, and finally **end-organ dysfunction**.

Bacteria can initiate SIRS in a variety of ways. Endotoxin, a lipopolysaccharide found in the cell wall of gram-negative bacteria, can trigger the production of vasoactive products (such as bradykinin) which can enhance endothelial permeability. Endotoxin also activates the coagulation and fibri-nolytic systems, disrupting the normal coagulation/lysis equilibrium, leading to microvascular thrombosis. Other inciting products include cell wall components of gram-positive bacteria (e.g., peptidoglycan and lipoteichoic acid), staphylococcal enterotoxin B, toxic shock syndrome toxin-1, *Pseudomonas* A, and the M protein of hemolytic group A streptococcus.

Systemic inflammation can result from any type of **infection**: viral, parasitic, bacterial, or fungal. Noninfectious etiologies include **trauma, burns, pancreatitis**, major blood loss such as occurs during major surgery or gastrointestinal bleeding, hepatic failure, and intracranial hemorrhage.

CLINICAL PRESENTATION

Signs of sepsis include the abrupt onset of fever, chills, tachycardia, tachyp-nea, and altered mental status. However, in some conditions, symptoms develop gradually over days, reaching a threshold in which severe illness manifests. Classically, skin may be warm ("warm shock") in early sepsis, reflecting massive systemic vasodilation. Later, skin becomes cool secondary to vasoconstriction, due to redirection of blood flow to core organs. Hypotension may occur in septic shock, from a loss of plasma volume into the interstitial space, decrease in vascular tone, and myocardial depression. Cutaneous signs include ischemic necrosis of peripheral tissue (fingers, toes). Purpuric lesions suggest meningococcemia, or in the summer with tick exposure, Rocky Mountain spotted fever. A bullous lesion surrounded by edema that undergoes central hemorrhage and necrosis is characteristic of *Pseudomonas* (ecthyma gangrenosum). Generalized erythroderma suggests toxic shock syndrome.

EVALUATION

Systemic inflammatory response syndrome is difficult to define clinically as it may have a variety of presentations and manifestations depending on the intensity of the inflammatory response and the presence of underlying conditions. Instead of precise criteria, most experts advocate for the recognition of the diverse signs and symptoms suggestive of SIRS and sepsis. For example, the parameters suggestive of sepsis reflect the body's variable response to infection:

1. Infection:
   - Documented or suspected and some of the following:
2. General parameters:
   - Fever >38.3°C
   - Hypothermia <36°C
   - Heart rate >90 or >2 SD above normal for age
   - Tachypnea >32/minute
   - Altered mental status
   - Significant edema, or positive fluid balance >20 mL/kg for 24 hours
   - Hyperglycemia (>110 mg/dL) in the absence of diabetes
3. Inflammatory parameters:
   - Leukocytosis (WBC >12,000/μL)
   - Leukopenia (WBC <4000/μL)
   - Normal WBC with >10% immature forms
   - Plasma C-reactive protein >2 SD above normal
   - Plasma procalcitonin >2 SD above normal
4. Hemodynamic parameters:
   - Arterial hypotension (systolic blood pressure [SBP] <90 mmHg, mean arterial pressure [MAP] <70 mmHg, SBP decrease >40 mmHg, SBP <2 SD below normal for age)
   - Mixed venous oxygen saturation (SvO_2) <70%
   - Cardiac index >3.5 L/min/m^2 body surface
   - Organ dysfunction:
     a. Pulmonary: PaO_2/FIO_2 <300
     b. Renal: acute oliguria (urine output [UOP] <0.5 mL/kg/h) or creatinine increase >0.5 mg/dL

    c. Coagulation: international normalized ratio (INR) >1.5 or partial thromboplastin time (PTT) >60

    d. Gastrointestinal: ileus

    e. Hematologic: thrombocytopenia (platelets <100,000/μL)

    f. Hepatic: total bilirubin >4 mg/dL

5. Tissue perfusion parameters:
   - Serum lactate >3 mmol/L
   - Decreased capillary refill/mottling

MANAGEMENT

Details of the comprehensive management of sepsis are beyond the scope of this textbook, but can be found and updated at: www.survivingsepsis.org. In general, initial resuscitation efforts should include **vigorous hydration with either colloid or crystalloids**, achieving a central venous pressure (CVP) of 8–12 mmHg, MAP ≥65 mmHg, UOP >0.5 mL/kg/h, and a mixed venous oxygen saturation ≥70% (see Chap. 4). As soon as possible, every septic patient should be evaluated for foci of infection amenable to **source control** (removal or drainage). In particular, vascular access devices suspected of infection should be removed as soon as alternative access is established. Cultures should be obtained before antibiotics are administered if possible. Blood cultures should always include at least two sets (one peripheral and one from each vascular access device). Additional cultures (e.g., lung, cerebrospinal fluid [CSF], and wound) should be obtained as clinically indicated. Antimicrobial therapy directed at the suspected organism should be started within 1 hour of diagnosis. However, antibiotics should be stopped if the process is discovered to be noninfectious SIRS. Vasopressor therapy may be required for patients who respond inadequately to adequate volume resuscitation. **Dopamine** and **norepinephrine** are first-line agents. Vasopressin is an alternative in patients who respond inadequately to first-line agents. If blood pressure remains low, inotropic therapy (dobutamine) should be combined with vasopressor therapy to increase cardiac output. IV hydrocortisone may be indicated in adequately volume-loaded patients on vasopressor therapy who remain in septic shock. Recombinant Human Activated Protein C (rhAPC; Xigris) is indicated in some patients with sepsis-induced organ failure or at high risk of death. Other therapies which should be considered include red blood cell and platelet transfusions, mechanical ventilation, tight glucose control in diabetics, and stress ulcer/deep vein thrombosis (DVT) prophylaxis.

    Predictors of mortality from SIRS and sepsis include the patient's underlying illness/comorbidity, type and extent of insult, response to therapy (including physiologic and biochemical markers), and degree of organ dysfunction.

INPATIENT ANTIBIOTIC CHOICE

Asha Ramsakal

SELECTION OF EMPIRIC ANTIBIOTICS

Most patients who present to the hospital with a known or presumed bacterial infection require empiric antibiotic therapy. Seldom do physicians initially know what bacteria are causing their infection. This requires a rational targeted approach to antimicrobial therapy beginning with broad coverage, which can be narrowed when culture results definitively identify an organism. When deciding on an empiric antibiotic regimen, a few basic considerations should be made:

1. **What are the most likely bacteria?** Consider broad categories such as gram positive (G+), gram negative (G–), or anaerobe.
2. **Where is the infection?** Antibiotics differ in the concentration which develops in different body spaces. For example, some antibiotics have poor penetration of the blood-brain barrier and should not be used if meningitis is suspected.
3. **How common are resistant organisms?** Resistance to a wide range of antibiotics is common among bacteria. Careful consideration of local resistance patterns is necessary when deciding on antimicrobial therapy.
4. **Does the patient have any comorbidities?** Antibiotics metabolized by the kidneys or liver may need to have dosage adjustments or may not be recommended. If the patient is pregnant, some antibiotics are contraindicated.
5. **What is the narrowest spectrum of effective antibiotics?** Because of the growing problem of resistance, if two antibiotics would both be effective for a patient's infection always choose the one with the narrowest spectrum (see Table 50-1).

Table 50-1 **Recommended Antibiotics for Particular Bacteria**

Bacteria	Antibiotic
C. difficile	Metronidazole
	Vancomycin
E. faecalis	Ampicillin ± gentamicin
	Vancomycin ± gentamicin
	Linezolid
E. faecium	Quinupristin/dalfopristin
	Linezolid
"HACEK"—Haemophilus, Actinobacillus, Cardiobacterium, Eikenella, and Kingella	Ceftriaxone or cefotaxime
Legionella pneumophila	Levofloxacin, gatifloxacin, or moxifloxacin
	Azithromycin
L. monocytogenes	Ampicillin
	TMP/SMX
Mycoplasma pneumoniae	Azithromycin or clarithromycin
	Levofloxacin, gatifloxacin, or moxifloxacin
N. meningitidis	PCN G
	Ceftriaxone, cefuroxime, or cefotaxime
P. jiroveci	TMP/SMX ± prednisone
	Pentamidine
	Clindamycin + primaquine
P. aeruginosa	Piperacillin or ticarcillin
	Imipenem or meropenem
	Ceftazidime, cefoperazone, or cefepime
	Tobramycin
	Ciprofloxacin
	(use β-lactam + tobra or Cipro for serious infections)
S. aureus (MRSA) serious infection	Vancomycin
	Linezolid
S. aureus (MRSA) skin or soft tissue infection	TMP/SMX
	Doxycycline
	Clindamycin
S. aureus (MSSA)	Nafcillin or oxacillin
S. pneumoniae	PCN G or ampicillin
	Ceftriaxone, cefuroxime, or cefotaxime
S. pneumoniae (PRSP)	Vancomycin ± rifampin
	Levofloxacin or gatifloxacin or moxifloxacin
Mycobacteria	See Chap. 16 in the First Exposure to Internal Medicine: Ambulatory Medicine

β-LACTAMS

This is a large class of antibiotics which have in common a central ring structure (β-lactam nucleus) and all inhibit cell wall synthesis. Otherwise, they have variable spectrums and resistance patterns. Resistance can develop through two distinct mechanisms:

1. **β-lactamase** production entails a protease which cleaves the β-lactam ring, common with G– enteric bacteria (*Escherichia coli, Proteus*), *Hemophilus influenzae,* and *Moraxella catarrhalis.* Recently, some β-lactamase production from G– organisms has been found to be resistant to most penicillins (PCNs), cephalosporins, and aztreonam, and is not inhibited by any of the currently available β-lactamase inhibitors (clavulanate, sulbactam, and tazobactam). Certain bacteria are known to have inducible production and are recognized under the mnemonic SPACE (Serratia, Pseudomonas, Acinetobacter, Citrobacter, and Enterobacter). Because of their inducible resistance, many physicians will cover these organisms with two antibiotics. *E. coli* and *Klebsiella* have also been found to produce a similar β-lactamase usually termed extended-spectrum β-lactamase (ESBL).
2. **Alteration of penicillin-binding proteins (PBPs)** which have a reduced affinity for β-lactams, common with *Staphylococcus* (methicillin-resistant *S. aureus* [MRSA]), *Streptococcus pneumoniae* (penicillin-resistant *S. pneumoniae* [PRSP]), and *Enterococcus.*

Penicillins

This is a group of antibiotics which have broad coverage of G+, G–, and anaerobic bacteria. PCNs cannot be used to cover atypical organisms (*Mycoplasma, Chlamydia,* and *Legionella*). PCNs have good penetration of most body compartments, but do require inflamed meninges to cross the blood-brain barrier.

All have substantial renal metabolism, except for the antistaphylococcal PCNs (nafcillin, oxacillin, dicloxacillin, and cloxacillin), and must have dose adjustments if renal dysfunction is present.

Natural PCNs: PCN VK (oral), PCN G (IV/IM):

- Spectrum of action includes G+ and anaerobes, but has limited indications in the inpatient setting because of high resistance patterns.
- Drug of choice for *Neisseria meningitidis* and *Treponema pallidum.*
- Also used for endocarditis from susceptible organisms (*Streptococcus*).

Aminopenicillins: amoxicillin (oral), ampicillin (IV):

- Have an extended spectrum of G+, G–, and anaerobes; however, still have limited inpatient indications because of resistance from β-lactamase production.

- Ampicillin is the drug of choice for *Enterococcus* and *Listeria monocytogenes*.
- Addition of β-lactamase inhibitors (amoxicillin/clavulanate or ampicillin/sulbactam) make these very useful antibiotics because of their broad coverage.

Antistaphylococcal PCNs: oxacillin, dicloxacillin, cloxacillin, and nafcillin:

- Resistant to β-lactamase-producing *S. aureus*, but have a narrow spectrum limited to G+ organisms only.
- Very effective against infections from *S. aureus* or *Streptococcus*.

Antipseudomonal PCNs: piperacillin ± tazobactam and ticarcillin ± clavulanate:

- Resistant to β-lactamase-producing G– bacteria, particularly *Pseudomonas*, *Proteus*, and *Enterobacter*, but in general have less activity against G+ organisms, particularly *Enterococcus*.
- Tazobactam and clavulanate expands activity versus β-lactamase-producing organisms, particularly anaerobes.
- Drug of choice for *Pseudomonas aeruginosa*.
- Note that ticarcillin provides a high sodium load (5.2 meq/g) and should be used with caution in patients with volume overload states (congestive heart failure [CHF], renal failure).

Cephalosporins

This is a broad class of β-lactams notable for their general resistance to β-lactamase production. Bacterial coverage depends on the generation, but all cephalosporins have poor coverage of *Enterococcus*, *Listeria*, coagulase negative *Staphylococcus* (CNS), and atypical organisms (*Chlamydia*, *Mycoplasma*, and *Legionella*). Most have excellent penetration of all body compartments. The major concern with the use of cephalosporins is their predilection to promote **bacterial resistance**. For example, patients exposed to cephalosporins are more likely to develop resistant *Enterococcus* species and resistant G– bacteria (through the production of ESBL).

First generation: cephalexin and cefazolin:

- Have **excellent G+ coverage**, but limited G– and no activity against anaerobes.
- Typically used for bone and soft tissue infections from *Staphylococcus* and *Streptococcus*.

Second generation: cefuroxime, cefoxitin, and cefotetan:

- **Less G+ and more G– coverage** than the first generation. Cefuroxime has greater activity against *H. influenzae*, whereas cefoxitin and cefotetan have added anaerobic coverage, particularly Bacteroides.

Third generation: ceftriaxone, cefotaxime, ceftazidime, and cefoperazone:

- Have **improved G– but less G+ coverage** and no coverage against anaerobes. Ceftriaxone and cefotaxime have excellent coverage of *S. pneumoniae*, but no coverage of *Pseudomonas*. Ceftazidime and cefoperazone have excellent coverage of *Pseudomonas*, but poor G+ coverage.

Fourth generation: cefepime:

- **Broader spectrum for G+ and G– bacteria** than the third generation and effective against *Pseudomonas*, but no anaerobic coverage.

Monobactam: aztreonam:

- Coverage is limited to only G– aerobes.
- Has adequate penetration of most body compartments.

Carbapenems: imipenem/cilastatin, meropenem, and ertapenem:

- Have the **broadest spectrum of any antibiotics**, G+, G–, and anaerobes. Plus, they are the only antibiotics that are known to be effective against G– bacteria which produce **ESBL**. Only gaps in coverage are MRSA, *Enterococcus faecium*, and atypical bacteria.
- Cilastatin protects against nephrotoxicity and prevents the inactivation of imipenem by renal dehydropeptidase I.
- Used as a last resort when other antibiotic choices are contraindicated or are limited due to resistant organisms.

FLUOROQUINOLONES

This is the only class of antibiotics which directly prevent DNA synthesis by inhibiting DNA gyrase and topoisomerase. They reach high concentrations in the kidneys and urine (renal excretion), but have poor blood-brain barrier penetration. In the past, their use has been avoided in children, because of a concern about cartilage destruction from animal studies. Currently, they are being used more widely in children without any additional side effects. Resistance has been of great concern because of its rapid development in certain bacteria.

First generation: Nalidixic acid (not routinely used)

Second generation: ciprofloxacin and ofloxacin:

- Excellent coverage of G– bacteria, with the best activity of any of the fluoroquinolones against *Pseudomonas* (especially ciprofloxacin), but G+ coverage is limited and they have no anaerobic activity.

Third generation: levofloxacin (single stereoisomer of ofloxacin):

- Same spectrum of action as ofloxacin with good coverage of *S. pneumoniae* (including PRSP) but less coverage of *Pseudomonas* when compared to ciprofloxacin.

Fourth generation: gatifloxacin and moxifloxacin:

- Similar to levofloxacin, but have improved coverage of G+ organisms (including MRSA and PRSP) and less activity against *Pseudomonas*. Moxifloxacin also has some anaerobic activity.

AMINOGLYCOSIDES: GENTAMICIN, TOBRAMYCIN

The aminoglycosides act by inhibiting bacterial protein synthesis via irreversible binding to the 30S ribosomal subunit. Their spectrum of activity is limited to **G− bacteria** only, including excellent coverage of *Pseudomonas*. However, the protein inhibitory effects are synergistic to the cell wall synthesis inhibition of β-lactams, and therefore aminoglycosides are sometimes used in combination with β-lactams to treat G+ infections (i.e., nafcillin and gentamicin for treatment of *S. aureus* endocarditis). They have poor penetration into the lungs and across the blood-brain barrier (unless the meninges are inflamed). Inhaled delivery of tobramycin is used to achieve high levels in bronchial secretions. This class is also **not effective to treat abscesses**, because their activity is limited by an acidic pH. The most substantial limitation of their use is toxicity, primarily **acute tubular necrosis** (ATN) and irreversible **ototoxicity**. Resistance to aminoglycosides is uncommon.

GLYCOPEPTIDES: VANCOMYCIN

Similar to β-lactams, vancomycin inhibits bacterial cell wall synthesis, but blocks peptidoglycan synthesis. Thus, vancomycin is not susceptible to β-lactamase production or PBP alteration. It has a narrow spectrum of activity limited to G+ organisms and is generally considered the drug of choice for serious infections caused by MRSA or PRSP. The only exception is that it does cover *Clostridium* and oral vancomycin can be used for recurrent *C. difficile* infections. It penetrates most body compartments well, but does require inflamed meninges to penetrate the blood-brain barrier. Toxicity is a concern, because of both nephrotoxicity and ototoxicity. Last, a common reaction to infusion can occur known as "Red Man Syndrome." This typically consists of flushing and pruritus caused by the release of histamine and can be treated by slowing the infusion and administering antihistamines.

FOLATE INHIBITORS: TRIMETHOPRIM/ SULFAMETHOXAZOLE (TMP/SMX)

This combination of two antibiotics effectively blocks bacterial folic acid synthesis. It has a generally broad spectrum of action including both G+ and G− organisms; however, widespread resistance often limits its use. The two most common indications are to treat *Pneumocystis jiroveci* pneumonia and nonserious soft tissue **MRSA** infections.

MACROLIDES: ERYTHROMYCIN, CLARITHROMYCIN, AZITHROMYCIN, AND TELITHROMYCIN

This class inhibits bacterial protein synthesis by binding to the 50S ribosomal subunit. They have good coverage against both G+ and G− organisms, but no activity against anaerobes. They are often used to treat pneumonia and respiratory tract infections, because they have coverage of *Pneumococcus*, *Haemophilus*, and *Moraxella* as well as coverage of atypical organisms (*Mycoplasma*, *Chlamydia*, and *Legionella*). In addition, azithromycin and clarithromycin are effective against Mycobacterium-avium complex.

TETRACYCLINES: TETRACYCLINE, MINOCYCLINE, AND DOXYCYCLINE

Similar to aminoglycosides, the tetracycline class also inhibits the 30S ribosomal subunit. This class has broad activity against many G+ and G− bacteria, but is often utilized because of its coverage of atypical organisms, particularly **Rickettsiae**, *Mycoplasma*, *Chlamydia*, *Borrelia*, *Coxiella*, and *Leptospira*. These drugs are not recommended in children under 8 years of age, because they may inhibit bone growth.

NITROIMIDAZOLE: METRONIDAZOLE

The mechanism of action of metronidazole is not clearly defined, but it seems to promote free radical production which is toxic to bacterial cells. It has activity only against anaerobes. It is used primarily for its **anaerobic** coverage, particularly for *C. difficile* **infections**. The most recognized side effect is a **disulfiram-type reaction** with the consumption of alcohol.

LINCOSAMIDE: CLINDAMYCIN

Similar to the macrolides, clindamycin also inhibits protein synthesis by binding to the 50S ribosomal subunit. It has a narrow spectrum of activity against G+ bacteria and anaerobes. Because of its inhibition of bacterial synthesis, it is often used against **toxin-producing organisms** (such as *S. aureus* and *S. pyogenes*) to prevent toxin-related complications. It is also effective in treating soft tissue infections caused by MRSA.

RIFAMYCIN: RIFAMPIN

Rifampin has a unique mechanism of action as it inhibits the DNA-dependent RNA polymerase. It has a broad spectrum of action against G+ and G– bacteria, and reaches high intracellular levels so has good coverage of *Chlamydia* and mycobacteria. However, most bacteria have a high rate of **inducible resistance** against rifampin, so it is rarely used for monotherapy. Its main indications are as **combination therapy** with vancomycin to treat serious MRSA infections (endocarditis, osteomyelitis). It is also used as prophylaxis for individuals exposed to a patient with *N. meningitidis*.

STREPTOGRAMIN: QUINUPRISTIN/DALFOPRISTIN

This combination of two naturally occurring compounds inhibits protein synthesis by binding to two different sites on the 50S bacterial ribosomal subunit. It has only G+ coverage and is indicated mainly for *E. faecium* and *S. aureus* infections which are resistant to vancomycin. Of note, it does not cover *Enterococcus faecalis*.

OXAZOLIDINONE: LINEZOLID

Linezolid is one of the newest antibiotics available and works through a novel mechanism, inhibiting the 23S ribosomal RNA of the 50S subunit during translation. Its coverage is limited to G+ bacteria and used almost exclusively to treat **infections from multidrug-resistant bacteria**. The most common indications are infections caused by vancomycin-resistant *Enterococcus faecium* (VRE), MRSA, and *S. pneumoniae* (including PRSP and other multidrug-resistant strains).

HEMATOLOGY-ONCOLOGY

APPROACH TO

ANEMIA AND

THROMBOCYTOPENIA

Sharon F. Green
Robert T. Means

KEY POINTS

- Anemia is a sign which requires diagnosis of the underlying cause.
- Anemias can be classified by red blood cell morphology (size) or by pathophysiology based on mechanism: decreased red cell survival or decreased production.
- The peripheral smear can be crucial in identifying both morphologic and pathophysiologic features of the anemia.
- Iron-deficiency anemia requires consideration of assessment of occult GI blood loss and may necessitate colonoscopy to rule out colon cancer or some other colonic pathology.
- Thrombocytopenia occurs from decreased bone marrow production, increased splenic sequestration, or accelerated destruction of platelets.

INTRODUCTION

Anemia is defined as the circumstance in which there are fewer than normal red blood cells or a decreased red blood cell mass. Since red cell mass is difficult to measure directly, the **hematocrit** (Hct, packed cell volume) and amount of **hemoglobin (HgB)** in specimens are used as surrogate measures. The Hct is roughly three times the HgB. Note that since the Hct and HgB are plasma dependent, values may be falsely elevated in periods of volume depletion (e.g., dehydration) and falsely lowered in periods of volume overload. Anemia is not a disease but a sign which is a manifestation of an underlying cause or disease process which must be identified.

PATHOPHYSIOLOGY

Red blood cells normally survive 100–120 days in the circulation. Hemato-poiesis, the process through which formed elements of the blood are pro-duced, begins in the bone marrow. Stem cells differentiate into hematopoietic progenitors, which in turn become committed to erythroid development and evolve into erythroid precursors under the regulatory influence of a number of cytokines and hematopoietic growth factors, the most important of which is erythropoietin (EPO). EPO is produced by the peritubular capillary cells in the kidney and maintains the committed erythroid progenitor during differ-entiation into erythroid precursors, which require iron, folate, and B_{12} to form the mature red blood cell. The key distinction in the pathophysiology of any anemia is whether the process involves increased destruction or decreased production of red blood cells.

CLINICAL PRESENTATION

Anemia may be discovered incidentally during routine laboratory testing in an otherwise relatively asymptomatic patient. When symptoms occur, a com-mon initial symptom is fatigue. Other symptoms may include dyspnea (HgB carries oxygen), dizziness, and pale skin. It is important to establish the time course of progression of symptoms to determine the acuity of the presenta-tion. Obviously, patients overtly losing blood (gastrointestinal [GI] bleed, trauma) may be anemic. More subtle symptoms of anemia could include fever, weight loss, anorexia, rash, night sweats, malaise, jaundice, diarrhea, melena, or changes in bowel habits. The past medical history should note any history of liver or kidney disease, cancer, or blood transfusions. The history must include a detailed discussion of nutrition and medications. Nutrition may be affected by age, alcohol use, and malabsorption. Chemotherapeutics, antibiotics, nonsteroidal anti-inflammatory drugs (NSAIDs), and anticonvul-sants are all broad categories of medications known to cause anemia for many reasons. In women, a detailed menstrual history should be obtained. Family history including geographic background and ethnic origin should be inves-tigated to determine risk of congenital disorders such as sickle cell anemia, thalassemias, and glucose-6-phosphate dehydrogenase (G6PD) deficiency. Social history must establish alcohol use and toxin exposures. Alcohol use or abuse can contribute to anemia at multiple levels. Alcohol suppresses bone marrow production and causes a macrocytic anemia. Many abusers of alco-hol have concomitant liver disease and poor nutrition which also contribute to anemia.

On physical examination, general presentation will vary from no discomfort to pallor, fatigue, and an ill appearance, depending on the severity and acuity of the anemia. Depending on the etiology of the anemia, the physical examination may reveal generalized pallor, decreased pigmentation of palmar creases, conjunctival pallor, petechiae, bruising, or jaundice, scleral icterus, dry mucous membranes, macroglossia, or lead lines, tachycardia, bounding pulses, a systolic flow murmur, tachypnea, splenomegaly and/or hepatomegaly, lymphadenopathy, peripheral neuropathy, and ataxia.

EVALUATION

Anemia is defined by a low HgB and Hct as measured on a peripheral blood sample. Anemias are classified by both pathophysiology and morphology. The first step in the evaluation is to differentiate between increased destruction and decreased production, which can be ascertained with the **reticulocyte count**. The reticulocyte count is the measure of immature red blood cells in the peripheral circulation. This provides information on the ability of the bone marrow to respond to the anemia. A high reticulocyte count indicates that the bone marrow has increased production either to compensate for blood loss or in response to therapy. Conversely, if there is decreased production, the reticulocyte count would be low or inappropriately normal in the presence of a severe anemia. The reticulocyte count is reported as a percentage of red blood cells, therefore, it must be corrected for both the degree of anemia and the longer life of prematurely released reticulocytes in the circulation. To correct for anemia: patient's Hct/45 (i.e., normal Hct) × patient's reticulocyte count = absolute reticulocyte count. In the presence of anemia and a normal marrow, reticulocytes are released earlier and are therefore present longer in the peripheral blood. This "shift" correction factor is 2 for moderate anemia (Hct about 25), 2.5 for Hct of 15, 3 for Hct of 10. Thus, to get the reticulocyte production index, divide the absolute reticulocyte count by the appropriate shift correction factor. Given that an adequate response to anemia would be an increase of red blood cell production to two to three times normal within 10 days, an appropriately adjusted reticulocyte count less than two to three times normal indicates an inadequate marrow response.

The next piece of information essential for distinguishing destruction from underproduction is examining the **peripheral smear**. The peripheral smear provides information about both pathophysiology and morphology. With hemolysis, red blood cell fragments may be present. From a morphologic standpoint, the peripheral smear provides information on red blood cell size (microcytic—see Fig. 51-1, normocytic, macrocytic), shape, and variation. Cell types such as sickled cells, target cells, spur cells, and others may also be present and provide diagnostic clues. Important information on neutrophils (hypersegmentation as in megaloblastic anemia, see Fig. 51-2) and

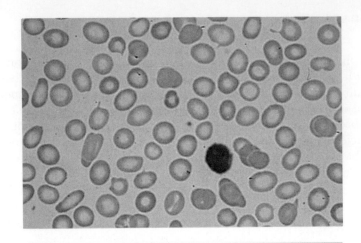

Figure 51-1 **Severe iron-deficiency anemia. Peripheral smear with microcytic (smaller than the nucleus of a lymphocyte) and hypochromic red cells associated with variation in size (anisocytosis) and shape (poikilocytosis).** (*Source:* Reproduced with permission from Lichtman MA, Beutler E, Kipps TJ, et al. *Williams Hematology,* 7th ed. New York: McGraw-Hill, 2006, Plate I-3.)

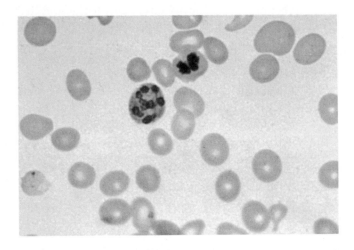

Figure 51-2 **Megaloblastic anemia. Peripheral smear with oval macrocytes, well filled with HgB, are admixed with lesser numbers of large red blood cells, some of which are teardrop-shaped. Note also hypersegmented granulocyte.** (*Source:* Reproduced with permission from Kasper DL, Braunwald E, Fauci AS, et al. *Harrison's Principles of Internal Medicine,* 16th ed. New York: McGraw-Hill, 2005, Figure 92-3.)

platelets (thrombocytopenia) can also be seen on the peripheral smear. Teardrop-shaped cells indicate red cell production outside the marrow, usually in the spleen. The presence of nucleated red blood cells in a patient with a functioning spleen indicates either severe hemolysis or replacement of the bone marrow by tumor or fibrosis.

Decreased red cell survival can be categorized into the categories of **blood loss** and hemolysis (**increased destruction**). Acute blood loss in most cases is fairly obvious (although there a few anatomic locations where significant acute blood loss can be difficult to detect such as the retroperitoneum or bleeding into the thigh). **Hemolytic anemias** are characterized by the absence of bleeding with an **elevated reticulocyte count**. Other lab data which suggest hemolysis include an **elevated serum bilirubin** and **lactate dehydrogenase (LDH)** in association with an **abnormally low haptoglobin** (levels drop because it binds to the HgB released from hemolyzed red cells). Hemolytic anemias can be either inherited or acquired and are classified by a molecular defect (hemoglobinopathy or enzymopathy) inside the cell, a cell membrane defect, or an environmental factor (mechanical trauma or autoantibody). Microangiopathic hemolytic anemias such as thrombotic thrombocytopenic purpura (TTP) and disseminated intravascular coagulation (DIC) are characterized by schistocytes (fragmented red blood cells) on peripheral smear. The peripheral smear may also reveal abnormalities caused by congenital intrinsic membrane defects such as sickle cell anemia (sickled cells), thalassemias (target cells), G6PD deficiency, and hereditary spherocytosis (spherocytes). **Immune-mediated hemolyses** are acquired disorders caused by IgG or IgM: IgG is often idiopathic and typically associated with a warm antibody hemolytic anemia, whereas IgM is usually associated with a cold antibody hemolytic anemia and is classically related to a mycoplasma infection or infectious mononucleosis. Either etiology may show red cell agglutinates on peripheral smear and are also characterized by a **positive direct Coombs' test**. The Coombs' reagent is a rabbit IgM antibody against human IgG or complement. The direct Coombs' test is performed by mixing the reagent with the patient's red blood cells, noting agglutination, which indicates the presence of antibody on the patient's red cell surfaces. The indirect Coombs' test consists of mixing the patient's serum with a panel of type O red blood cells. After incubation, the Coombs' reagent is added. A positive agglutination suggests the presence of antibody in the patient's serum.

Hemolytic anemias also can be classified by where the hemolysis occurs. **Intravascular hemolysis** is less common, but occurs when red blood cells are broken down directly in the blood vessels, such as in trauma from a mechanical heart valve, overwhelming complement activation as in ABO incompatible blood transfusions, in states of DIC, or when red cells are abnormally sensitive to complement, such as in paroxysmal nocturnal hemoglobinuria. Tests suggesting intravascular hemolysis include the presence of urine-free

HgB and hemosiderin in shed renal tubular cells (positive urine hemosiderin). **Extravascular hemolysis** is much more common, with abnormally shaped cells (e.g., spherocytes) lysed in the reticuloendothelial cells of the liver and spleen.

Decreased production can be caused by either (1) **hypoproliferation**, which is usually a problem in the bone marrow affecting stem cell or progenitor proliferation and differentiation; or (2) a **maturation defect**, either nuclear (B_{12} or folate deficiency, toxic effect from a drug, or myelodysplasia) or cytoplasmic (iron deficiency, globin or heme synthesis). A **normal or low reticulocyte count in the setting of anemia indicates decreased production**.

To differentiate causes of decreased production of red cells, one must review the **red blood cell indices**. These provide morphologic information related to size and variation. The **mean corpuscular volume (MCV)** is a measure of red blood cell size, expressed in femtoliters. This helps classify the anemia as **microcytic** (MCV <80), **normocytic** (MCV 80–100), or **macrocytic** (MCV >100). A low **mean corpuscular hemoglobin concentration** (MCHC) indicates that the red cells are hypochromic and helps distinguish microcytic anemia due to iron deficiency from that associated with thalassemia. The **red cell distribution width (RDW)** provides additional quantitative information about the variability of the size of the cells (anisocytosis). A low RDW indicates that most of the cells are of the same size. A high RDW indicates variability in size.

Causes of **microcytic anemia** include iron-deficiency anemia, thalassemia, lead poisoning, and sideroblastic anemia. Iron deficiency is the most common cause (Fig. 51-1), and therefore iron studies should be performed (serum iron, total iron binding capacity [TIBC], and ferritin). **In iron-deficiency anemia, serum iron levels will be low while TIBC will be high**; the Fe/TIBC ratio is usually <10%. Serum **ferritin**, a marker of whole body iron stores, will be **low**. Iron deficiency in adults is rarely from poor nutrition or malabsorption, and is much more commonly from blood loss. Iron deficiency may occur in a young woman with heavy menstrual periods. In all other patients, a source of possible blood loss should be identified, which usually mandates colonoscopy (for colon cancer) and occasionally upper endoscopy. Thalassemia should be suspected in patients of Mediterranean origin, especially when the MCV is extremely low (in the 60–70 range) with a fairly preserved Hct (in the 30s). Target cells may be seen on peripheral smear. Lead poisoning more often occurs in pediatric patients, but may be seen in patients drinking moonshine whiskey from lead-based stills or drinking from lead-based glazed pots or jugs. Other findings may include abdominal pain, motor neuropathy, gout, and chronic interstitial kidney disease leading to renal insufficiency. The smear classically shows basophilic stippling.

Normocytic normochromic anemias are classified as hypoproliferative as they result from decreased red blood cell production. This may be due to many of the conditions described above, or to marrow damage such as infiltration by tumor or granulomas, fibrosis, or aplasia. In addition, they may be caused by systemic illnesses such as multiple myeloma or decreased EPO production seen in renal disease (seen when the creatinine clearance is <45 mL/min). Early iron deficiency can have a normal MCV, so iron studies are indicated; this will also help differentiate iron-deficiency anemia from **anemia of chronic disease (ACD)**, a common cause of normocytic normochromic anemia. ACD is found in chronic inflammatory disorders such as chronic infections (HIV, TB, osteomyelitis), malignancies, and other inflammatory diseases (rheumatologic diseases such as lupus or rheumatoid arthritis; inflammatory bowel disease). Note the noninflammatory chronic diseases (diabetes with normal renal function, heart disease, chronic obstructive pulmonary disease [COPD], and hypertension) do NOT cause ACD. The underlying chronic disorder causes increased production of the cytokines (tumor necrosis factor [TNF], interleukin [IL]-1, and interferons) that mediate the immune or inflammatory response. These cytokines are responsible for contributing to ACD by decreasing red cell survival, decreasing EPO production, decreasing erythroid colony response to EPO, and impairing mobilization of reticuloendothelial iron stores. Consequently in ACD, the **serum iron level will be low** (unable to mobilize stored iron) and the **TIBC will also be low** or inappropriately normal. Transferrin saturation will therefore be normal or only slightly low (usually >16%). In contrast to iron deficiency, the serum **ferritin** level is typically **normal or high**. However, ferritin is an acute phase reactant and therefore may be elevated for other reasons.

Macrocytic anemia classically occurs from B_{12} and folate deficiency, with striking elevations in the MCV at times. The MCV of a reticulocyte approaches 160, so a situation of marked reticulocytosis can elevate the MCV. Myelodysplastic disorders, medications, chronic liver disease/alcohol abuse, and hypothyroidism can also cause macrocytosis. Folic acid is present in most fruits and vegetables (especially green leafy ones) and a balanced diet meets daily requirements. Body stores of folate are sufficient for 2–3 months (although folate requirements increase in pregnancy and with chronic hemolytic diseases). **Folate deficiency** occurs in malnourished persons, alcoholics with poor diets, anorectic patients, and those who overcook their food. In contrast, dietary **B_{12} deficiency** occurs rarely, usually in strict vegetarians who also avoid dairy products. B_{12} is present in all foods of animal origin. After ingestion, B_{12} is bound to intrinsic factor (IF), a protein secreted by gastric parietal cells. The B_{12}-IF complex is absorbed in the terminal ileum. Therefore, other causes of B_{12} deficiency include postgastrectomy (no parietal cells), competition for B_{12} by bacteria (blind loop syndrome) or the fish tapeworm (*Diphyllobothrium latum*; perhaps in anchovies or other undercooked fish), or diseases of the terminal ileum resulting in malabsorption (postresection; Crohn's terminal ileitis). The most common cause of B_{12} deficiency in older patients is **pernicious anemia**, characterized by lack of IF.

Patients with B_{12} deficiency also have neurologic defects, often involving the dorsal columns, with impaired proprioception and balance, and a positive Romberg's sign, as well as the peripheral nerves, with paresthesias and dysesthesias. More profound nervous system deficits can be seen with advanced disease, including neuropsychiatric symptoms and dementia. For macrocytic anemia, the peripheral smear can again be quite valuable, with oval macrocytes and hypersegmented neutrophils in B_{12} deficiency (Fig. 51-2) and round macrocytes with target cells or stomatocytes in liver disease and excess ethanol consumption. Macrocytosis may also be caused by myelodysplastic syndromes with a distinctive blood smear displaying hypogranular or hypolobulated neutrophils and blast cells along with other abnormalities. Serum B_{12} and folate levels should be obtained with macrocytic anemia. A low normal B_{12} level (200–350) does not rule out B_{12} deficiency. If clinical suspicion of B_{12} deficiency is high, a methylmalonic acid and homocysteine levels should be ordered. These levels will be increased with tissue B_{12} deficiency, since B_{12} is instrumental in the synthesis of methionine from homocysteine, and the conversion of methylmalonyl coenzyme A to succinyl coenzyme A. Anti-IF antibodies will be found in 60% of patients with pernicious anemia and can aid in diagnosis.

MANAGEMENT

Management of anemia depends on treatment of the underlying condition, and given the breadth of conditions causing anemia, is beyond the scope of this chapter. Obviously, patients with hemodynamic instability or symptoms secondary to anemia may need transfusion (see Chap. 52). As mentioned, iron-deficiency anemia mandates a workup to detect a source of bleeding. When iron is replaced, it is generally replaced orally, which is sometimes difficult because of side effects (nausea, epigastric pain, bowel changes) and that it is ideally taken on an empty stomach. The first sign of response will be a reticulocytosis, usually evident by 7–10 days. In pernicious anemia, B_{12} may not be orally absorbed, and is therefore given intramuscularly.

THROMBOCYTOPENIA

Thrombocytopenia is caused by decreased bone marrow production, increased splenic sequestration, or accelerated destruction of platelets. **Decreased production** occurs from disorders that injure or prevent the proliferation of stem cells, such as aplastic anemia, hematologic malignancies, or myelodysplasia. Generally, these conditions are recognizable since all cell lines are affected to varying degrees, with accompanying leukopenia and anemia. Occasionally, thrombocytopenia will be the presenting finding in these disorders; bone marrow examination will show decreased megakaryocytes, in addition to the underlying disorder (marrow aplasia, fibrosis, or infiltration). After platelets leave the marrow space, about one-third are sequestered in the spleen, while the other two-thirds circulate for 7–10 days. Therefore, **splenic sequestration** will reduce the platelet count by 30% or more. Causes include portal hypertension and splenic infiltration from tumor cells in myeloproliferative or lymphoproliferative disorders. **Accelerated destruction** can occur in conditions such as hemolytic-uremic syndrome, TTP, or in cases of DIC. A common condition seen on internal medicine services is **heparin-induced thrombocytopenia (HIT)**, which occurs to some degree in 10–15% of patients receiving heparin. Type I HIT is a mild thrombocytopenia that occurs 1–2 days after starting heparin, caused by heparin directly agglutinating platelets, and is rarely of clinical consequence. More serious is type II HIT, which occurs in 0.3–3% of patients receiving heparin, especially perioperatively. It is autoimmune in origin, and occurs from an immune complex formed between heparin and the platelet-derived heparin-neutralizing protein, platelet factor 4 (PF 4). Platelet counts begin to drop 5–14 days after heparin has begun, decreasing to <50% of the preheparin value (usually to levels of 60,000/μL, usually no lower than 20,000/μL). However, this heparin/PF 4 complex is profoundly thrombotic, so morbidity arises from venous and sometimes arterial thrombosis. Such complications can occur postdischarge and up to 100 days after heparin exposure. Care must be taken that platelet counts are not dropping on heparin during a hospitalization. Diagnosis can be affirmed by demonstrating HIT antibodies (against heparin/PF 4). Therapy entails more than simply stopping the heparin, as immune complexes may be circulating for weeks to months. Direct thrombin inhibitors such as lepirudin or argatroban are used. Low molecular weight heparins (LMWH) are less likely to induce HIT, but once HIT occurs, 80–90% of the antibodies generated against unfractionated heparin cross-react with LMWH, making them not usable in HIT. These antibodies don't retain an amnestic response, and it is generally safe to give heparin to patients with a history of HIT if the episode was more than 3 months earlier.

Idiopathic thrombocytopenic purpura (ITP) occurs acutely most often in children after a viral or respiratory infection, and most patients recover. In contrast, chronic ITP occurs in adults, especially women 20–40 years of age. In this autoimmune disorder, antibodies form against platelet antigens, such as the antigens on glycoprotein IIb/IIIa. Platelets are not destroyed by direct lysis, but rather, destruction takes place in the spleen, where splenic macrophages with Fc receptors bind to antibody-coated platelets. Platelet counts can be profoundly low, sometimes <5000/μL. Initially patients are treated with high-dose prednisone, to decrease the affinity of splenic macrophages for the antibody-coated platelets. IV immunoglobulin is sometimes used when platelet counts are extremely low, for temporary phagocytic blockade. Platelet transfusions are ineffective in ITP, as the transfused platelets are destroyed within a few hours of administration. In contrast to acute ITP, most adults with chronic ITP require lifelong therapy, and many require splenectomy. In all patients with chronic ITP, immunization against encapsulated bacteria (*Streptococcus pneumoniae, Neisseria meningitidis, Haemophilus influenzae*) should be administered 2 weeks before splenectomy. In addition, some require lifelong immunosuppressive therapy, such as with the anti-CD20 monoclonal antibody rituximab.

ISSUES IN BLOOD
TRANSFUSIONS

Mark M. Udden

KEY POINTS

- Transfusions, whether RBCs, platelets, or plasma, are generally given only to treat symptoms not laboratory values.
- Adverse effects of transfusion include infectious and immunologic complications, as well as volume and/or iron overload.
- Infectious complications are rare; platelets are the most prone to bacterial contamination.
- Hemolytic transfusion reactions can be acute or delayed; delayed hemolytic reactions are the most common complication of RBC transfusions.

INTRODUCTION

Transfusions are an important part of medical care resulting in the use of 10–12 million units of blood annually in the United States. Although the blood supply has never been safer, complications do occur, and therefore blood products should be used only when necessary and the fewer units given, the better. **Transfusions require consent which includes warnings about risks**: death, renal failure (usually red cells), febrile reactions, transmission of hepatitis, and HIV. Many states require the physician to make the patient aware of the availability of alternatives such as self (autologous) donation of blood prior to elective procedures. In emergencies, however, the physician may transfuse blood without consent. One should also remember that some patients object to the use of blood on religious grounds.

The safety of the blood supply is based on collection of blood from volunteers who must answer questions that establish likelihood of carrying a transmissible disease. Blood obtained is subjected to serologic and antigenic screening tests to establish the presence of HIV1 and 2, HTLV1 and 2, hepatitis B and C, and syphilis. Nucleic acid screening strategies for detecting Parvovirus and West Nile virus are recently being employed.

Some important questions to ask the patient before you transfuse are: Have you ever received a blood transfusion? Did you have any complications or reactions? Did your doctors have difficulty finding blood of your type? The hepatitis C serology of patients who received blood products before 1991 should be assessed. In addition, transfusions must be justified in the clinical record. Numbers such as the hematocrit, prothrombin time (PT), partial thromboplastin time (PTT), or platelet count seldom justify a prophylactic transfusion without some description of the clinical circumstances and goals. The results of a transfusion must be described in the notes. These include adequacy of response, and whether there were any complications.

All whole donated units are centrifuged in a stepwise fashion to separate platelets and plasma so that each donation typically results in three units of blood product for transfusion. During this process white blood cells are usually removed by filtration. Plasma does not require filtration to remove white cells. The packed red blood cell (RBC) unit obtained contains about 180 mL of red cells, 40 mL of plasma, and 100 mL of additive in a total volume of 320 mL and are stored at 1–6°C for up to 42 days. Specifics of each transfusion component will be discussed separately below.

RED BLOOD CELLS

In general, blood is transfused **only to treat symptoms** and furthermore, symptom relief determines the amount of blood transfused. Obviously, patients who are actively hemorrhaging will require transfusion to compensate for acute blood loss. In addition, transfusion is appropriate for those exhibiting symptoms of anemia (refractory to initial therapy with crystalloid), such as syncope, dyspnea, postural hypotension, tachycardia, angina, and transient ischemic attacks. RBC units should be given on a unit-by-unit basis. Patients should never be transfused with the goal of obtaining a normal hemoglobin. To continue to give additional units once a patient is asymptomatic or above a critical hemoglobin value is to risk volume overload, and indeed, most patients will have adequate tissue delivery of oxygen with a hemoglobin of 7 g/dL. An important exception is the patient with severe cardiovascular disease, who is at increased risk for myocardial ischemia, congestive heart failure, or stroke when his or her hemoglobin falls below 10 g/dL. Patients who are chronically anemic may require transfusions on a regular basis because of their disease, or because of treatments such as chemotherapy. Erythropoietin treatment has greatly reduced the burden of anemia as well as transfusion needs for these patients. In conditions which do not respond to erythropoietin, the typical transfusion requirement is 1 unit per week of packed RBCs.

Each unit of packed red cells contains 180–200 mL of red cells. One can calculate the expected rise in hematocrit from transfusing a unit of blood. For example, a 70-kg person may be presumed to have a total blood volume of 70 mL/kg, or 4900 mL. Therefore, each unit of blood consisting of 200 mL of red cells will raise the hematocrit 200/4900 mL, or about 4%.

PLATELETS

Single donor (pheresis) units are the main source of platelets in large centers. The typical transfusion order is for 6 units of platelets obtained from individual donor whole blood units or one pheresis unit. Under ideal circumstances, the platelet count will rise approximately 5–10,000/μL for each unit—an increment of 30–60,000/μL for a typical transfusion. Fever, infection, disseminated intravascular coagulation (DIC), splenomegaly, and alloimmunization will blunt the response to platelet transfusions. Platelet transfusions do not require a crossmatch, but the recipient's ABO Rh blood type has to be determined so that compatible units are given.

Bleeding risk increases when the platelet count drops below 10,000/μL and risk is significant when below 5000/μL; therefore, transfusions are usually reserved for patients whose platelet count ≤10,000/μL. Platelets are transfused to reach higher targets in special circumstances like bleeding or for a procedure. Patients do well with procedures or with hemorrhage if the platelet count is above 30–50,000/μL. Bleeding seldom occurs in the absence of a platelet disorder or other hemostatic defect (such as prolonged PT, PTT) when the platelet count is above 50,000/μL. In idiopathic thrombocytopenia (ITP), platelet transfusions have a limited role when the destructive process exceeds the capacity to transfuse. Thus, transfusions for patients with ITP are used only in desperate circumstances, or just prior to major surgery. Platelets are contraindicated in the treatment of thrombocytopenia associated with thrombotic thrombocytopenia (TTP), as neurologic symptoms and renal failure may worsen, presumably due to new or expanding thrombi as the infused platelets are consumed.

PLASMA AND PLASMA FRACTIONS

Plasma is usually obtained as fresh frozen plasma (FFP) from single units of red cells with a volume of 200–250 mL or as larger units from pheresis donors in which the volume is usually 400 or 600 mL. FFP contains all the coagulation factors and other proteins in the original unit of blood. Most transfusion guidelines recommend administering 10–15 mL/kg for liver disease or DIC. Remember that patients receive about 1 unit of FFP per 6 units of platelets or one pheresis platelet unit. The greatest use of plasma is in the treatment of patients with the coagulopathy associated with liver disease and DIC, but actually there are no studies to support this practice in terms of reducing morbidity or mortality. Other situations in which to consider administering FFP include: the replacement of factor V deficiency (other factors are replaced with the specific component), reversal of warfarin effect when patients are actively bleeding or require surgery before treatment with vitamin K can be reasonably expected to reverse anticoagulation, in conjunction with massive blood transfusion (1–1.5 × blood volume in a few hours) who are still bleeding, to replace antithrombin III, and in the treatment of TTP. **Cryoprecipitate** is obtained by thawing FFP at 1–6°C to produce a cold precipitate which contains 80–120 units of factor VIII and von Willebrand factor. Cryoprecipitate also contains 200–250 mg of fibrinogen. It is used in treatment of von Willebrand's disease and mild hemophilia.

COMPLICATION OF TRANSFUSIONS

Infectious Complications

Table 52-1 outlines the principal risks of blood transfusion. Most striking is the concern of bacterial contamination of platelets and RBCs. Screening of donor units by serologic or polymerase chain reaction (PCR) techniques for viral DNA or RNA has greatly reduced the chance of a donor contributing a unit of blood with a virus. Platelet transfusions are most likely to contain a

Table 52-1 **Some Risks of Blood Transfusion**

Risk Factor		Risk/Unit	Deaths/10^6 Units
Viral infection	Hep A	1/1,000,000	0
	Hep B	1/50,000–170,000	0–0.14
	Hep C	1/200,000	<0.5
	HIV	1/2,000,000	<0.5
	HTLV1 and 2	1/19,000–80,000	0
	Parvovirus B19	1/10,000	0
Bacterial	Red cells	1/500,000	0.1–0.25
contamination	Platelets	1/12,000	21
Immune	Acute hemolytic	1/250,000–1,000,000	0.67
	Delayed hemolytic	1/1000	0.4
	Allergic	2–3/100	?
	Anaphylactic	1/20,000–50,000	?
	TRALI	1/50,000–200,000	?
	TA-GVHD	1/500,000–1,000,000	?

bacterial contaminant. When transfused, a unit with bacterial contamination will cause fever, hypotension, and may cause DIC. The transfusion should be stopped and returned to the blood bank for Gram stain and culture. The patient should have blood cultures taken and broad-spectrum antibiotic coverage should be initiated. Gram-negative bacteria and skin flora are the most common bacterial contaminants; *Yersinia enterocolitica* is commonly implicated, as it is able to grow in refrigerated storage. Other potential infectious risks include malaria, Babesia, Chagas disease (*Trypanosoma cruzi*), Lyme disease, cytomegalovirus (CMV), Epstein-Barr virus (EBV), and West Nile virus. Transmission of prion disease (variant Creutzfeldt-Jakob disease [vCJD]) is also considered to be a potential risk of blood transfusions.

Immunologic Complications

To prevent **acute hemolytic transfusion reactions**, the ABO blood type and presence or absence of Rh D are determined before transfusion, as well as the presence of clinically significant antibodies (e.g., anti-Kell, Duffy). Yet, despite these blood bank safeguards, acute hemolytic transfusion reactions (ABO mismatch) continue to occur, and can usually be traced to simple human errors such as mislabeling the blood tube sent for crossmatch. Hemolysis from intravascular lysis of the incompatible red cells is quite rapid. The typical presentation is fever, hypotension, flank pain, and change in urine. The urine output may suddenly decrease and the urine may appear brown or concentrated due to the presence of hemoglobin. Acute renal failure can ensue despite treatment with fluids. DIC is also a complication. Once the possibility of a hemolytic transfusion reaction is entertained, the blood bank and the pathologist on call should be notified immediately. If problems are recognized during the transfusion, it should be immediately stopped, and the blood returned to the blood bank as part of the transfusion reaction workup. The amount of damage done correlates with the amount transfused. The treatment is supportive.

Delayed hemolytic transfusion reactions are events due to the acquisition of a warm IgG antibody in a patient previously exposed to blood. Exposure may be through transfusion, pregnancy (including miscarriage or elective termination), or sharing needles for injection drug use. The hemolysis is extravascular and takes place at a slower rate, with the development of jaundice, fever, joint pain, and anemia usually 5 or more days after transfusion. An alloantibody (i.e., anti-Kidd, Kell, Duffy) is then discovered completing the picture of a delayed hemolytic transfusion reaction. Management is generally supportive, with any future transfusions providing compatible, antigen-negative units.

Febrile, nonhemolytic transfusion reactions occur less often now that most blood banks remove white blood cells at the blood bank. Pheresis units of platelets or plasma are also leukocyte poor. These reactions are felt to occur because of cytokines derived from donor leukocytes, or recipient antibodies against donor leukocyte antigens. Patients develop fever and chills within 12 hours of the transfusion. Because hemolysis does not occur, the hematocrit rises posttransfusion as expected. Treatment includes stopping the transfusion, with steroids reserved for severe symptoms. **Allergic** and even **anaphylactic reactions** can occur with transfusion. Allergic reactions occur when plasma proteins behave as allergens, reacting with the patient's IgE on mast cells, causing pruritus, urticaria, and occasionally mucosal edema, with wheezing and frank anaphylaxis. The allergic reaction can be immediate or delayed, and occurs more often with FFP and platelet transfusions than RBC. Patients who are IgA deficient may develop these reactions because of antibodies to IgA, and subsequent transfusions should be with IgA-deficient blood. Treatment of allergic reactions involves the administration of antihistamines, steroids, or both; if anaphylaxis ensues, epinephrine, steroids, and cardiopulmonary support may be needed. **Transfusion-related acute lung injury** (TRALI) is another serious complication in which the recipient develops rapid onset of fever, dyspnea, and a noncardiogenic pulmonary edema. These reactions generally occur after FFP; one should suspect this order in a patient who develops frank adult respiratory distress syndrome following a transfusion. The presence of human leukocyte antigen (HLA) or leukocyte antibodies in the donor plasma may be the cause of these reactions. Units from that donor can be quarantined. Antibodies in the patient's plasma may also be the problem—use of leukocyte poor products will help to prevent future lung injury. Proinflammatory cytokines and lipids originating from cellular degradation in the transfused units are thought to be the cause of TRALI when antileukocyte or HLA antibodies cannot be identified. **Transfusion-associated graft versus host disease** (TA-GVHD) is a rare but uniformly fatal event in a recipient caused by lymphocytes in a donor unit. This can occur when the recipient is severely immunocompromised as in transplant settings. Patients die from irreversible bone marrow failure leading to thrombocytopenia and neutropenia. Irradiation of units of RBCs and platelets prevents transfusion GVHD. Irradiated units are recommended for transplant patients, neonates, and patients who are severely immunocompromised. Many cancer centers routinely irradiate blood products given to patients undergoing chemotherapy. In addition, first-degree relatives have a higher likelihood of being HLA-haploid identical, promoting engraftment, and therefore directed family donor units should be irradiated before transfusion.

    Volume overload is a complication of RBC or plasma transfusion. For example, in patients with chronic anemia, plasma volume expands to compensate for reduced red cell mass. Transfusing an asymptomatic patient with chronic anemia therefore risks volume overload. **Iron overload** is an important consequence of chronic transfusion in the absence of bleeding. There is approximately 1 mg/mL packed RBCs of iron or 200 mg/unit of packed RBCs. Patients should be instructed to avoid iron-containing multivitamins and vitamin C (which enhances iron absorption).

ONCOLOGIC

EMERGENCIES

Kanchan Kamath

KEY POINTS

- Cancer-related complications can occur from the cancer itself or its treatment.
- Spinal cord compression can result in irreversible neurologic impairment.
- Elevated ICP from brain tumors can cause cerebral herniation.
- Tumor lysis syndrome is most often associated with treatment of lymphomas and leukemias.
- Infection is a common cause of neutropenic fever, thus empiric antibiotics should always be prescribed.

SPINAL CORD COMPRESSION

Tumors metastatic to the spine, particularly **breast, lung, and prostate cancer** most commonly result in spinal cord compression. Cord compression most often ensues when a metastatic vertebral tumor expands into the epidural space. Alternatively, a pathologic vertebral fracture from metastatic disease can also result in cord compression. The most commonly affected areas of the spine are the thoracic followed by the lumbosacral region then the cervical (directly proportional to the number of vertebral bodies in each region).

Clinical Presentation

Depending on the degree of compression, symptoms can range from asymptomatic to severe neurologic symptoms. The hallmarks of cord compression are pain, weakness, sensory loss, and autonomic dysfunction. Pain is usually the first and most consistent symptom and is described as a progressively increasing localized back pain which worsens with recumbency.

With progression, the pain may radiate into the limbs. On physical examination, patients may have localized tenderness over vertebral bodies, pain with straight leg raise or neck flexion, and diminished sensation to pinprick, vibratory, or position sense. Lhermitte's sign, an electric sensation radiating down the spine with flexion of the neck, may occur with cervical cord compression. As compression progresses, motor weakness and sensory deficits including numbness and paresthesias develop. On examination, patients have brisk deep tendon reflexes and spasticity in addition to weakness. Cauda equina involvement is signified by the loss of anal wink or bulbocavernosus reflex. Loss of bladder or bowel function is generally a late finding and portends a poor prognosis.

Evaluation

The diagnosis should be confirmed with **magnetic resonance imaging (MRI)** which allows evaluation of the entire spinal cord. As many as one-quarter of patients will have epidural metastases evident on MRI which have significant management and prognostic implications.

Management

Spinal cord compression is a medical emergency requiring prompt therapy, which should not be delayed awaiting imaging results. The majority of ambulatory patients have a complete recovery, but once paraplegia or bowel and bladder incontinence occur, fewer than 10% recover. Symptomatic treatment includes: initiation of high-dose corticosteroids (dexamethasone 24 mg IV every 6 hours) and pain control with opiate analgesics. Definitive treatment typically involves continued high-dose corticosteroids combined with radiation therapy to the affected area. Surgery such as vertebral tumor resection presents another alternative.

ELEVATED INTRACRANIAL PRESSURE

Although primary brain tumors are relatively uncommon, one-quarter of patients who die of cancer have intracranial metastases. The tumors most likely to metastasize to the brain are **lung cancer, breast cancer, and melanoma**. Metastases are important to detect and treat as they result in substantial morbidity and mortality. The cranial vault has a fixed volume and increase in the mass within this fixed space leads to deleterious elevations in intracranial pressure (ICP). This, in turn, causes decreased cerebral perfusion, brain-stem herniation, and irreversible damage to the neuronal cells.

Clinical Presentation

The initial presenting symptoms of increased ICP include headache, nausea, vomiting, and focal neurologic signs. As ICP continues to increase, patients will develop somnolence and confusion progressing to coma. Papilledema and neck stiffness are classic physical examination findings of elevated ICP. Occasionally, patients may have Cushing's triad, a combination of hypertension, bradycardia, and respiratory depression which is an ominous sign of impending herniation.

Evaluation

The diagnosis of increased ICP is generally based on clinical presentation and is confirmed by either computed tomography (CT) or MRI of the brain. CT with contrast is the most appropriate initial study as it can be performed quickly and is reliable.

Management

Any patient suspected of having elevated ICP should receive immediate treatment prior to imaging studies. Dexamethasone (10 mg IV every 6 hours) is the initial treatment of choice. Patients suspected of having imminent brain herniation should be immediately intubated and hyperventilated (PCO_2 of 25–30 mmHg results in vasoconstriction thus diminishing intracranial blood volume) and receive mannitol to decrease ICP.

TUMOR LYSIS SYNDROME

Tumor lysis syndrome results from the rapid destruction of malignant cells, which causes the abrupt release of intracellular contents into the extracellular space. It typically follows initiation of chemotherapy for lymphoproliferative malignancies; however, it can occur spontaneously or after initiating treatment in any patient with a large tumor burden.

Clinical Presentation

The syndrome typically develops 48–72 hours after the initiation of chemotherapy. Characteristic laboratory results include hyperuricemia, hyperphosphatemia, hyperkalemia, and hypocalcemia, with concomitant acute renal insufficiency. **Hyperuricemia** is the most common clinical abnormality and often the cause of complications. **Hyperphosphatemia** results in hypocalcemia from the precipitation of calcium phosphate. **Hypocalcemia** if severe may cause severe neuromuscular irritability and tetany. **Hyperkalemia** is particularly dangerous with concomitant renal failure as levels may become significantly elevated and cause ventricular arrhythmias. **Acute renal failure** is a common consequence of tumor lysis and is classically multifactorial. A preglomerular component is often related to decreased effective circulating volume. Renal tubules are affected by decreased perfusion, toxins (including chemotherapy agents), and blockage of tubules by precipitating urate and calcium phosphate. Last, the collecting system can become obstructed from urate and calcium phosphate as well.

Management

Once tumor lysis syndrome has developed, management is difficult, so the best practice is to prevent its development. Patients with lymphoprolifera-tive diseases who are beginning chemotherapy should be aggressively hydrated and receive allopurinol. Volume depletion must be avoided as it will only increase the risk of precipitation and renal failure. Allopurinol is used to decrease uric acid formation. Alkalinization of the urine was for-merly a standard procedure because it converts uric acid to the more soluble urate salt thus diminishing the precipitation of uric acid. However, it also worsens hypocalcemia by promoting calcium phosphate deposition. If sodium bicarbonate is used, it should be titrated to a urinary pH >7.0 and should be discontinued when hyperuricemia resolves. If tumor lysis syn-drome does develop, the above procedures should be initiated immediately and electrolytes, particularly hypocalcemia and hyperkalemia, should be aggressively corrected. In severe cases, hemodialysis may be necessary to correct electrolyte abnormalities until renal function improves.

NEUTROPENIC FEVER

Neutropenia is a common complication with cytotoxic chemotherapy or with malignancies which involve the bone marrow. Neutrophils are the immune cells primarily responsible for host defense against bacteria and fungi. Thus, the degree and duration of neutropenia are directly related to the susceptibility for infection with these microbes. In general, susceptibility increases when the absolute neutrophil count (ANC) falls below 1000 cells/μL. Patients with an **ANC <500** are at risk for infection from endogenous flora (e.g., bacterial colonization of the gastrointestinal [GI] tract) and patients with an ANC <200 cannot mount an inflammatory response. Approximately 40% of individuals with a fever and an ANC <500 will have a defined infection. The cause for the remainder is unknown, but is often presumed to be from a viral infection.

The major source of infection remains colonized microorganisms, thus the main bacteria are gram-positive skin flora and gram-negative GI tract flora. *Candida* infections are also possible, particularly of the skin and oral mucosa. Last, reactivation of latent infections may occur, such as herpes sim-plex, varicella zoster virus, Epstein-Barr virus, cytomegalovirus, or *Mycobacterium tuberculosis*. Additional risk factors for infection should be identified in all patients with neutropenic fever. Patients undergoing chemotherapy frequently have indwelling catheters or surgical wounds which are primary sites of infection. Further, both the chemotherapy and the malignancy itself may result in mucosal breakdown or tissue damage. Although all cancer patients are immunosuppressed, certain factors must be considered in susceptibility. Malignancies such as multiple myeloma and chronic lymphocytic leukemia are associated with hypogammaglobulinemia which increases the susceptibility to encapsulated organisms, particularly *Streptococcus pneumoniae*, *Haemophilus influenzae*, and *Neisseria meningitidis*. Further, patients receiving long-term steroid therapy have impaired cellular immunity and are more at risk for fungal infections, *Pneumocystis jiroveci* pneumonia, and reactivation tuberculosis.

Evaluation

Neutropenic fever is typically defined as a temperature of **>101°F** in a patient with an **ANC <500**. The initial approach centers on identifying a source for infection with a thorough history and physical examination as well as certain requisite workup including:

- Complete blood count and differential
- Blood cultures ×2 (including from a vascular device if present)
- Urinalysis and urine culture
- Chest x-ray
- Liver and renal function (to help classify risk—see later)

Management

Any identified infection should be treated as deemed necessary (inpatient vs. outpatient). However, most patients will not have a clear infection and will require empiric treatment. Empiric therapy is based on that patient's risk for infection and complications (see Table 53-1). High-risk patients must

Table 53-1 **Low- and High-Risk Variables for Individuals Presenting With Neutropenic Fever**

	Low Risk	High Risk
Initial presentation	Outpatient	Inpatient
Expected duration of neutropenia	<10 days	>10 days
Comorbid illness	None	Hypotension Dehydration Altered mental status Respiratory compromise Uncontrolled pain
Renal and hepatic function	Normal	Impaired
Malignancy	In remission	Uncontrolled
Others	Age 60 years or younger	ANC <100

be hospitalized, but low-risk patients can be managed either as an inpatient or outpatient. Therapy should include coverage of gram positives as well as gram negatives, including *Pseudomonas*. Vancomycin should only be started in those patients who are at high risk for gram-positive infections, such as clinically apparent catheter-related infections, extensive mucosal damage, or severe symptoms (shock). Recommended regimens are:

- Low-risk outpatient → ciprofloxacin and amoxicillin/clavulanate
- Low- or high-risk treated as an inpatient → cefepime, ceftazidime, imipenem, meropenem, or piperacillin/tazobactam ± aminoglycoside

Regardless of where the patient is managed, daily follow-up on culture results and patient status is necessary. Most patients will remain febrile for 2–5 days regardless of the efficacy of the initial antibiotics. After a patient becomes afebrile, antibiotics are continued until the ANC recovers to above 500. Patients with persistent fever for over 5 days should be completely re-evaluated and a change in the antimicrobial regimen should be considered, particularly the addition of empiric antifungal therapy.

SUPERIOR VENA CAVA SYNDROME

External compression of the superior vena cava (SVC) typically occurs from malignant tumors of the mediastinum. The two most common causes are **lung cancer** (particularly bronchogenic carcinoma) and **lymphoma**. The symptoms are typically caused by the formation of venous collaterals around the SVC compression. Patients will most commonly complain about **dyspnea** or **facial swelling** (which worsens with bending forward or lying down). Physical examination demonstrates **engorged venous collaterals** over the chest wall and neck, and **facial edema**. Treatment should be directed at the underlying malignancy and decreasing tumor size.

HYPERVISCOSITY SYNDROME

Hyperviscosity syndrome results from abnormally high levels of parapro-teins, leukocytes, or erythrocytes. The elevated serum viscosity results in vascular sludging with resultant decreased perfusion of the microcirculation which can cause significant organ dysfunction, particularly of the central nervous system (CNS), the visual system, and cardiopulmonary system. This syndrome is classically seen in **Waldenstrom's macroglobulinemia**, but has also been noted in multiple myeloma, leukemias, and polycythemia. The classic triad of symptoms includes **visual impairment**, **neurologic symp-toms**, and **bleeding**. Visual disturbances occur from venous engorgement of retinal vessels, visible on retina examination as "boxcar segments." The neu-rologic symptoms are typically **headaches**, somnolence, vertigo, and per-haps seizures. Bleeding occurs from reduced platelet function and is typically mucosal. The presence of increased plasma volume can lead to symptoms of congestive heart failure. The only effective treatment is to treat the underlying condition to prevent further episodes. Symptoms can be managed by decreasing the serum viscosity with plasmapheresis, leuko-pheresis, or phlebotomy (depending on the underlying condition).

LEUKEMIA, LYMPHOMA, AND MULTIPLE MYELOMA

Mark M. Udden

LEUKEMIA

Key Points

- ALL predominates in childhood.
- AML is the most common acute leukemia in adults.
- CML is characterized by the presence of the Philadelphia chromosome.
- CLL should be suspected in patients with absolute lymphocytosis >10,000/μL.

Leukemia, lymphoma, and multiple myeloma are neoplasms of hematopoietic cells. Leukemia is a malignant proliferation of progenitor cells whereas multiple myeloma is a proliferation of plasma cells, both arising in the bone marrow. By contrast, lymphomas are malignant proliferations of leukocytes arising in lymph nodes, thymus, or bone marrow.

Introduction

Leukemias are malignant clonal proliferations of myeloid or lymphoid progenitor cells arising in the bone marrow. Leukemias are generally classified according to the clinical course (acute or chronic) and according to the progenitor cells affected (lymphocytic or myelogenous). Acute leukemia is an aggressive and rapidly progressing disease usually characterized by a predominance of immature white blood cell (WBC) precursors (blasts), whereas chronic leukemia has a more indolent course and a predominance of relatively mature WBCs. The breakdown of leukemia in adulthood is: 36% chronic lymphocytic leukemia (CLL), 32% acute myelogenous leukemia (AML), 18% chronic myelogenous leukemia (CML), and 14% acute lymphocytic leukemia (ALL). ALL is the most common form in children accounting for 80% of all cases of leukemia, whereas CML peaks between the ages of 50 and 60.

Pathophysiology

The underlying problem in leukemia is a series of genetic changes within the bone marrow progenitor cells which allow them to proliferate. Certain gene abnormalities are common in each type of leukemia. For example, the translocation t (9;22), also known as the Philadelphia chromosome, occurs in virtually all cases of CML. Acute leukemias are characterized by proliferation without appropriate differentiation and resistance to apoptosis. The accumulation of immature malignant cells, myeloblasts in AML and lymphoblasts in ALL, eventually replace the bone marrow and circulate in the blood. AML can affect any cell in the myeloid lineage and is usually classified according to the type and morphology of the cells. Chronic leukemias are characterized by an increased proliferation of WBC lines with the early release of cells into the circulation and infiltration of other organs. The cells typically reflect the entire spectrum of differentiation without a predominance of blasts.

Clinical Presentation

In acute leukemia, the pace of disease is rapid and most patients present with complications resulting from bone marrow replacement, such as anemia, thrombocytopenia, and absence of normal WBCs, with symptoms and signs of fatigue, bleeding, and infection. Lymphadenopathy and splenomegaly are common in ALL, but rare in AML. Central nervous system (CNS) involvement is also more common in ALL than in AML and is a frequent site of relapse in ALL. Routine blood counts reveal equal numbers of patients with low, normal, and high leukocyte counts. The peripheral smear almost always shows immature blast cells. Anemia is common and may be severe in patients with significant bleeding. Most patients have severe thrombocytopenia and disseminated intravascular coagulation is particularly common in acute promyelocytic leukemia.

The chronic leukemias are much more indolent disorders and patients are more likely to be detected when abnormalities are found on routine screening labs. Chronic leukemias are characterized by high white counts, mild anemia, thrombocytosis (CML), and thrombocytopenia (CLL). Autoimmune hemolytic anemia is also commonly observed in association with CLL. The most common physical examination findings in chronic leukemia include lymphadenopathy and/or splenomegaly. CML may develop into an acute blast crisis which resembles acute leukemia and is heralded by an increase of myeloblasts (usually >30%) in the peripheral blood. CLL is characterized by an absolute lymphocytosis in the peripheral blood with total counts usually >10,000/µL.

Evaluation

The most essential step in the diagnosis of any leukemia is bone marrow examination with cytogenetic analysis to assess the maturity and types of WBCs. Patients with ALL are further classified according to the type of lymphocyte with 80% having B-cell leukemia (and a worse prognosis) and the remaining have T-cell leukemia. AML is further classified according to the myeloid lineage that is abnormal (e.g., myeloid, promyelocytic, monoblastic, and erythroblastic).

Management

The standard treatment of acute leukemias is combination antineoplastic therapy to induce remission. Remission is defined by normalization of the complete blood count (CBC), the presence of fewer than 5% blasts in the bone marrow, and absence of cytogenetic abnormalities. After remission, consolidation therapy is provided for all patients to eliminate any undetectable disease. Chemotherapy commonly results in prolonged pancytopenia often requiring intensive-transfusion and recombinant granulocyte colony-stimulating factor (G-CSF) therapy. Patients must also be closely monitored for complications of therapy including tumor lysis syndrome during induction and neutropenic fever (see Chap. 52). Patients with poor prognostic factors or who relapse should be considered for allogeneic bone marrow transplantation.

Because CML follows a slow indolent course, the goals of therapy are to suppress proliferation of malignant cells, normalize blood counts, and delay the onset of blast crisis. The standard treatments are hydroxyurea and interferon-α. Both are effective in normalizing cell counts. However, neither effectively suppresses the malignant clone and patients still progress to develop acute blast crisis. Young patients, under the age of 40, with a matched allogenic donor should receive bone marrow transplantation, because this results in the best long-term outcomes. Once patients develop a blast crisis, they should be treated similarly to AML. Most patients with CLL do not require treatment and are more likely to die of other causes. Patients require treatment if their leukemia is advanced or if they are symptomatic with fever, weight loss, severe fatigue, massive hepatosplenomegaly, pancytopenias, or severe lymphocytosis (>100,000/μL).

LYMPHOMA

Key Points

- The most common presentation is asymptomatic lymphadenopathy.
- Lymph node biopsy should be considered for large (>2 cm) nodes or nodes which persist for over 4–6 weeks.
- Hodgkin's disease has a better prognosis than NHL.

Introduction

Lymphomas are malignant proliferations of cells arising in lymph nodes, thymus, or bone marrow. Lymphomas are classified according to the cell line involved, with over 90% derived from B cells, 9% from T cells, and <1% from natural killer cells or monocytes. Lymphomas are also classified as Hodgkin's lymphoma, a B-cell lymphoma which spreads regionally and has characteristic Reed-Sternberg cells on histology, or non-Hodgkin's lymphoma (NHL). In the United States, approximately 7500 new cases of Hodgkin's lymphoma and 55,000 new cases of NHL are diagnosed each year. Hodgkin's disease has a bimodal distribution with peaks in the third and sixth decades. NHL varies by subtype, but indolent, usually follicular, lymphomas are seen in older patients and more aggressive large cell lymphomas are seen in younger patients.

Pathophysiology

A clonal proliferation of a single cell type is responsible for all lymphomas. The etiologies behind this proliferation are complex, but there are important predisposing factors, such as immunosuppression (including HIV/AIDS), chronic antigenic stimulation, and infections (e.g., Epstein-Barr virus [EBV] and Burkitt's lymphoma). These predisposing factors cause genetic abnormalities which allow uncontrolled proliferation and resistance to apoptosis. Most cases of NHL result from the activation of proto-oncogenes or the formation of chimeric proteins from chromosomal translocations, similar to the leukemias. By contrast, the etiology of Hodgkin's disease is less clear.

Clinical Manifestations

Patients most commonly present with lymph node enlargement that may be palpable on physical examination or discovered on computed tomography (CT) scans of neck, chest, abdomen, and pelvis. Approximately half of patients will also complain of systemic symptoms, weight loss, fevers, night sweats, and malaise, also referred to as "B" symptoms (see staging section below). These symptoms occur more commonly with more aggressive lymphomas or with extranodal involvement of the bone marrow, liver, or spleen. A unique symptom associated with Hodgkin's lymphoma is pain which follows the consumption of alcohol; pruritus is common in patients with Hodgkin's lymphoma. Patients should also be evaluated for other sites of spread including the gastrointestinal tract, skin, Waldeyer's ring (tonsils, base of the tongue, and nasopharynx), and the testes. In general, patients with Hodgkin's disease have localized disease which spreads only to contiguous lymph nodes with 80% of cases presenting with lymphadenopathy only above the diaphragm. Disseminated lymphadenopathy is more typical of NHL.

Occasionally, patients may present with abnormal laboratory findings such as anemia, leukopenia, or thrombocytopenia from bone marrow involvement.

Hypersplenism from splenic involvement can also cause thrombocytopenia and anemia. Liver function tests are usually normal. Hypercalcemia can develop with spread to bone or secondary to a paraneoplastic syndrome.

Evaluation

Diagnosis most often requires **excisional biopsy** of the node. Fine needle aspiration (FNA) is not sensitive and a proper histologic diagnosis usually requires excisional biopsy. In particular, FNA is not sufficient to make a diagnosis of Hodgkin's lymphoma, because the characteristic Reed-Sternberg cell is usually surrounded by an array of reactive lymphocytes, plasma cells, and eosinophils. Most patients also require bone marrow examination, particularly if the patient has a cytopenia or systemic symptoms. Morphology and cell surface markers in the bone marrow may further define the histologic type of lymphoma.

Staging of lymphoma is important as it helps determine prognosis and treatment along with histology. It involves routine blood work (CBC, chemistries, liver function tests), imaging of the chest (x-ray or CT), abdomen and pelvis as indicated, and a lumbar puncture if there is high likelihood of CNS disease. In addition, most will obtain a lactate dehydrogenase (LDH), which is part of risk stratification because it correlates with prognosis.

Management

Prognosis and treatment for lymphomas depends on their grade and presentation. In general, the indolent lymphomas (e.g., small lymphocytic, mycosis fungoides, and follicular lymphomas) are difficult to cure but have a good prognosis, whereas the aggressive lymphomas (e.g., Burkitt's and peripheral T-cell lymphoma) have a poor prognosis but a cure is possible. Most indolent lymphomas present with disseminated disease and may be observed until symptoms occur. If patients do present in an early stage with localized disease, radiotherapy is typically the best option. No clear consensus exists on the best therapy for low-grade lymphomas. Options include monotherapy or combination chemotherapy. Aggressive lymphomas should be aggressively treated with a goal of cure. Patients with localized disease should be treated with a combination of rituximab (if a B-cell lymphoma) and chemotherapy with cyclophosphamide, doxorubicin (hydroxydaunomycin), vincristine (Oncovin), and prednisone (R-CHOP). Patients with high-grade lymphomas or who relapse after initial therapy should be considered for autologous stem cell transplantation.

Hodgkin's lymphoma is a highly treatable form of lymphoma and decisions regarding treatment are based on stage. Localized disease may be treated by radiotherapy alone. Advanced stage with diffuse disease is treated with chemotherapy with adriamycin, bleomycin, vinblastine, and dacarbazine (ABVD). Combined modality therapy with radiation and ABVD is usually favored for patients in intermediate stages.

MULTIPLE MYELOMA

Key Points

- MM is suggested by the presence of increased immunoglobulins in the serum or urine.
- Renal failure is a common complication of MM.
- MM produces lytic bone lesions which are not detectable on bone scan.

Introduction

Multiple myeloma (MM) is a proliferation of malignant plasma cells which secrete a monoclonal immunoglobulin protcin (M-protein). It accounts for 1% of all malignancies and 10% of all hematologic malignancies. It is predominantly a malignancy of older adults with a median age of 65 years.

Pathophysiology

Multiple myeloma is a B-cell malignancy, specifically a proliferation of a single clone of plasma cells, which produces a monoclonal immunoglobulin. The clonal cells proliferate in the bone marrow and invade adjacent bone, producing the characteristically widespread bony destruction. The plasma cells also secrete interleukin (IL)-6 which activates osteoclasts, resulting in lytic bone lesions and hypercalcemia. The replacement of normal bone marrow along with humoral suppression of stem cell differentiation produces anemia and eventual bone marrow failure. The elevated monoclonal immunoglobulins are filtered by the kidney and can result in renal failure through the formation of casts within the nephron tubules (myeloma kidney). Deposition in tissues may lead to amyloidosis and high circulating levels may result in hyperviscosity. Patients with myeloma do not produce normal antibodies in response to antigens, so are particularly susceptible to infections by encapsulated organisms, especially *Streptococcus pneumoniae*.

Clinical Presentation

Most patients with MM will have systemic complaints including bone pain (most commonly of the back, chest, or extremities), weakness, fatigue, and weight loss. Clinicians should also inquire about symptoms related to the complications of MM including hypercalcemia, renal failure, or amyloidosis. Fever is uncommon and when present should be considered a sign of infection. Physical findings are nonspecific with the most common symptom being pallor. Occasionally, patients will present with a solitary plasmacytoma, which can appear as a large purple subcutaneous mass.

Most patients will develop a normocytic, normochromic anemia and the peripheral smear shows rouleaux formation (because of the increase in positively charged immunoglobulins causing red blood cell [RBC] adhesion). Less commonly, patients will develop leukopenia or thrombocytopenia. The presence of elevated immunoglobulins (which are positively charged) in the blood is often suggested by a high total protein level and a small anion gap. Patients are also at risk for renal failure, most commonly from cast nephropathy and hypercalcemia. Because the routine urinalysis detects only the protein albumin, this is a poor screen for kidney involvement.

Evaluation

The initial evaluation for MM usually involves the identification of an M-protein in the blood or Bence-Jones (B-J) proteins in the urine, by ordering serum protein electrophoresis (SPEP) and urine protein electrophoresis (UPEP), respectively. The heavy chain class and light chain type is determined by immunoelectrophoresis. IgG and IgA are the most common M-proteins in MM, followed by light chain disease in 15–20% of cases. Light chain disease produces a significant amount of B-J proteinuria, but without a detectable M-protein spike on SPEP. This is one example of why both SPEP and UPEP must be ordered as it is possible for one to be normal and still have MM. Not all M-protein spikes reflect MM. In fact, the most common diagnosis is **benign monoclonal gammopathy** of uncertain significance (MGUS) which can precede the development of MM.

Definitive diagnosis of MM ultimately requires the identification of increased plasma cells in the bone marrow or the presence of a plasmacytoma (Table 54-1). Evaluation of the patient also includes a skeletal survey (plain x-rays of the whole body), determination of renal function, and a calcium level. Bone involvement results in lytic lesions detectable on plain films but not on bone scan (detects only osteoblastic processes). Bony destruction may also result in osteoporosis, pathologic fractures, and hypercalcemia. The β_2-microglobulin level is elevated in most patients and high levels portend a poor prognosis. Amyloid may be seen as eosinophilic material in tissue and more specifically identified by apple green birefringence on Congo red staining of tissue.

Table 54-1 **Criteria for the Diagnosis of MM**[*]

1. Bone marrow plasma cells of >10%
2. Plasmacytoma
3. M-protein in serum >3.0 g IgG
4. Light chains in urine >1.0 g/dL
5. Lytic bone lesions
6. Plasma cells circulating in peripheral blood

[*]Diagnosis: criteria 1 and 2 OR 1 or 2 + 3, 4, 5, or 6.

Management

Patients with minimal disease (smoldering MM) may be safely observed, but once symptoms develop, treatment must be initiated. Unfortunately, the best chemotherapeutic regimen has not been determined. Once a response to a chemotherapeutic regimen has been demonstrated (usually 50% or greater decline in M-protein and/or B-J protein), patients who are under age 70 are referred for autologous bone marrow transplantation. The bisphosphonates are used to stabilize bone disease and to treat hypercalcemia. Localized radiotherapy is also palliative in patients with bone pain or pathologic fractures.

MUSCULOSKELETAL

INFECTIOUS ARTHRITIS

Erica Friedman

KEY POINTS

- Septic arthritis presents as an acute, monoarticular large joint arthritis in patients with risk factors, most commonly persistent bacteremia or damaged joints.
- The most common cause of infectious arthritis in individuals under age 40 is DGI.
- Synovial fluid findings consistent with septic arthritis include WBC >50,000 cells/μL with predominately neutrophils and a low synovial fluid glucose (<50% serum glucose).
- Parenteral antibiotic treatment must be initiated immediately to prevent joint destruction.

INTRODUCTION

Infections cause three main types of arthritis. **Septic arthritis** is caused by direct invasion of a joint cavity by bacteria that remain viable within the joint. **Immune complex arthritis** is caused by the deposition of circulating immune complexes generated by the immune response to an infectious agent, and is best typified by disseminated gonococcal infection (DGI). **Reactive arthritis** is caused by an immune response to an infectious agent. The immune response may be to a fragment of an infectious agent or because of alterations within the joint that expose neoantigens and generate an immune response to them. The fragment of the infectious agent may remain in the joint, but no viable infectious agents persist within the joint. This most commonly occurs after an infection with *Shigella* or *Chlamydia*.

Acute bacterial nongonococcal arthritis typically occurs in patients with an underlying predisposition, particularly persistent bacteremia, immunosuppression, or damaged joints. For example, patients with rheumatoid arthritis have the highest incidence of septic arthritis due to their joint damage and concomitant use of immunosuppressive medications. Certain organisms which are considered arthrotropic tend to predominate. Gram positives (especially *Staphylococcus aureus*) are the most commonly implicated, accounting for 80% of all septic arthritides. Gram negatives account for approximately 15% and anaerobes only 5%.

As opposed to septic arthritis, most individuals with gonococcal arthritis are otherwise healthy. The arthritis occurs as part of a DGI and always follows a mucosal gonococcal infection (cervicitis, urethritis, pharyngitis, or proctitis). The infection is more common in women and often occurs during menses or pregnancy. Gonococcal arthritis is the most common cause of septic arthritis under the age of 40 years.

PATHOPHYSIOLOGY

Nongonococcal infectious arthritis infection occurs via one of three mechanisms: hematogenous spread secondary to bacteremia, contiguous spread from a local infection (such as osteomyelitis), or direct inoculation from trauma or surgery. The most common route is hematogenous spread via synovial capillaries which lack a basement membrane allowing free flow of bacteria from the bloodstream into the synovium. Once bacteria enter the synovial fluid, they attach to articular cartilage. Within hours an inflammatory process begins with the influx of neutrophils, complement activation, and release of chemokines. The combined effects of infection and inflammation lead to cartilage degeneration within 48 hours. If the infection is not treated promptly, cartilage destruction will ensue with further spread of bacteria and inflammation into subchondral bone.

The initial event in gonococcal arthritis is a mucosal infection with *Neisseria gonorrhoeae*. Approximately 1% of individuals will then develop a hematogenous infection (gonococcemia) which allows dissemination to joints as well as skin. The resultant joint pathology can either be a tenosynovitis, presumably caused by the deposition of circulating immune complexes, or a purulent monoarthritis, presumably caused by the direct invasion by *N. gonorrhoeae*.

CLINICAL PRESENTATION

The classic presentation of septic arthritis is an acute monoarticular arthritis, which occurs in over 80% of cases. Patients typically present within 24–48 hours of onset of symptoms because of the severity of the pain, which occurs at rest and increases with movement and weight bearing. The **knee** is the most commonly affected joint, followed by the ankle, wrist, shoulder, hip, elbow, and sacroiliac joint in descending order of frequency. Systemic symptoms of anorexia, weight loss, fatigue, fever and chills, rash, and other organ dysfunction are often associated as well. Physical examination for the acute monoarthritis typically reveals a warm, erythematous, swollen joint with a large joint effusion, pain on palpation, and decreased active and passive range of motion (ROM). Patients with septic arthritis of the hip typically have no apparent swelling, but will complain of groin pain which worsens with activity.

Less commonly, patients can present with an insidious onset with joint findings (swelling) that are often out of proportion to the patients' complaints (massive effusion with minimal complaints). Similar to the acute monoarthritis, it usually affects large joints (knees, hips, elbows). This presentation occurs more commonly in individuals infected with atypical bacteria, such as *Borrelia burgdorferi* (Lyme disease) or *Mycobacterium tuberculosis*, or with fungal infections, most commonly *Coccidioides immitis* and *Blastomycosis dermatitides*. Clues to the infectious agent can often be obtained on history. For example, patients with Lyme disease commonly have cranial nerve palsies, heart block, or a history of an erythema migrans rash. Patients with tuberculosis frequently report weight loss, fever, and night sweats. Last, fungal infections often have concomitant pulmonary symptoms or erythema nodosum.

The classic triad for **DGI** is **dermatitis**, **tenosynovitis**, and **polyarthritis**. Although preceded by a mucosal gonorrhea infection, most patients are asymptomatic from that source. Patients will initially complain of migratory polyarthralgias typically involving the wrist, knee, ankle, and/or elbow. Thereafter, 60% of patients will develop a tenosynovitis and 40% will develop a purulent monoarthritis, most commonly involving the knee. Patients with DGI and tenosynovitis will also have warm erythematous joints, but classically do not have effusion and only have pain on movement of the involved tendons. Patients should also be evaluated for extra-articular sites of infection and evidence of a local or diffuse skin rash. Two-thirds of patients will also develop the classic skin lesion of small necrotic pustules on the palms and soles (Fig. 55-1).

EVALUATION

Synovial fluid analysis is essential to make the diagnosis of septic arthritis (Table 55-1). Synovial fluid should be sent for cell count, differential, glucose, analysis for crystals, Gram stain, and culture. The culture is essential in establishing the diagnosis; however, even classic nongonococcal septic arthritis will have negative cultures in 10–30% of patients. Thus, a negative culture does not completely exclude septic arthritis. If DGI is suspected, the synovial fluid culture should include chocolate agar as 40% of cases will have a positive culture. Other lab tests are not as helpful, although the presence of renal or liver dysfunction may suggest sepsis. Blood cultures

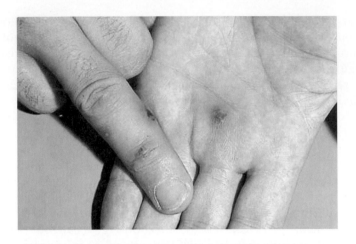

Figure 55-1 **Disseminated gonococcal infection. Hemorrhagic, painful pustules on erythematous bases on the palm and the finger of the other hand.** (*Source:* Reproduced with permission from Wolff K, Johnson RA, Suurmond D, et al. *Fitzpatrick's Color Atlas & Synopsis of Clinical Dermatology*, 5th ed. New York: McGraw-Hill, 2005, Figure 27-17.)

in individuals with DGI are positive in 40% if tenosynovitis is present but rarely if they have acute monoarthritis. The most useful tests for suspected DGI are cultures of the throat, urethra, cervix, and rectum as one is positive in 80% of patients. Radiographs are usually nonspecific early in the course of the arthritis.

Other conditions to consider in the differential diagnosis include crystal-induced arthritis (gout or pseudogout), traumatic arthritis (especially

Table 55-1 **Synovial Fluid Studies in the Most Common Causes of an Acute Monoarthritis**

	Septic Arthritis	DGI	Inflammatory	Traumatic
Appearance	Cloudy	Cloudy	Translucent	Bloody
WBC	>50,000	>50,000	5000–50,000	<5000
Polymorphonuclear cells (PMNs)	>90%	>90%	>50%	<25%
Culture	90% positive	40% positive	Negative	Negative

hemarthrosis), Still's disease, reactive arthritis, or other inflammatory arthritides (rheumatoid arthritis). With the exception of traumatic arthritis, these are inflammatory and often have a similar presentation to septic arthritis. Thus, the diagnosis depends on the synovial fluid analysis (Table 55-1). The most common cause of monoarticular arthritis remains crystal-induced disease (gout or pseudogout), so these must be excluded.

MANAGEMENT

Treatment of an infected joint requires antibiotics and **adequate joint drainage**. Initial joint aspiration is usually sufficient, but repeat arthrocenteses may be necessary if effusion persists. Open surgical drainage may be required for difficult joint aspirations (shoulder or hip), inadequately drained joints, or persistently positive cultures despite appropriate antibiotic and drainage. If a prosthesis becomes infected, it usually needs to be removed, and an antibiotic-impregnated spacer placed. A new prosthesis can be placed after 2–6 weeks of IV antibiotics.

Pharmacologic treatment should be initiated immediately after appropriate cultures are taken (before culture confirmation or sensitivities) as delays in treatment can cause permanent cartilage damage or spread the infection to other sites. Empiric antibiotics are usually guided by the initial Gram stain results.

- Gram positive: cefazolin or nafcillin/oxacillin
- Gram-negative cocci (presumed *Neisseria*): ceftriaxone or cefotaxime
- Gram-negative rods: cefepime or piperacillin/tazobactam

If the Gram stain does not yield any organisms, then broad coverage with antibiotics active against both gram-positive and gram-negative bacteria are necessary. The addition of **vancomycin** should be considered if the infection is hospital acquired or in communities with a high rate of community-acquired methicillin-resistant *S. aureus* (MRSA). Once a specific bacterium is isolated in culture, specific antibiotic coverage can be directed (see Chap. 50). Parenteral antimicrobials are usually given for 3–4 weeks followed by oral antimicrobials for 2–4 weeks. The total duration of treatment depends on the host immune status, organism, susceptibilities, and the presence of a prosthetic joint.

NEUROLOGIC

ALTERED MENTAL STATUS

Christopher A. Feddock

KEY POINTS

- Delirium is a common but often unrecognized complication in hospitalized elderly patients.
- Recognition of risk factors is essential to preventing delirium.
- Haloperidol is the drug of choice for patients with severe behavioral symptoms.

INTRODUCTION

The term **mental status change** refers to a large range of symptoms including changes in the level of consciousness and the content of consciousness. **Delirium** is a more specific term referring to an acute confusional state. The risk of delirium increases with severity of illness and age, occurring in 25–50% of elderly hospitalized patients. Delirium can be a sign of serious illness such as myocardial infarction or infection and carries a poor prognosis. Patients who have delirium during a hospitalization are more likely to have a prolonged hospitalization, functional decline, and be institutionalized. The 1-year mortality following a diagnosis of delirium is 40%. Unfortunately, delirium is commonly missed by nurses and physicians and not appropriately managed.

PATHOPHYSIOLOGY

The underlying pathophysiology of delirium has yet to be delineated. Delirium is felt to be a final common pathway of global cerebral dysfunction caused by a range of insults. Symptoms develop because of reduced cerebral oxidative metabolism and impaired neurotransmitter systems. Classic delirium develops in patients given **anticholinergic** and **dopaminergic** medications. Further, patients with delirium from anticholinergics generally respond to cholinesterase inhibitors. Likewise, the most effective drugs for treating the symptoms of delirium are dopamine antagonists.

CLINICAL PRESENTATION

Delirium has an **acute onset** usually over a period of hours to days. The **symptoms fluctuate** throughout the day and are characteristically worse at night with lucid periods occurring during the day. Patients often have **difficulty focusing their attention** and following conversation and commands. Cognitive deficits range from **disorganized thinking** to memory deficits and impaired language. Some patients may also develop an **altered level of consciousness** from hyperactive (agitation) to hypoactive (lethargy) or a combination of both (Table 56-1). Another characteristic feature of delirium is **disturbance of the sleep wake cycle** with daytime somnolence and nighttime insomnia. Last, about 30% of patients will have hallucinations, which are usually visual. Auditory hallucinations may also occur, but are more suggestive of psychotic etiologies. The duration of delirium can be highly variable. Symptoms typically resolve as the underlying disorders are managed and the patient improves; however, some symptoms can persist for weeks to months.

EVALUATION

The first step is to confirm that the patient has delirium. The **confusion assessment method** provides a simple set of diagnostic criteria. Individuals are diagnosed with delirium if they have an **acute onset of fluctuating**

Table 56-1 **Levels of Consciousness**

Hyperalert	Awake, anxious and agitated, or restless
Normal	Awake, cooperative, oriented, and tranquil
Lethargic	Awake but responds to commands only
Obtunded	Appears asleep (this is not true sleep) but responds briskly to a light glabellar tap or a loud auditory stimulus
Stuporous	Appears asleep, and responds only sluggishly to a light glabellar tap or a loud auditory stimulus
Coma	Appears asleep, with no response to stimuli

symptoms marked by inattention and either disorganized thinking or an altered level of consciousness. In elderly patients, delirium may be difficult to differentiate from dementia. Although the manifestations are often similar, delirium is marked by an acute onset and patients with dementia do not typically develop altered level of consciousness and hallucinations unless they are in the end-stage of dementia. A careful history of baseline mental status and abilities is essential. Further, patients with dementia are at great risk of developing delirium and, in fact, 30–50% of all patients with delirium have underlying dementia.

The next step is to determine the underlying cause of the delirium. This multifactorial condition typically occurs in patients who have predisposing factors and then develop an insult which precipitates the acute change. **Common predisposing conditions include age (over 65 years), immobility, visual or hearing impairments, a history of neurologic disease (dementia, stroke, and so forth), polypharmacy, alcohol or drug abuse, renal disease, and hepatic disease**. All of these conditions make patients prone to develop delirium with even seemingly minor conditions. Common causes of delirium are listed in Table 56-2. Three causes account for the majority of cases— drugs, underlying infections, and alcohol withdrawal.

Because of the multitude of possibilities causing delirium, there is no established algorithm, so the evaluation should be customized to each individual. A thorough history and physical will often reveal predisposing conditions and causes that need to be addressed. Some basic laboratory tests may be informative such as **electrolytes** (including calcium, magnesium, and phosphorous), **glucose**, **renal function**, **hepatic function**, and **urinalysis**. Pulse oximetry should be checked in all patients to exclude hypoxia. Elderly patients should be evaluated for infection as delirium may be the only sign of a serious infection. Patients should have an ECG and cardiac biomarkers checked. Patients should have a chest x-ray and cultures from urine, blood and possibly CSF. Neuroimaging is often obtained, but rarely leads to a diagnosis. Selective use of neuroimaging is recommended targeting patients with a history of trauma or focal neurologic signs or those without an apparent etiology. Electroencephalogram (EEG) is only helpful if seizures are suspected. The only EEG finding in delirium is nonspecific diffuse slow-wave activity, which is not present in 20% of patients with delirium.

MANAGEMENT

Prevention is the key to the management of elderly patients at risk for developing delirium during their hospitalization. **Medications should be minimized** with careful attention to avoid those with psychotropic properties. In the process of decreasing medications, wean unnecessary medications which have withdrawal potential (e.g., benzodiazepines, opiates, and selective

Table 56-2 **Most Common Conditions Causing Delirium**

Metabolic	Volume depletion
	Hepatic failure
	Hypoglycemia
	Hyperglycemia
	Hyponatremia
	Hypernatremia
	Hypercalcemia
	Hypoxemia
	Uremia
Infectious	Urinary tract infection
	Pneumonia
	Cellulitis
Drugs or toxins	Alcohol abuse
	Alcohol withdrawal
	Anticholinergics
	Anticonvulsants
	Antihistamines
	Benzodiazepines
	Corticosteroids
	Digoxin
	H_2-receptor antagonists
	Opiates
	Sedatives
Cardiovascular	Congestive heart failure
	Myocardial infarction
	Shock
Neurologic	Cerebrovascular accident
	Encephalitis
	Intracranial hemorrhage
	Meningitis
Environmental	Bladder catheters
	Pain
	Restraints
	Sleep deprivation

serotonin reuptake inhibitors [SSRIs]). Studies have shown a fourfold increase in delirium when more than three medications are started on admission and a 14-fold increase in patients who are taking over six medications. **Mobilization** should be encouraged and the use of restraining devices (physical restraints and bladder catheters) should be minimized. Every effort should be made to preserve sleep schedules and avoid sleep deprivation. **Communication** with the patient is essential, particularly orienting the patient to their location and reason for admission. Ensure that patients have the necessary hearing and visual aids to facilitate orientation and communication. Last, any potential causes of delirium should be promptly addressed and treated.

Once patients develop delirium, the goals of management are to provide supportive care, prevent complications, and treat behavioral symptoms. The most effective care measures are to reorient the patient in a calm comfortable environment and to avoid physical restraints. Keeping clocks, calendars, and familiar objects from home in plain site can often aid in comforting and reorienting the patient. Family members and friends can often be soothing influences for patients with delirium as well.

Pharmacologic management should be reserved for patients who are at risk of harming themselves or others despite conservative management. **Haloperidol** is the preferred agent at doses of 0.5–1 mg orally every 4 hours or intramuscularly every hour as needed to manage symptoms. Although haloperidol is often dosed in shorter intervals, this can result in overdose as the time to peak effect is 4 hours with oral dosing and 1 hour with intramuscular dosing. Intravenous haloperidol should be avoided because of the short half-life and a greater risk of side effects, particularly QT prolongation and hypotension. Older patients are also more likely to develop extrapyramidal side effects, especially if given doses over 5 mg daily. Alternatives include the atypical antipsychotics (olanzapine, risperidone, and quetiapine) because of the lower incidence of extrapyramidal side effects, but they are costly and offer no other advantages. Benzodiazepines should generally be avoided except in alcohol withdrawal delirium for which they are the preferred agents. Although they have a rapid onset of action, benzodiazepines cause sedation and disorientation, which tend to prolong and worsen the symptoms of delirium.

SEIZURES

Meriem Bensalem-Owen

KEY POINTS

- The diagnosis of a seizure is a purely clinical diagnosis, mainly based on history.
- Identification of the seizure type is essential for appropriate treatment.
- Although most are idiopathic, patients should be evaluated for specific etiologies.
- Be familiar with the potential side effects of the most commonly used AEDs.
- SE is a medical emergency.

INTRODUCTION

Seizures result from an abnormal, sudden, synchronous discharge of a population of cerebral neurons. The particular site of the brain affected determines the clinical expression of the seizure. Seizures are commonly classified as either partial (focal) or generalized depending on their onset. Epilepsy is a chronic neurologic condition in which recurrent (two or more) seizures occur unprovoked by systemic or neurologic insults. In the United States, epilepsy affects approximately 2.5 million individuals, with an estimated 125,000–181,000 new cases diagnosed each year.

PATHOPHYSIOLOGY

Neurotransmission is accomplished by the conduction of electrical impulses from the neuronal body to the axon, where neurotransmitters are released into the synaptic cleft and stimulate the depolarization of the next neuron. At rest, neurons have a high concentration of intracellular K^+ whereas Na^+ and Ca^{2+} predominate outside of the cell. In this resting state, extracellular

Na$^+$ flows into the cell and intracellular K$^+$ flows out, but the resting cell potential is maintained by a Na-K pump which continually pumps K$^+$ back in and Na$^+$ back out. When the cell membrane is depolarized, Na$^+$ channels open allowing ions to flow intracellularly which creates the action potential. This is followed by the efflux of K$^+$ which repolarizes the cell membrane. When this action potential reaches the axon terminal, Ca^{2+} channels open allowing ion influx which stimulates the release of neurotransmitters into the synaptic cleft. Neurotransmitters are classified into excitatory (glutamate and aspartate) if they stimulate depolarization of the next neuron or inhibitory (gamma-aminobutyric acid [GABA]) if they inhibit it.

Seizures occur from an imbalance in these inhibitory and excitatory stimuli, which reduces the threshold for neuronal depolarization within a group of neurons causing paroxysmal discharges. These discharges may remain localized and restricted in focus (simple partial seizures) or may spread to other areas of the brain (generalized seizures). Depending on the size of the discharging area and the area of brain involved, behavioral changes and physical signs may occur. When these abnormal neuronal discharges are recorded by an electroencephalogram (EEG) from the scalp, the paroxysms appear as spikes or sharp wave potentials, known as epileptiform discharges.

Seizures can occur in normal individuals under conditions which shift the balance toward excitability. For example, fever, electrolyte disturbances, drugs, and toxins can all cause seizures in otherwise normal patients. Alternatively, a pathologic change can take place in the brain that converts a normal neural network into one that is hyperexcitable. An example of this is penetrating head trauma, after which 50% of patients will have seizures. The pathophysiology of epileptic disorders is not very well understood, but they are caused by some change that results in a hyperexcitable neural network. Structural abnormalities of neurotransmitter receptors and ion channels, cortical remodeling, and loss of inhibitory neuronal activity have all been implicated as possible mechanisms.

CLINICAL PRESENTATION

Most seizures are short periods (<2 minutes) of transient cerebral dysfunction. The period during which the seizure actually occurs is referred to as the **ictal period**. After a seizure, a **postictal period** occurs lasting a few minutes to several hours. This period is characterized by unresponsiveness, fatigue, agitation, speech difficulties, or focal limb weakness, known as Todd's paralysis. Seizures are classified according to the characteristics of the ictal period as either partial (focal) or generalized (Table 57-1).

Partial seizures occur from localized paroxysmal electrical activity, so are characterized by focal motor, sensory, autonomic, or psychic symptoms. Patients may develop only a subjective sensation (usually the same symptom in a given patient), known as **aura** without any objective findings. More

Table 57-1 **Classification of Primary Seizure Disorders**

Seizure Type	Key Feature	Initial Treatment
Partial Seizure		
Simple	Focal motor or somatosensory symptoms with preservation of consciousness	Carbamazepine Phenytoin Oxcarbamazepine
Complex	Focal symptoms preceded, accompanied or followed by impaired awareness	
Generalized Seizure		
Absence	Abrupt episodes of altered consciousness	Ethosuximide Valproic acid
Myoclonic	Single or multiple quick muscular jerks usually with preserved consciousness	Valporic acid Clonezepan
Tonic-clonic	Sudden loss of consciousness with rigidity followed by jerking	Phenytoin Valproic acid

commonly, patients will develop a variety of focal neurologic findings. Motor features can include focal tonic or clonic activity, vocalizations, speech arrest, or involuntary movements of the head or eyes. Sensory symptoms can include a variety of somatosensory, auditory, visual, olfactory, gustatory, or vertiginous sensations. Autonomic findings include piloerection, pallor, sweating, or flushing. Last, psychic experiences include "déjà vu," illusions or hallucinations. Partial seizures can be further subdivided into **simple partial**, where awareness is not impaired and **complex partial seizures**, which are characterized by impairment of awareness, but not necessarily loss of consciousness. Patients may also develop a generalized seizure following their focal symptoms if the electrical discharge becomes generalized. For example, a patient may experience a seizure arising from the olfactory cortex, and may report a "funny smell" (simple partial seizure). This experience may be followed by staring and manual automatisms, such as wringing clothes, and observers may report that the patient is not responding to them (complex partial seizure). If the patient subsequently falls to the ground and has tonic posturing followed by clonic movements, the seizure is said to have secondarily generalized.

Generalized seizures occur when the abnormal electrical discharge starts over both hemispheres at the same time. The most common type of generalized seizures is the **generalized tonic-clonic seizure,** previously called "grand mal" seizure. It is characterized initially by a tonic phase lasting 10–15 seconds during which the jaw snaps shut, the entire body is overcome by a tonic spasm, and cyanosis can be noted. This phase is followed by rhythmic generalized muscle contractions lasting 1–2 minutes. During the terminal phase of the seizure breathing resumes although the patient remains unconscious. At times, patients can bite their tongue, and lose bladder or sometimes bowel control (all clues that a seizure has occurred). **Absence seizures** are a type of generalized seizure, during which patients do not experience an aura or a postictal phase. This type of seizure usually lasts a few seconds, and is characterized by behavioral arrest, impaired awareness, staring, and sometimes repetitive blinking. Occasionally, patients will also have mild clonic, tonic, or atonic episodes as well. The onset and cessation of these episodes is quite abrupt, and many patients do not realize that they have had a seizure.

Status epilepticus (SE) is a life-threatening condition defined as a prolonged seizure or repetitive seizures between which the patient does not fully recover. Since most seizures end within 2 minutes, any patient presenting with a seizure lasting longer than 5 minutes should be presumed to have SE. Although most individuals have generalized tonic-clonic SE, any type of partial or generalized seizure can develop into SE. The generalized tonic-clonic SE is the most concerning, because it can be life threatening.

EVALUATION

When evaluating a patient with a suspected seizure, the first goal is to confirm that the episode actually was a seizure. In most cases, the diagnosis of a seizure is a **purely clinical diagnosis** with most tests providing little confirmatory information. Common conditions that can be mistaken for seizures include syncope, movement disorders, migraine headaches, sleep disturbance and parasomnias, panic attacks, and psychogenic spells (pseudoseizures) which can occur in patients with conversion disorder.

The history is the most important diagnostic tool to determine if the episode is consistent with a seizure. Patients should be specifically asked to describe any recurrent stereotypic sensations or experiences, which could constitute an aura. Observers of the episode should be asked to describe the characteristics and duration of the seizure and postictal phase. Although most seizures occur unpredictably, a few patients will have seizures which are provoked by specific stimuli, such as sleep deprivation or flashing lights. The neurologic examination is often normal unless the patient has a structural brain lesion or suffered a cerebral insult. In the postictal period, patients may have some decrease in awareness or focal abnormalities, such as weakness or asymmetric and brisk deep tendon reflexes.

An **EEG** is frequently obtained after a new-onset seizure; however, the EEG is quite limited diagnostically. Specifically, a normal EEG does not exclude seizures or epilepsy. Prolonged EEG with video monitoring can be very helpful if a patient has frequent events suspicious for seizures. If a patient has a seizure during the EEG, a specific diagnosis can often be made. For example, absence seizures have a very characteristic pattern of generalized 3 Hz spike and wave discharges. Less than one-third of patients with partial seizures have no obvious changes on EEG even when they are actively seizing, because the area of cerebral cortex involved is small and not detected on the scalp EEG.

Most seizures (60%) are idiopathic, but every patient should be evaluated for potential etiologies with a first seizure (Table 57-2). A past history of seizures or febrile convulsions is an important clue to underlying epilepsy. Past conditions such as head trauma, stroke, or brain tumors are potential etiologies and also have prognostic implications. Careful questioning as to alcohol intake and cessation, and drug use are crucial. Patients should be carefully questioned and examined for symptoms or signs of meningitis or encephalitis. A careful skin examination may reveal evidence of neurocutaneous disorders, such as neurofibromatosis (café au lait spots and axillary freckling) or tuberous sclerosis (shagreen patch, subungual fibromas, and hypopigmented spots). Limb asymmetry may be a clue to perinatal brain injury which may predispose to seizures.

Table 57-2 **Known Causes of Seizures in Adults**

Metabolic	Drug	Illness	Neurologic
Hyponatremia	Alcohol withdrawal	Eclampsia	Central nervous
Hypernatremia	Theophylline	Hypertensive	system (CNS)
Hypoglycemia	Phenothiazines	encephalopathy	vasculitis
Hyperglycemia	Lidocaine	Liver failure	Meningitis
Hyperosmolality	Meperidine	Polyarteritis	Encephalitis
Hypocalcemia	Isoniazid	nodosa	Acute head
Respiratory	Amitriptyline	Porphyria	trauma
alkalosis	Haloperidol	Renal failure	Stroke
Uremia	Cyclosporine	Sickle cell	Brain abscess
	Cocaine (crack)	disease	Brain tumor
	Phencyclidine	Syphilis	Alzheimer's
	Amphetamines	Systemic	disease
	Phenytoin	lupus	Neuro-
	Carbamazepine	erythematosus	degenerative
		Thrombotic	diseases
		thrombocytopenic	
		purpura	
		Whipple's disease	

Patients with a first unprovoked seizure should have a basic laboratory and imaging workup. Laboratory tests, as indicated by the history, may include electrolytes, urine drug screen, renal function, white blood cell count, and hepatic panel. **Magnetic resonance imaging (MRI)** of the brain with temporal lobe protocol (thin coronal slices through the hippocampi) should be ordered if the patient had a focal seizure or an abnormal neurologic examination. Alternatively, a computed tomography (CT) of the head may be obtained, although an MRI is more sensitive for detecting subtle lesions. If meningitis or encephalitis is suspected, a lumbar puncture should be performed.

MANAGEMENT

Antiepileptic drug (AED) therapy may not be necessary in patients presenting with a new-onset seizure. A careful evaluation may reveal etiologies which are reversible. Even in individuals without a clear etiology, AEDs can be safely withheld if they have had a short uncomplicated seizure as they do not affect prognosis. AED therapy should be started in patients with a high chance of recurrence such as patients with structural brain abnormalities (i.e., trauma, tumor, or stroke), focal neurologic findings, an abnormal EEG, or who have partial seizures. Overall, monotherapy or combination therapy can achieve control of seizures in over 70% of patients. Patients who do not achieve control after two different trials of monotherapy and a trial of combination therapy are considered medically refractory and other treatment modalities should be considered such as epilepsy surgery, vagus nerve stimulator implantation, and ketogenic diet.

Most AEDs target the presumed pathophysiology of seizures (Table 57-3). The classes of medication are targeted toward the sodium, potassium, or calcium channels to reduce the propagation of the action potential, or block neurotransmission by enhancing GABA activity or antagonizing glutamate activity. Patients are usually started on low-dose monotherapy with a drug of choice. The dosage is gradually increased until the patient no longer experiences seizures, the maximum dosage is attained, or side effects prevent further dose adjustment. If the patient continues to experience seizures, a second drug preferably with a different mechanism can be added and the first drug gradually withdrawn. The choice between first- and second-generation AEDs can be difficult as most second-generation AEDs have considerable advantages. All AEDs have comparable efficacy, but the newer drugs have fewer drug interactions and generally better safety profiles. Unfortunately, most of the newer AEDs are also considerably more expensive.

SE is a medical emergency that must be aggressively treated. Initial management should be directed at securing an airway and maintaining good oxygenation. Routine labs are drawn to check for reversible metabolic disturbances. Glucose is administered in case hypoglycemia is responsible.

Table 57-3 **Antiepileptic Medications**

	Mechanism	Adverse Effect
First-Generation AEDs		
Phenytoin	Na	Rash, ataxia, hirsutism, gingival hypertrophy, osteoporosis
Carbamazepine	Na	Rash, diplopia, sexual dysfunction, osteoporosis
Valproic acid	Multiple	Weight gain, tremor, hair loss, pancreatitis, hepatotoxicity, encephalopathy, polycystic ovaries
Ethosuximide	Na, GABA	Nausea, vomiting, anorexia, rash
Second-Generation AEDs		
Gabapentin	Unknown	Weight gain, edema, myoclonus
Lamotrigine	Na, glutamate	Rash
Levetiracetam	Unknown	Behavioral changes, asthenia
Oxcarbazepine	Na, Ca	Hyponatremia, diplopia, rash
Tiagabine	Na	Encephalopathy
Topiramate	Multiple	Renal stones, speech difficulties, paresthesias, weight loss, acidosis, closed-angle glaucoma
Zonisamide	Multiple	Renal stones, weight loss, paresthesias, sulfa allergy
Pregabalin	Unknown	Dizziness, somnolence, edema, weight gain

If thiamine deficiency is a concern, administer thiamine intravenously before glucose administration in adults to avoid precipitating or exacerbating Wernicke's encephalopathy. The initial drug of choice for the treatment of SE is a benzodiazepine, usually lorazepam or diazepam. Regardless of the response, all patients should be loaded on intravenous fosphenytoin. If seizures persist, the patient should be intubated and given phenobarbital. Once seizures are controlled, the patient should be admitted to the intensive care unit, and have an EEG to evaluate for subclinical seizures.

Any patient with a seizure should have his or her driving privileges suspended for several (3–12) months; the exact length varies depending on the state. Patients should be counseled to avoid baths and take showers instead because of the risk of drowning if the patient seizes in the bathtub. In addition, patients should avoid working with heavy machinery or working at heights. Women of childbearing age should take folic acid daily because of the association between many AEDs and fetal neural tube defects.

STROKE

Sibu P. Saha
M. Salik Jahania

KEY POINTS

- Stroke is the third most common cause of death in the United States, and is a leading cause of severe, long-term disability.
- Strokes are generally classified as ischemic (80% of strokes) and hemorrhagic.
- CT scan without contrast is the preferred initial diagnostic study.
- Hypertension is the most prevalent and modifiable risk factor for stroke.

INTRODUCTION

Stroke refers to a constellation of neurologic symptoms and deficits caused by disruption of blood flow to a portion of the brain, with subsequent neuronal cell injury or death. In contrast, **transient ischemic attack (TIA)** is the term used for neurologic deficits lasting <24 hours (usually symptoms are <5 minutes) from a temporary disruption of blood flow, with subsequent spontaneous restoration of blood flow and reversal of the neurologic deficits. TIAs are ominous harbingers of impending stroke in the near future. Stroke is the third leading cause of death in the United States and is the leading cause of adult neurologic disability, affecting nearly 700,000 people each year. Indirect and direct costs for stroke are estimated to be about $53 billion per year. Stroke is not just an older person's disease: 28% of strokes happen in persons under age 65.

PATHOPHYSIOLOGY

Strokes are generally classified into two broad categories: **ischemic** strokes and **hemorrhagic** strokes. Over 80% of strokes are ischemic, with blood flow disrupted to the brain despite intact blood vessel integrity. Ischemic strokes can occur from thrombosis, such as from a ruptured atherosclerotic plaque, or arterial intimal dissection. Emboli can also cause ischemic strokes, with emboli arising from the carotid bulb, the aortic arch, and the heart. Ischemic strokes can also occur from hypoperfusion, such as from hypotension, especially in the setting of significant carotid atherosclerosis. An important subset of ischemic strokes are lacunar infarctions, which are small, deep ischemic lesions in the basal ganglia, pons, cerebellum, or internal capsule most often related to intrinsic small vessel disease (lipohyalinosis), seen frequently in patients with hypertension and/or diabetes.

Hemorrhagic strokes occur when a blood vessel supplying the brain ruptures. Spontaneous intracerebral hemorrhage is most often related to hypertension. Other causes of hemorrhagic strokes include subarachnoid hemorrhages, ruptured aneurysms, and ruptured arteriovenous malformations (AVMs). In younger patients (<45) with strokes, one should suspect less common etiologies, such as vasculitis or hypercoagulable states (lupus anticoagulant, antiphospholipid antibody syndrome, hyperhomocysteinemia). Other causes to consider include drug-induced (cocaine, methamphetamine), sickle cell disease, and hyperviscosity syndromes (polycythemia vera, multiple myeloma).

Hypertension is the most prevalent modifiable risk factor for stroke. Hypertensive patients have a risk of stroke that is four to six times higher than their peers. Other risk factors include advanced age, carotid arteriosclerosis, atrial fibrillation, diabetes, hyperlipidemia, and smoking.

CLINICAL PRESENTATION

Symptoms of a stroke may be acute, gradual, or recurrent. Frequent symptoms include weakness and numbness on one side of the body or face, dysphasia, visual deficits, and loss of balance. **Amaurosis fugax** is described by patients as a curtain being pulled down over the visual field of one eye, reflecting retinal emboli from ipsilateral carotid artery disease. Strokes can cause hemodynamic instability, coma, or even death. On the other hand, some patients can have a "silent stroke," where brain damage occurs without any obvious clinical symptoms.

Timing of symptoms can be helpful in determining the etiology of the stroke. Classically, major embolic strokes present suddenly, with maximal deficit occurring immediately, perhaps slowly improving over ensuing days. Thrombotic strokes often present in a stuttering fashion, with deficits worsening or fluctuating over several days. Intracerebral hemorrhage usually has gradual progression of deficits over minutes to hours. A subarachnoid hemorrhage is often described as "the worst headache of my life," accompanied by neck stiffness.

Certain clinical findings suggest involvement of different arteries:

- **Anterior cerebral artery**: contralateral foot and leg weakness, contralateral grasp reflex and sucking reflex, behavioral changes, confusion, abulia (akinetic mutism, manifesting as lack of initiative), urinary incontinence, impairment of gait and stance (gait apraxia)
- **Middle cerebral artery (MCA)**: contralateral face, arm, and leg weakness and sensory loss, homonymous hemianopsia (absence of half a visual field, on the same side in both eyes) with eyes deviated to the side of the lesion, expressive (Broca's) and receptive (Wernicke's) aphasia. (Most people are left-brain dominant, so left MCA strokes result in aphasia whereas right MCA strokes cause defects in visual or spatial functions, manifesting as unilateral neglect of a limb, or difficulty recognizing objects by feel, "stereognosis.")
- **Posterior circulation (vertebrobasilar artery)**: vomiting, vertigo, ataxia, dysarthria, discrete cranial nerve palsies, diplopia, weakness, or sensory disturbances in some or all of the limbs

Certain conditions should be considered in the differential diagnosis depending on the patient presentation. Patients presenting with altered mental status or coma can represent a large differential diagnosis (see Chap. 56). **Bell's palsy** is sometimes mistaken for stroke, presenting with unilateral facial weakness. In Bell's palsy, the patient will not be able to contract the muscles of the forehead on the side of the facial weakness; in contrast, because of contralateral and ipsilateral central innervation of the frontalis muscle, a conscious patient with a stroke will be able to contract the muscles of the forehead. **Hemiplegic migraines** can present with focal motor deficits. **Todd's paralysis** is a transient focal motor deficit that occurs after a seizure, resolving spontaneously. **Multiple sclerosis** can cause vague stroke-like symptoms (optic neuritis presenting as acute loss of vision, sometimes confused with amaurosis fugax), but the neurologic findings will not be consistent with any cerebral vasculature distribution.

EVALUATION

The diagnosis of acute stroke is usually made with a computed tomography (CT) without contrast of the brain. CT is preferred to MRI because of its rapid availability and better detection of intracranial hemorrhage than MRI within the first 48 hours of a bleed (although the CT scan of a patient with ischemic stroke may be normal in the first 6 hours; Fig. 58-1). Once the patient is stabilized, other studies are often performed to look for the etiology of the stroke, especially treatable causes (e.g., carotid stenosis, vasculitis). An MRI can provide more detail particularly with smaller cortical infarctions.

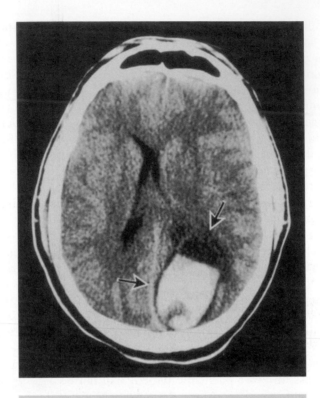

Figure 58-1 **Intracerebral hemorrhage (arrows). Note compression of ventricles.** (*Source:* Reproduced with permission from Lichtman MA, Beutler E, Kipps TJ, et al. *Williams Hematology*, 7th ed. New York: McGraw-Hill, 2006, Figure 115-10.)

An MR-angiogram can show evidence of vasculitis. An ECG may reveal atrial fibrillation, and an echocardiogram a mural thrombus. Duplex carotid ultrasound can demonstrate significant stenosis. When hypercoagulable states or vasculitis is suspected, other labs may be appropriate (e.g., erythrocyte sedimentation rate [ESR], rapid plasma reagin [RPR], antinuclear antibody [ANA], and antiphospholipid antibody).

MANAGEMENT

Initial management entails stabilizing the patient by ensuring a patent airway and effective ventilation. Blood pressure should not be lowered precipitously, as an adequate mean arterial pressure will be necessary to maintain cerebral perfusion (see Chap. 10). Patients presenting within 3 hours with an acute ischemic stroke and moderate neurologic symptoms should be considered for thrombolytic therapy. Rehabilitation and physical therapy is a significant component in the management of stroke patients. The goal of rehabilitation is to regain as much function as possible. It is a long-term process and it is important to manage the patient's depression and pain (such as neuropathic pain). In general, about one-third to two-thirds of patients who survive a stroke regain independence, and up to 80% of these patients retain or regain the ability to walk.

Given the severe consequences of a stroke, primary prevention is important particularly in patients with multiple risk factors. Prevention involves aggressive control of hypertension and hyperlipidemia, smoking cessation, and anticoagulation for patients with atrial fibrillation. In addition, patients with symptoms referable to the carotid artery and >60% stenosis of the vessel can benefit from prophylactic carotid endarterectomy. Carotid artery stenting is gaining in popularity though still currently recommended only for patients considered high-risk such as those with recurrent stenosis, severe cardiopulmonary compromise, or with a history of neck irradiation or dissection. Asymptomatic patients with significant stenosis (>60%) may benefit from endarterectomy, but the benefits are less clear. In an experienced surgeon's hands (<3% operative complication rate), stroke risk is decreased, but it's unclear whether risk of permanently disabling stroke or death is less with endarterectomy in asymptomatic patients. Secondary prevention of stroke entails antiplatelet therapy with aspirin or occasionally clopidogrel. Warfarin is indicated for patients with atrial fibrillation.

SYNCOPE

Jennifer R. Kogan
Susan Day

KEY POINTS

- Syncope results from a decrease in cardiac output (decreased stroke volume, decreased heart rate), a decrease in systemic vascular resistance, decreased cerebral perfusion, or nutrient poor cerebral blood flow.
- Neurally mediated syncope, cardiac syncope, and orthostasis are the most common causes of syncope.
- A careful history and physical examination is important since together they can identify a possible cause in up to 45% of patients presenting with syncope in whom a diagnosis can be made.
- The presence of suspected heart disease on history, physical examination, and/or ECG is a strong predictor for a cardiac cause of syncope and warrants further evaluation.

INTRODUCTION

Syncope is defined as a **sudden, transient loss of consciousness associated with loss of postural tone followed by spontaneous recovery**. Syncope is a common problem with as many as 20–37% of "normal" patients having lost consciousness at some point in their lives. Additionally, syncope is responsible for 3–5% of all emergency room visits and 1–3% of all hospital admissions.

Patients in whom the initial episode of syncope is attributed to a cardiac cause are at high risk for increased overall mortality as well as for sudden death; however, this risk is largely related to the patient's underlying cardiac disease rather than the syncope per se. In contrast, young healthy individuals without heart disease and a normal ECG and patients with vasovagal syncope appear to have a benign prognosis. Patients with syncope of unknown cause represent a heterogeneous group of patients and are at intermediate risk of death compared to groups with cardiac and vasovagal syncope.

PATHOPHYSIOLOGY

Syncope occurs when there is transient, insufficient blood flow or nutrient flow to parts of the brain responsible for consciousness (reticular-activating systems and bilateral cerebral hemispheres). This occurs secondary to (1) decreased cardiac output secondary to mechanical outflow obstruction, arrhythmia, or loss of preload, (2) decreased systemic vascular resistance, (3) focal or generalized decrease in cerebral perfusion by cerebrovascular disease, or (4) preserved but nutrient poor cerebral blood flow (hypoglycemia and hypoxia).

The pathophysiology of vasovagal syncope is incompletely understood. One theory involves the Bezold-Jarisch reflex, in which increased or excessive venous pooling causes decreased ventricular volume and an increase in ventricular inotropy. This activates left ventricle mechanoreceptors (cardiac C fibers) which paradoxically stimulate vagal afferent output to the brainstem. Therefore, sympathetic output to the vasculature decreases (vasodilation) and parasympathetic activity increases (bradycardia) leading to hypotension and loss of consciousness.

CLINICAL PRESENTATION

There are many causes of syncope (Table 59-1) although the most common causes are neurally mediated syncope, orthostatic hypotension, and cardiac arrhythmias. The clinical presentation of syncope will, in part, be determined by the underlying cause of the syncopal event (Table 59-2).

EVALUATION

The initial evaluation of a patient with syncope should focus on (1) determining the cause of the patient's syncope and (2) identifying those few patients with clinically serious conditions who will need further diagnostic evaluation and treatment. A careful history (from both the patient and witnesses to the event) and physical examination can suggest a diagnosis in 45% of patients who are diagnosed (Table 59-2). The history should focus on precipitating factors, the specific situation during which the syncope occurred, and any associated neurologic symptoms (e.g., associated with seizure, transient ischemic attack [TIA]). A past medical history of cardiac disease, psychiatric illness, or certain medications (e.g., antihypertensives, antiarrhythmics) may also suggest a certain diagnosis. A family history of sudden death suggests inherited conditions such as hypertrophic cardiomyopathy or long QT syndrome. Excessive use of alcohol or other drugs of abuse may also result in syncope and should be inquired about. The essential

Table 59-1 **Causes of Syncope**

Cardiac—structural	Aortic stenosis, mitral stenosis, left atrial myxoma, aortic dissection, acute myocardial infarction, pericardial tamponade, pulmonary embolism, hypertrophic obstructive cardiomyopathy, pulmonary hypertension
Cardiac—arrhythmias	Tachyarrhythmias: ventricular tachycardia, supraventricular tachycardia, torsades de pointes Bradyarrhythmias: sinus node disease, heart block
NMS	Vasovagal (neurocardiogenic) Carotid sinus Situational (cough, micturition, defecation, swallow)
Neurologic	Seizure disorder, TIA, subclavian steal, normal pressure hydrocephalus
Metabolic	Hypoxia, hypoglycemia, hyperventilation
Psychiatric	Somatization, hysteria, panic disorder
Orthostatic/postural hypotension	
Medications	
Idiopathic	

components of the physical examination include an assessment of the level of alertness, orthostatics, pulse rate, blood pressure, and oxygen saturation. Syncope which is reproduced by a unilateral carotid massage suggests carotid body hypersensitivity. A thorough cardiovascular, pulmonary, and neurologic examination may also have findings which suggest a definitive diagnosis.

Diagnostic evaluation should be focused and tailored to the patient's symptoms and likelihood for underlying disease. For example, in most patients with a classic history suggesting vasovagal syncope, no further evaluation is needed. Electrocardiogram should be ordered in all patients to identify tachy or bradyarrhythmias, conduction disturbances, a prolonged QT interval, chamber enlargement, or ischemia/infarction. A normal ECG lowers the probability of occult arrhythmia or ischemic disease. Whether the evaluation should be performed in the outpatient or inpatient setting depends on the individual patient and the presenting symptoms. Patients who require admission to the hospital for further diagnostic evaluation include those with structural heart disease (such as known coronary artery disease [CAD], valvular disease, physical examination findings such as

Table 59-2 **Clinical Features Suggestive of a Specific Cause of Syncope**

Symptom or Finding	Diagnosis to be Considered
Lacerated tongue, sense of déjà vu or jamais vu, head turning, unusual posturing or jerking limbs no memory of episode afterward, confusion or after episode	Seizure
Episode occurs when going to standing position	Orthostatic hypotension
Episode after cough, micturition, defecation, swallowing	Situational syncope
Prodromal symptoms of nausea, diaphoresis, lightheadedness, and blurred vision and a "washed out" feeling after the event. Episodes associated with preceding fear, pain, unpleasant event, or prolonged standing	Vasovagal syncope
Event occurs with head turning or pressure on the carotid sinus (i.e., tight neckwear, tight collars). Symptoms reproduced by carotid sinus massage	Carotid sinus syncope
Sudden, transient loss of consciousness without prodrome; underlying heart disease (left ventricular dysfunction); palpitations, serious injuries like broken bones can occur	Arrhythmia
Family history of syncope or prolonged QT on ECG	Long QT syndrome
Syncope with exertion	Coronary artery disease, aortic stenosis, hypertrophic obstructive cardiomyopathy, pulmonary hypertension, mitral stenosis
Frequent syncope with somatic symptoms but no heart disease	Psychiatric illness
Medications that prolong QT, cause hypotension, or bradycardia	Medication-associated syncope
Associated vertigo, dysarthria, diplopia	TIA

those of hypertrophic obstructive cardiomyopathy [HOCM] or aortic steno-sis), symptoms suggestive of arrhythmias or ischemia (exertional syncope, chest pain), ECG abnormalities, older age, and focal neurologic findings.

In patients at risk for structural heart disease, an echocardiogram and electrocardiographic (ECG) monitoring are essential. Echocardiography should be ordered for patients with syncope from valvular heart disease, hypertrophic cardiomyopathy, or known or suspected underlying cardiac disease including low left ventricular function. In patients without sus-pected cardiac disease based on history, physical examination, and electro-cardiogram, the yield of echocardiography is very low. Several approaches to monitoring for cardiac arrhythmias include 24- and 48-hour Holter mon-itoring, patient-triggered event recorders, and implantable loop recorders (ILR). In patient-activated event recorders with memory loops, the patient activates the monitor after symptoms occur which freezes in memory the readings from the past 2–5 minutes and subsequent 60 seconds. However, patient compliance and technical difficulties associated with the event recorders can limit their usefulness. ILR are implanted subcutaneously in the left pectoralis region and are used to detect cardiac arrhythmias for a period as long as 18–24 months. ILR can be useful in high-risk patients with recur-rent events. An **electrophysiologic study (EPS)** may be required for high-risk patients in whom preliminary data suggest a high risk of life-threatening cardiac syncope. EPS is usually reserved for patients in whom noninvasive tests fail to provide a cause of syncope because it is both expensive and inva-sive. It can provide important therapeutic and prognostic information in patients with structural heart disease or specific conduction system disease.

In patients who have no risks of structural heart disease and a normal ECG, and have recurrent or severe syncope requiring therapy, a **head-up tilt-table testing (HUTT)** may be helpful. HUTT is widely used to diagnose vasovagal syncope; however, the interpretation of findings and clinical applicability are difficult secondary to issues of reproducibility, sensitivity, and specificity. HUTT is generally used for patients with one or more of the following: (1) recurrent syncope, including exercise-induced syncope after exclusion of organic heart disease, (2) a single episode of syncope associated with injury or motor vehicle accident, (3) a single syncopal event in a high-risk setting (airline pilots), and (4) syncope of another established cause whose treatment might be affected by vasovagal syncope. The first phase of a HUTT is a 10- to 60-minute period of passive upright tilt-table testing at 60–80°. The study is often repeated with pharmacologic agents such as iso-proterenol, nitroglycerin, adenosine, or clomipramine to provoke a response.

In patients with focal neurologic findings, a computed tomography (CT) or magnetic resonance imaging (MRI) of the brain is warranted, but these studies should not be used routinely because of their low yield in the gen-eral evaluation. Although transcranial or carotid Doppler ultrasound is often ordered in the evaluation of syncope, these studies are not recommended unless the patient has neurologic findings or symptoms suggestive of transient ischemia referable to the carotid or vertebrobasilar arteries. Any patient with a history suggestive of seizure should have an electroencephalography (EEG) ordered.

MANAGEMENT

Treatment for syncope involves treating the underlying cause of the syncopal event. Single or infrequent episodes of vasovagal syncope do not require intervention other than patient counseling and observation. Treatment of recurrent vasovagal syncope is largely empirical. Management can include increasing preload (hydration, salt intake, mineralocorticoids), vasoconstrictors, anticholinergic agents, negative cardiac inotropes (beta-blockers), central agents, and in rare instances, pacemaker therapy to prevent bradycardia. Psychiatric problems such as generalized anxiety disorder, panic disorder, somatization disorder, and major depression are common in patients with syncope. Psychiatric evaluation should be considered for patients who have recurrent, unexplained syncope.

OTHER

ALCOHOL WITHDRAWAL

Christopher A. Feddock

KEY POINTS

- Alcohol withdrawal seizures occur between 8 and 48 hours after cessation.
- Alcohol withdrawal delirium (AWD) begins 48–96 hours after abstention.
- AWD is marked by mental confusion, agitation, and fluctuating levels of consciousness in addition to autonomic hyperactivity.
- Only benzodiazepines have proven efficacious in the treatment and prevention of mild to moderate alcohol withdrawal, alcohol withdrawal seizures, and AWD.

INTRODUCTION

Approximately 5% of all alcoholics will experience withdrawal symptoms at some point in their lives. Although this seems like a relatively small number, the comorbidities associated with alcoholism result in a large number of hospitalizations. Thus, 15–20% of hospitalized patients have alcohol dependence and are at risk for symptomatic withdrawal.

PATHOPHYSIOLOGY

Individuals at risk for withdrawal symptoms typically have abrupt cessation of alcohol after a prolonged, sustained intake. However, even among individuals with substantial long-term intake, withdrawal severity varies widely. Although some mechanisms behind withdrawal have been elucidated, the reasons for these disparities remain unclear. Acute signs of alcohol intoxication reflect its generalized depressant effects on the central nervous system. Alcohol has been shown to interact with many neurotransmitter systems, including γ-aminobutyric acid (GABA), glutamate, serotonin, and norepinephrine. Alcohol potentiates the effects of GABA (the major inhibitory neurotransmitter) and inhibits N-methyl-D-aspartate (NMDA) receptors which bind glutamate (the major excitatory neurotransmitter). These effects are responsible for the classic signs of intoxication, disorientation, confusion, ataxia, and decreased level of consciousness. With chronic alcohol use, GABA receptors are downregulated and NMDA receptors are upregulated to modulate the depressive effects of alcohol. With sudden abstention from alcohol, the brain of an alcoholic has blunted inhibitory neurotransmission and increased excitatory neurotransmission, both of which have been implicated in causing the symptoms of withdrawal. This is also the rationale for treating alcohol withdrawal with benzodiazepines which will enhance GABA activity.

CLINICAL PRESENTATION

Alcohol withdrawal has a wide spectrum of manifestations. Most individuals experiencing withdrawal will have only minor symptoms; however, 25% of alcoholics will experience a withdrawal seizure and approximately 5% will develop alcohol withdrawal delirium (AWD).

Mild to Moderate Alcohol Withdrawal

Most patients who experience withdrawal have symptoms within the first 48 hours after cessation of alcohol intake. Mild to moderate withdrawal symptoms generally begin within 6–8 hours after cessation (or marked decrease) of alcohol intake and peak in intensity on day 2 or 3. The hallmark of early withdrawal is autonomic nervous system hyperactivity, including diaphoresis, tachycardia, tachypnea, fever, and hypertension. Other typical symptoms include hand tremors, insomnia, nausea and vomiting, hallucinations, agitation, and anxiety. Hallucinations are most commonly visual, but auditory, olfactory, and tactile hallucinations have been reported. Despite the hallucinations, patients with uncomplicated withdrawal have a completely clear sensorium, which differentiates them from individuals with AWD. Most patients have complete resolution of their symptoms by day 4 or 5, although a protracted abstinence syndrome is possible with persistent symptoms for over 6 months.

Withdrawal Seizures

Alcohol withdrawal seizures occur early in the course of withdrawal, typically within 24 hours of cessation of alcohol. Over 90% occur within 48 hours of alcohol cessation. Seizures are generalized tonic-clonic and typically self-limited although multiple seizures can occur.

Alcohol Withdrawal Delirium—Delirium Tremens (DTS)

Major alcohol withdrawal refers to the presence of delirium (mental confusion, agitation, disorientation, and fluctuating levels of consciousness) in addition to extreme autonomic hyperactivity and tremulousness. AWD can occur as early as 48 hours after abstinence, but typically occurs 3–4 days after alcohol cessation. Symptoms are typically present for 72 hours; however, prolonged cases lasting 2 weeks have been described. Risk factors for delirium include: age >30, history of sustained drinking, history of previous alcohol withdrawal (particularly prior delirium or seizures), and concurrent illness. AWD is a life-threatening complication with mortality of 15% without treatment and 1% with adequate treatment.

EVALUATION

Any patient with recent cessation of alcohol use needs to have a thorough history and physical examination. The goals are to: (1) determine the presence and severity of any withdrawal symptoms; (2) consider other conditions that mimic the manifestations of alcohol withdrawal; (3) search for evidence of any complications from alcoholism (Table 60-1). The differential diagnosis of alcohol withdrawal is complex and depends on the patient's particular symptoms. Autonomic hyperactivity can be caused from cocaine or amphetamine intoxication, opioid withdrawal, hyperthyroidism, hypertensive encephalopathy, anticholinergic poisoning, or even infection. Alcoholic hallucinosis must be differentiated from intoxication with hallucinogenic agents, anticholinergic poisoning, or other acute paranoid states such as amphetamine psychosis or paranoid schizophrenia. The differential diagnosis for delirium is extensive (see Chap. 56) and other etiologies must be strongly considered when AWD is suspected.

Table 60-1 **Medical Complications of Heavy Alcohol Use**

Cardiovascular	Atrial fibrillation, dilated cardiomyopathy, hypertension
Gastrointestinal	Esophagitis, Mallory-Weiss tear, cirrhosis, gastritis, hepatitis, pancreatitis (acute or chronic)
Nutritional	Vitamin B_{12} deficiency, folate deficiency, thiamine deficiency, obesity, malnutrition
Hematologic	Macrocytosis (B_{12} deficiency, folate deficiency, or direct toxic effects of alcohol), anemia, leukopenia, thrombocytopenia (usually mild)
Neurologic	Hemorrhagic stroke, subdural hematoma, Wernicke's encephalopathy, Korsakoff dementia, peripheral neuropathy, cerebellar degeneration
Metabolic	Hypoglycemia, hypokalemia, hypophosphatemia, hypomagnesemia
Musculoskeletal	Myositis, osteoporosis

Patients presenting with a history of alcohol abuse should also be evaluated for complications of alcoholism (Table 60-1). Two disorders deserve special consideration given their frequent association with alcohol abuse. **Wernicke's encephalopathy** and **Korsakoff dementia** represent a continuum of disorders resulting from a nutritional deficiency of thiamine (the spectrum is also referred to as Wernicke-Korsakoff syndrome). Wernicke's encephalopathy consists of a classic triad of symptoms: (1) **altered mental status**, (2) **ataxia**, and (3) **ophthalmoplegia** (most commonly nystagmus and bilateral lateral rectus palsies). Unfortunately, only a minority have all three manifestations (<1%), so thiamine deficiency should be suspected in any alcoholic with any of the symptoms. Korsakoff dementia causes prominent anterograde amnesia and a variable milder retrograde amnesia with relative preservation of other cognitive functions (most have a normal IQ). Affected individuals have intact long-term memory, but a profound inability to learn or establish new memories and often confabulate when asked about the recent past.

MANAGEMENT

The first step in the management of any patient with alcohol withdrawal is supportive care and rest. Any patient with AWD should be admitted to an intensive care unit for close monitoring, whereas patients with less severe symptoms can be managed in a calm, quiet hospital room. All patients must be closely monitored with frequent neurologic examinations to track the progression of symptoms using a standardized withdrawal assessment.

The second step in treating withdrawal is to offer adequate nutrition and supplementation. As discussed previously, the prompt administration of **thiamine** is critical to the treatment of Wernicke-Korsakoff syndrome. Although thiamine often fully reverses delirium rapidly (within hours), it takes several weeks to show only a partial improvement in memory impairment. Thiamine administration must precede any other glucose-containing solutions or resumption of diet. Administration of glucose without concomitant thiamine may precipitate or worsen encephalopathy. Thiamine should be administered either IV or IM at a dose of 50–100 mg and should be continued parenterally for several days. Patients should also receive a multivitamin and folate supplementation as well. Most individuals with alcohol withdrawal are volume-depleted because of the concomitant diaphoresis, tachycardia, vomiting, or fever. Therefore, most patients should receive hydration with isotonic fluids with dextrose (after or with thiamine administration). A standard practice at many institutions is to administer a "rally pack," which consists of a 1 L bag of IV fluids with variable contents, possibly including magnesium, thiamine, multivitamins, and folic acid. Practitioners must realize that no standard formula for a rally pack exists and should be aware of their own institution's preferences.

Benzodiazepines are the drugs of choice for all alcohol withdrawal, regardless of severity. Benzodiazepines not only lessen the severity of autonomic symptoms and hallucinations, but are the only agents proven to prevent seizures and AWD. Other agents, such as neuroleptic agents, clonidine, beta-blockers, baclofen, and carbamazepine, do reduce the symptoms of mild to moderate withdrawal, but may actually complicate management. The neuroleptic agents frequently cause delirium and reduce the seizure threshold, clonidine and beta-blockers have both been implicated in causing delirium, and baclofen reduces the seizure threshold. The longer-acting benzodiazepines (diazepam and chlordiazepoxide) are usually preferred; however, both of these agents undergo hepatic metabolism and can have prolonged effects if hepatic dysfunction is present. Patients with suspected hepatic dysfunction are generally treated with either lorazepam or oxazepam, which have minimal hepatic metabolism.

Several regimens have been proposed for the prevention and treatment of withdrawal symptoms (Table 60-2). Benzodiazepines can be dosed on a fixed dose schedule, front-loaded dosing, or symptom-triggered dosing. Using a fixed dose schedule, benzodiazepines are given regularly with a tapering dose over several days. This regimen typically results in greater amounts of drugs, longer sedation, and longer hospital stays, without an improvement in symptom control compared to the other regimens for most patients. Front-loaded dosing delivers a high dose of a long-acting benzodiazepine early in the course of withdrawal which then self-tapers over time. The advantages of this regimen are that frequent monitoring of symptoms is limited to the initial period of withdrawal and symptoms are usually alleviated the quickest. Patients are dosed every 1–2 hours until symptoms subside. For asymptomatic patients, a single loading dose can be given. Symptom-triggered dosing requires frequent monitoring of withdrawal symptoms with dosing only when a patient is symptomatic. This regimen results in the lowest dosing of medication and the greatest protection against over sedation. However, it does require close frequent monitoring, as often as every 1–2 hours in the initial

Table 60-2 **Recommended Benzodiazepine Doses to Treat Mild to Moderate Alcohol Withdrawal**

Agent	Front-Loaded Dosing	Symptom-Triggered Dosing	Half-Life (h)
Diazepam	20 mg IV/PO	5–20 mg IV/PO	30–100
Chlordiazepoxide	100 mg PO	25–100 mg PO	5–30
Lorazepam	2 mg IV/IM/PO	1–4 mg IV/IM/PO	10–20
Oxazepam	Not recommended	15–60 mg PO	5–15

presentation. In practice, front-loaded dosing and symptom-triggered are often combined into a single regimen. Patients will initially receive a high dose of a long-acting benzodiazepine and then will receive subsequent doses based on symptoms. Dosing of benzodiazepines for AWD is based purely on controlling the patient's symptoms and should not be limited by arbitrary maximum daily dosages. Medications should be titrated until the patient maintains a light somnolence.

Several adjuncts are recommended in to control symptoms which persist despite benzodiazepine administration. Haldol (0.5–5 mg IV/IM q 1 h or 0.5–5 mg PO q 4 h) is effective in reducing the agitation and hallucinations. Beta-blockers (atenolol 50–100 mg PO qd) and clonidine (0.1–0.2 mg PO bid) are beneficial in patients with persistent hypertension or tachycardia despite adequate doses of benzodiazepines.

OVERDOSE AND
TOXICOLOGY

Ashutosh J. Barve

KEY POINTS

- Intentional or unintentional overdose of medicines or ingestion of poisons result in a significant number of ER and hospital admissions.
- Identification of the offending substance by a detailed history, physical examination, and lab tests is critical.
- If the entire ingested toxin has not entered the bloodstream, initial management consists of elimination of the noxious foreign substance before it enters the circulation (e.g., GI decontamination).
- Definitive management involves either inhibition of the metabolic activation of the substance, antagonism at its site of action with a specific pharmacologic antagonist, or acceleration/facilitation of its detoxification and elimination from the body.
- Management should include the evaluation and treatment of the circumstances that led to the overdose.

ACETAMINOPHEN

Introduction

Acetaminophen overdose is the leading cause of inpatient admissions for acute liver failure in the United States. The extensive therapeutic use and over-the-counter availability in multiple formulations makes it readily accessible to the public. Acetaminophen toxicity presents in two distinct forms. More common is acute toxicity from overdose seen in deliberate or inadvertent ingestion of a supratherapeutic dose. Another scenario is that of therapeutic misadventure, such as a therapeutic dose in a patient with alcoholism resulting in fulminant liver failure a few days after the use of the drug.

Pathophysiology

Acetaminophen is metabolized by the liver through multiple pathways. When a small amount of acetaminophen is taken, >90% of the drug is glucuronidated or sulfated to produce harmless metabolites which are excreted by the kidney. About 5% is metabolized by the cytochrome P-450 mixed function oxidase system (CYP 2E1, 3A4, and 1A2) to yield a highly reactive electrophilic metabolite called **N-acetyl-p-benzoquinone imine (NAPQI)**. At therapeutic doses, all of the NAPQI is detoxified by the enzyme glutathione S-transferase via conjugation with glutathione. However, at toxic doses (e.g., overdose), the glucuronidation and sulfation pathways are overwhelmed and more acetaminophen becomes available to the cytochrome P-450 system. Alternatively, if the cytochrome P-450 enzymes are induced (e.g., by chronic alcohol abuse) or the glucuronidation pathway suppressed (e.g., recent fasting), a larger share of the acetaminophen in the hepatocyte is metabolized by the cytochrome P-450 system producing more NAPQI. As the amount of NAPQI increases, **glutathione stores are depleted** and the reactive metabolite increasingly binds to sulfhydryl groups on cellular proteins, presumably disrupting their function. In alcoholics or malnourished individuals who already have low hepatic glutathione, even a slight increase in the amount of NAPQI can be deleterious to the hepatocyte. It is interesting to note that on histopathologic examination, acetaminophen hepatotoxicity manifests as classical centrilobular (zone 3) necrosis, that is, necrosis in the region of the liver where there is the highest concentration of cytochrome P-450 enzymes.

Clinical Presentation

Patients presenting with acetaminophen overdose may present with a history of voluntary ingestion of a large dose of the drug as in suicide attempts. Alternately, an inadvertent overdose may be revealed during the interview. Most patients are initially asymptomatic, but some nonspecific symptoms such as nausea, vomiting, diaphoresis, pallor, lethargy, and malaise may be present. Overt hepatotoxicity develops about 24 hours after the toxic dose and is manifested by right upper quadrant pain which progresses to jaundice, confusion (hepatic encephalopathy), and bleeding diathesis over 3–4 days. Symptoms of acute renal failure such as oliguria develop in 25% of patients with significant liver toxicity and more than half of those with frank liver failure. While some patients succumb to liver failure, patients who survive beyond 4 days usually make a complete recovery with no chronic liver sequelae. Another common presentation is often described as a "therapeutic misadventure" in which patients with alcoholism develop massive liver injury about 2–3 days after taking acetaminophen with therapeutic intent. The initial signs and symptoms of this type of acetaminophen poisoning are very insidious, vague, and nonspecific and can easily be confused with an alternate diagnosis like a viral syndrome. By the time these patients present for medical attention, significant amount of liver injury has occurred despite a serum acetaminophen concentration in the nontoxic range. Persons with risk factors for acetaminophen toxicity such as chronic alcohol abuse, malnutrition, recent fasting, or use of cytochrome P-450-inducing drugs are at an increased risk for this type of acetaminophen toxicity which is sometimes referred to as "chronic overdose."

Aspartate aminotransferase (AST) and **alanine aminotransferase (ALT)** values rise markedly (>3000 IU/L) and can often exceed 10,000 IU/L in severe injury. Elevation of **bilirubin** and **international normalized ratio (INR)** are other signs of liver toxicity. Severe liver injury can also cause **hypoglycemia**, **lactic acidosis**, and **hyperammonemia**. If the patient develops acute renal failure (generally acute tubular necrosis), serum creatinine and blood urea nitrogen (BUN) will increase and urinalysis may show proteinuria, hematuria, and granular casts.

Evaluation

The clinical evaluation involves: (1) suspecting and establishing that the poisoning has occurred; (2) determining the identity, time, and dose of the offending drug; (3) assessing severity; (4) predicting toxicity; and (5) evaluating and addressing the underlying cause of the overdose.

In all patients with suspected acute acetaminophen overdose, a detailed history should be obtained regarding the identity of the drug formulation, dose, time elapsed, and comorbid conditions that predispose to increased hepatotoxicity (e.g., history of alcohol abuse, malnutrition, recent fasting, and use of cytochrome P-450-inducing drugs). **Serum acetaminophen** should be measured. The risk of hepatotoxicity can be best predicted by correlating the serum acetaminophen concentration to the time elapsed since ingestion of the drug using the **Modified Rumack-Matthew nomogram** (see Fig. 61-1). This nomogram is most useful in directing further management decisions in cases of acute overdose. The cause and circumstances of the overdose should also be elicited and for cases of intentional overdose or given unreliable history, toxic screening of blood and urine for other drugs should be considered. The Rumack-Matthew nomogram is not very useful in the evaluation of victims of therapeutic misadventure or chronic overdose since the serum acetaminophen levels are generally in the nontoxic range. Evaluation of this type of overdose requires an astute history and recognition of risk factors for acetaminophen toxicity and clinical and laboratory findings consistent with hepatotoxicity.

Management

After ingestion of an acute acetaminophen overdose, the most effective method of gastrointestinal (GI) decontamination is a single dose of **activated charcoal** (1 g/kg). It has been shown to work better than gastric lavage or syrup of ipecac. Activated charcoal avidly adsorbs acetaminophen and

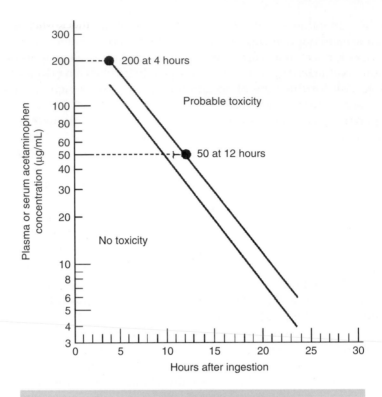

Figure 61-1 **Modified Rumack-Matthew nomogram.** (*Source:* Modified and reproduced with permission from Rumack BH, Matthew H. Acetaminophen poisoning and toxicity. *Pediatrics* 1975;55:871.)

reduces its absorption from the GI tract by 50–90%. It should be given within 2 hours of ingestion, but may be useful if more time has elapsed when the patient has coingested substances that retard acetaminophen absorption or slow GI motility, or taken an extended release preparation.

The antidote of choice in acetaminophen overdose is **N-acetylcysteine (NAC)**. It is a glutathione precursor and promotes the formation of hepatic glutathione which detoxifies NAPQI. It can also directly bind to NAPQI as a glutathione substitute. Apart from that it enhances the nontoxic sulfation of acetaminophen. It is highly effective if used within 10 hours of the overdose but accumulating data suggest that it may be moderately helpful even beyond 10 hours. Its efficacy in late treatment of acetaminophen toxicity is probably due to its anti-inflammatory and antioxidant actions possibly through the modification of cytokine production and quenching of free radicals. Classically, NAC is indicated in acute overdose if the serum acetaminophen concentration lies above the "possible hepatic toxicity" line on the Rumack-Matthew nomogram. Other indications include any significant overdose (>7.5 g), inability to obtain a serum concentration within 10 hours of the ingestion, or if the time of ingestion is not known and the serum acetaminophen level is >10 μg/mL. Guidelines are unclear for cases of chronic overdose or therapeutic misadventure, but treatment with NAC should be considered for all patients with liver tenderness, elevations of aminotransferases, or serum acetaminophen concentrations >10 μg/mL. The Food and Drug Administration (FDA) approved oral dose of NAC is a 72-hour regimen consisting of a 140 mg/kg loading dose followed by 17 doses of 70 mg/kg every 4 hours (total dose 1330 mg/kg). Common side effects are nausea and vomiting due to its "rotten egg" taste and odor. This may necessitate the use of antiemetic agents or even a nasogastric tube. Recently, an IV preparation was approved in the United States for use in patients in whom the oral dosing is not feasible. Liver transplant is a final modality in the treatment of acetaminophen overdose but is reserved for patients who develop fulminant hepatic failure and necessitates urgent referral to a transplant hepatologist.

All cases of intentional overdose require a psychiatric evaluation with appropriate management of resultant diagnoses. On the other hand, victims of unintentional overdose or therapeutic misadventure need extensive counseling about the indications, dosage, adverse effects, and drug interactions of acetaminophen.

OPIOIDS

Opioids or narcotics are frequently used in clinical practice to treat severe acute and chronic pain. Further, narcotic drug abuse is a prevalent health problem in the United States and drug abusers may be more susceptible to overdose due to the varying bioavailability of active ingredients in illegally obtained street drugs. Opioid drugs bind to opiate receptors in the central nervous system (CNS), causing inhibition of ascending pain pathways, altering the perception of and response to pain. Opioids also act on several other CNS neurotransmitter systems, including dopamine, gamma-aminobutyric acid (GABA), and glutamate. Their overall effect is to produce generalized CNS depression. The signs and symptoms of an **acute opioid overdose** include **abnormal mental status** (somnolence, confusion, stupor, coma) **substantially decreased respiration**, hypotension, bradycardia, **miotic pupils**, apnea, and pulmonary edema. Combination with sedative-hypnotics or other CNS depressants potentiates the toxicity of opioids. The respiratory depression can lead to hypoxia and severe respiratory acidosis. The altered mental status can result in an inability to protect the airway predisposing to aspiration. Evaluation involves recognizing the signs of an opioid overdose and assessing the severity of respiratory and CNS depression. Initial management consists of securing an adequate airway and stabilizing the respiratory and cardiac status. Patients who are breathing adequately without assistance can be monitored, but those with compromised respiration are administered an opioid antagonist. If patients respond to this antidote, endotracheal intubation and mechanical ventilation may not be necessary. Intravenous **naloxone** is the antidote of choice for opioid overdose. It is a relatively pure opioid antagonist that is highly lipid soluble, has a rapid onset of action, and is well absorbed intravenously, intramuscularly, subcutaneously, or via endotracheal tube. Patients with an acute overdose can be given 0.4 IV push, but caution should be exercised in opioid-dependent patients. Patients on chronic opioids can develop acute withdrawal with naloxone administration, so they should be started on a low dose to reverse respiratory depression (0.1–0.2 mg). If the first dose is not effective, it can be repeated with escalating doses up to 2 mg every 3 minutes to a maximum of 10 mg. Most patients improve with low doses of naloxone; however, patients taking pentazocine, propoxyphene, methadone, or fentanyl may require higher doses. It is important to note that its duration of action is 1–2 hours while most narcotic drugs have a duration of action of 4–6 hours (that of methadone is 24–36 hours). Hence, the patient must be monitored for recurrence of symptoms as naloxone wears off. If needed, naloxone can be administered every 20 minutes or given as an IV drip.

COCAINE

Cocaine is a sympathomimetic, stimulant drug which is the second most common illicit drug used in the United States. Its pharmacologic action is mediated by the inhibition of synaptic reuptake of norepinephrine by sympathetic neurons. Since reuptake is the major mechanism by which the neurotransmitter is removed from its active receptor sites, this inhibition results in a potentiation of the natural activity of the sympathetic nervous system. Cocaine may also enhance the release of catecholamines from central and peripheral stores. Acute cocaine overdose presents with symptoms of dizziness, tremor, hyperreflexia, hyperpyrexia, **mydriasis**, tachypnea, seizures, tachycardia, and hypertension. Behavioral changes include euphoria, grandiosity, hypervigilance, restlessness, aggression, impaired judgment, and acute psychotic reaction. The most common reason cocaine users seek medical care is for **chest pain**, 5–10% of which are secondary to a **myocardial infarction**. The different mechanisms suggested explaining these cardiac symptoms include increased coronary demand; coronary artery vasoconstriction and spasm; and platelet activation. The risk of myocardial infarction is the highest during the first hour after the cocaine use and it is important to closely monitor the patient during this time. Treatment is generally supportive due to the short duration of action of cocaine. Acute psychotic episodes can be treated with antipsychotic agents like haloperidol. Patients with cocaine-induced chest pain should be managed differently than patients with classic angina: **beta-blockers should be avoided**, because of concern that the resulting unopposed alpha-adrenergic activity will exacerbate cocaine-induced vasoconstriction and cause hypertensive crisis. **Benzodiazepines** are the preferred agents for patients who are hypertensive, tachycardic, or anxious since they reduce blood pressure and heart rate. All patients should also receive aspirin and nitrates as is standard for angina. Aspirin prevents thrombus formation and nitrates can reverse cocaine-induced coronary artery vasoconstriction. Oxygen administration should be considered to limit ischemia. In spite of this, if the patient continues to have chest pain or ischemic changes, calcium channel blockers and alpha-blockers can be used.

BENZODIAZEPINES

Benzodiazepines, like diazepam, temazepam, alprazolam, and midazolam, are the most commonly prescribed sedative-hypnotics. They are used as sedatives, anxiolytics, and for conscious sedation during minor surgical procedures. They bind to the alpha subunit of the GABA-benzodiazepine chloride ionophore receptor complex on the postsynaptic neurons at several sites within the CNS including the limbic system and reticular formation. When GABA, a naturally occurring inhibitory neurotransmitter, binds to the beta subunit of the receptor, the chloride channel opens and causes an influx of chloride ions into the postsynaptic neuron thus hyperpolarizing the neuron and rendering it relatively refractory to excitatory stimuli. Binding of benzodiazepines to the alpha unit of the receptor changes its configuration and results in a greater influx of chloride ions when GABA binds to the same receptor. So benzodiazepines essentially potentiate the effect of GABA at its receptor. They are safer than barbiturates which are a class of drugs that benzodiazepines have replaced in clinical practice but they do have abuse potential and potential for misuse as an agent of suicide. Patients with an overdose present with symptoms of neurologic depression, such as drowsiness, dizziness, slurred speech, ataxia, and confusion, but can progress to stupor and coma. Benzodiazepines may also have a disinhibiting effect on patients leading to inappropriate behavior and impaired judgment. Benzodiazepines are often coingested with other substances and rarely lead to significant morbidity or mortality on their own, so ingestion of other substances should always be considered. Initial management of benzodiazepine overdose is supportive with maintenance of an adequate airway, respiration, and cardiovascular status. For oral overdoses, GI decontamination can be attempted by a single dose of 50 g of activated charcoal typically mixed with water or sorbitol administered as a slurry orally or via nasogastric tube. Activated charcoal not only inhibits absorption of the drug but also prevents reabsorption of active metabolites through enterohepatic recirculation. A benzodiazepine antagonist is available for acute treatment, but **flumazenil should only be administered to patients with a known acute overdose** (i.e., procedural sedation). Flumazenil does not have serious side effects of its own, but has precipitated seizures in patients dependent to benzodiazepines. Furthermore in cases of mixed poisoning with tricyclic antidepressants, flumazenil could precipitate tricyclic antidepressant-induced arrhythmias that were otherwise suppressed by the sedative. Hence, it should not be routinely administered to a comatose patient if the identity of the overdosed drug is not known.

PAIN MANAGEMENT IN

THE HOSPITALIZED

PATIENT

Winifred G. Teuteberg

KEY POINTS

- Pain is highly prevalent and often undertreated in hospitalized patients.
- Pain should be addressed daily in all hospitalized patients, not just those specifically admitted for pain control.
- Pain is always subjective and many patients experiencing pain show no physical signs of pain. Clinicians must accept a patient's report of pain.
- Understanding the etiology of a patient's pain is essential in providing appropriate therapy.
- Follow a stepwise approach to pain management and titrate the dose using equianalgesic ratios.

INTRODUCTION

It is estimated that between 45 and 75% of all hospitalized patients report pain. The majority of these patients report that their pain is moderate to severe. Although some of these patients are admitted specifically for pain control, most are admitted for other reasons. It is the responsibility of those caring for hospitalized patients to **question all inpatients about pain** and evaluate and treat their pain appropriately. This chapter will focus on pain management for hospitalized patients. Evaluation of patients with certain pain syndromes (e.g., chest pain, abdominal pain) can be found in their respective chapters.

Table 62-1 **Types of Physical Pain and Treatment**

Pain Type	Examples	Mechanism	Character	Therapy
Somatic Soft tissue	Arthritis, soft tissue metastasis, cellulitis	Activation of nociceptors by tissue injury from trauma, thermal injury, tumor infiltration, or ischemia	Usually gnawing or aching, occasionally cramping, usually well localized	NSAIDs, acetaminophen, opiates, hot or cold compresses, physical therapy, massage
Somatic Bone	Bone metastases, fracture	Activation of nociceptors in the periosteum by trauma or tumor infiltration	Usually gnawing, aching, stabbing, well localized	Anti-inflammatories (steroids or NSAIDs), opioid analgesics, surgical or external fixation, radiation therapy, IV bisphosphonates for osteolytic metastases
Visceral	Pancreatitis, biliary obstruction, ischemic bowel	Activation of visceral nociceptors by distention, compression, infiltration, or ischemia of organs such as the lungs, heart, or GI tract	Aching, squeezing, often cramping, generally poorly localized, occasionally referred, can be well localized, if adjacent somatic tissue has been involved in injury process	Opioid analgesics, anti-cholinergics, surgical, endoscopic or percutaneous decompression of obstructed viscus
Neuropathic	Spinal stenosis, herpes zoster, diabetic neuropathy, trigeminal neuralgia	Destruction, inflammation, compression, or chemical damage of a peripheral or central nervous tissue	Burning, radiating, occasionally sharp or stabbing, occasional paroxysmal shooting pain, hyperalgesia sometimes present	Opioid analgesics, tricyclic antidepressants, anticonvulsants, interventional procedures (epidural catheter or nerve block)

PATHOPHYSIOLOGY

Pain is an unpleasant sensory or emotional experience resulting from actual or potential tissue damage. Pain generally begins with physical injury, but can persist or become aggravated by spiritual or psychosocial factors such as anxiety, depression, financial or interpersonal stressors, and spiritual distress resulting from coping with a serious or life-threatening illness. Different types of physical pain include somatic pain, visceral pain, and neuropathic pain. Understanding the primary underlying mechanism of the patient's pain can help tailor therapy, as described in Table 62-1, realizing that many patients have elements of more than one type of pain.

CLINICAL PRESENTATION

Pain is always subjective and many patients experiencing pain show no physical signs of pain. Clinicians must accept a patient's report of pain. Assess the **severity** of pain each day using a pain scale. Several types of pain scales exist, depending on the capabilities of the patient (Fig. 62-1). Some patients are unable to assign numbers to their pain and find a word scale more useful. A visual analogue scale can be useful for nonverbal patients. Although severity of pain is rarely helpful in diagnosis, daily measurements using the same scale provide reliable and important information about response to therapy.

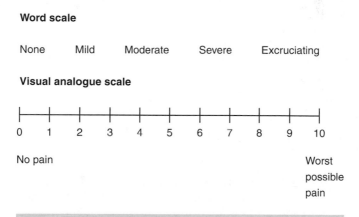

Figure 62-1 **Pain assessment scales.**

MANAGEMENT

A variety of medications and therapies are available for the treatment of pain in the hospital. Therapy should be tailored as much as possible to the etiology and severity of the patient's pain (Table 62-1). Pharmacologic therapies for treating pain in the hospital include nonopioid and opioid analgesics, as well as adjuvant medications. Acetaminophen and nonsteroidal anti-inflammatory drugs (NSAIDs) are used for mild pain, and sometimes as an adjuvant to narcotics. For example, NSAIDs are especially effective in the adjuvant treatment of pain from bone metastases. NSAIDs should be used with caution in older patients, those with renal insufficiency, those with decreased effective circulatory volume (i.e., heart failure, ascites), and those at risk of gastrointestinal (GI) bleeding. Other adjuvant therapies useful in certain situations include tricyclic antidepressants and anticonvulsants (gabapentin, carbamazepine) for neuropathic pain, and bisphonates (pamidronate) for pain from bone metastases. The cornerstone of the management of moderate to severe pain in the hospitalized patient is narcotics, examples of which are presented in Table 62-2.

Route of delivery depends on the patient's underlying condition. For example, quick pain control is best achieved IV. Patients who need long-acting narcotics and cannot swallow or absorb sustained release tablets may benefit from a transdermal patch preparation (although these take a day or two to reach steady state, and other medicines should be prescribed in the interim). **Patient-controlled anesthesia (PCA)** is appropriate for many patients with moderate to severe pain (postoperative, sickle cell pain crisis). In PCA, patients can receive a bolus of medication by pushing a button, with set limits on dosing intervals and total number of doses delivered in a set period of time to avoid overdosing. Advantages to PCA are that it allows the patient to control the amount of pain medication, thus avoiding over or under dosing, and allows for rapid access because the patient does not need to wait for staff to bring medication. This is a poor choice in patients who are confused, uncoordinated, or have difficulty understanding how to use it.

DOSING, TITRATION, AND SELECTION OF ANALGESICS

Once the appropriate mode of delivery for the patient is determined, select which type of analgesic to use. When treating a patient with medication for pain, the **World Health Organization** recommends a stepwise approach, as outlined below.

Table 62-2 *Commonly Used Opioid Analgesics and Relative Potencies*

| Drug | Indication | Relative Potency(mg) | | Starting Oral Dose (mg) | Note/Formulation |
		PO	IV		
Codeine	Mild to moderate pain	200	—	30–60	Available in combination with acetaminophen (Tylenol #3)
Fentanyl	Moderate to severe pain	—	0.1	—	Available as transdermal patch (Duragesic), trans-mucosal lozenge (Actiq); 25 µg transdermal patch equivalent to 50 mg of oral morphine per day
Hydromorphone	Moderate to severe pain	7.5	1.5	4–8	
Hydrocodone	Mild to moderate pain	30	—	5–10 mg	Available in combination with acetaminophen (Vicodin, Lortab)
Meperidine	—	300	75		**Not recommended for pain management**. CNS excitation from metabolite accumulation
Methadone	Moderate to severe pain	20 (2–4)*	10 (2–4)*	15–30	Long half-life for CNS effects and respiratory depression cause significant risk for overdosing. Dose titrations by pain specialists only
Morphine	Moderate to severe pain	30	10	15–30	Available as oral sustained release (MS Contin, Oramorph SR, Kadian, Avinza), concentrated SL liquid (Roxanol)
Oxycodone	Moderate to severe pain	20	—	10–20	Available in combination with acetaminophen for mild to moderate pain (Percocet, Tylox), as oral sustained release tablets (Oxycontin), as concentrated SL liquid (Oxyfast)

*Chronic use.

459

STEP 1: Mild to Moderate Pain

Initiate a nonopioid ± adjuvant medication (acetaminophen or an NSAID), scheduled on an as-needed (prn) basis. Treat concurrent symptoms that exacerbate pain, and/or provide independent analgesic activity for specific types of pain.

STEP 2: Mild to Moderate Pain Uncontrolled After Step 1

Initiate a short-acting prn opioid for mild or moderate pain ± nonopioid scheduled around the clock (ATC) ± adjuvant medication. Note that codeine, hydrocodone, and oxycodone are available in combination with acetaminophen. Remember the maximum daily dose of acetaminophen is 4000 mg, so take care not to exceed this when prescribing opioid/acetaminophen combination tablets. **Initiate a bowel regimen (i.e., stool softeners +/– a laxative) when starting opiates**.

STEP 3: Moderate to Severe Pain Uncontrolled After Step 2

Initiate an opioid for moderate to severe pain ± nonopioid scheduled ATC ± adjuvant medication. If using codeine or hydrocodone, switch to an opioid for moderate to severe pain. If using hydromorphone, morphine, or oxycodone, increase the dose by 50–100%. If still no response, rotate to a different opioid for moderate to severe pain and assess mode of delivery for efficacy (e.g., poor response to an oral medication could indicate poor absorption in the GI tract).

OPIOID DOSES CONVERSIONS

The need to change from one opioid to another or from one route to another is common. One can carry out dose conversions by calculating the 24-hour usage of the prescribed opioid. For example, a patient taking six doses of 30 mg PO morphine would have a 24-hour morphine usage of 180 mg (six times 30 mg = 180 mg). Then determine the equivalent 24-hour dose of the new medication or formulation using the equianalgesic ratio, which is the **relative potency** between two drugs or two formulations of the same drug. For example, from Table 62-2, 30 mg PO morphine = 10 mg IV morphine. Therefore, 180 mg PO morphine in 24 hours × 10 mg IV morphine/30 mg PO morphine = 60 mg of IV morphine in 24 hours.

Next, calculate the dosing interval or infusion rate. For intermittent dosing, divide the desired dosing interval into 24 hours. For example, for q2 hour dosing, there are 24 divided by 2 or 12, 2-hour dosing intervals in 24 hours. Therefore, 60 mg IV morphine in 24 hours/12 dosing intervals = 5 mg IV morphine q2 hours. For conversions between medications, calculate the equianalgesic 24-hour dose as above; however, because of incomplete cross-tolerance to side effects between different opiates, it is recommended to then decrease the 24-hour equianalgesic dose by 25–50%. For example, in converting between PO morphine and PO oxycodone, 180 mg PO morphine in 24 hours × 20 mg PO oxycodone/30 mg PO morphine × 0.75 = 90 mg PO oxycodone in 24 hours.

SUSTAINED RELEASE OPIATES

Acute pain such as postsurgical or trauma pain tends to resolve in several days and these patients seldom require more than short-acting prn opiates. Patients with chronic pain or cancer pain, however, often require the addition of a sustained release opioid. If a patient with chronic or cancer pain requires three to four doses of short-acting opioid daily for several days, a sustained release formulation should be added.

Once a long-acting formulation has been started, it is important to provide a short-acting medication on a prn basis for **breakthrough pain**. This is pain that occurs, or "breaks through," despite the long-acting medication. Often, patients experience breakthrough pain with activity or interventions such as dressing changes or positioning in bed. They can also experience breakthrough pain from inadequate dosing of sustained release opioid or from progression of their disease. When writing prn orders for breakthrough pain, avoid writing an interval range such as q2-4 hours as this creates unnecessary confusion and may result in your patient not getting the medication frequently enough.

Side effects of opiates are common but often manageable. They rarely warrant cessation of opioid therapy. The most common side effect is constipation, hence the need for a bowel regimen. Tolerance to side effects such as sedation or nausea usually occurs during the first few days, and then subsides. Sometimes patients with intractable pain, such as severe cancer pain, require large doses of narcotics to control their pain, to the point of respiratory depression. There is no maximum dose for narcotics and respiratory depression and sedation are usually the limiting factors. However, when treating patients with end-of-life pain, it is important not to sacrifice pain control for respiratory rate.

INTERVENTIONAL OR NONPHARMACOLOGIC THERAPIES

Other therapies for pain include radiation therapy for bone metastases, internal or external fixation of fractures or sprains, and surgical, endoscopic, or percutaneous decompression of an obstructed viscous or interventional anesthesia such as an epidural catheter or nerve block. These procedures should be used whenever possible to maximize the patient's comfort while minimizing the need for systemic medical therapies and their side effects. It is important not to overlook simple interventions like hot or cold compresses, massage, and gentle physical therapy particularly for somatic, soft tissue pain.

PSYCHOSOCIAL AND SPIRITUAL ASPECTS OF PAIN

This chapter focused on evaluating and treating physical pain. It is important to note that psychosocial and spiritual distress can exacerbate and sometime perpetuate a patient's pain. Types of psychosocial and spiritual distress are often related to coping with a serious or life-altering illness. They include anxiety, depression, financial stressors, interpersonal stressors, and spiritual distress. When evaluating a patient for pain, be certain to address how the illness is affecting the patient's life and the lives of any close family members or loved ones. Also assess the patient for depression and anxiety. If a psychosocial or spiritual aspect to the patient's pain is identified, treat depression/anxiety and/or refer to social work or chaplains if indicated.

NUTRITION IN THE

HOSPITALIZED PATIENT

Cortney Youens Lee
Paul Kearney

KEY POINTS

- Many hospitalized patients are malnourished or will be by the time of discharge.
- Nutritional status affects morbidity and mortality.
- Prealbumin is the best test to assess nutritional status (predicts outcome).
- Daily caloric needs can be estimated by 25 × weight (kg).
- Parenteral nutrition (TPN) is a last resort.

INTRODUCTION

Malnutrition is common among patients admitted to the hospital and the nutritional status of most patients will worsen during their hospitalization. Further, nutritional status is directly linked to patient outcomes and length of stay. Malnutrition results in poor wound healing, increased susceptibility to infection, and an increased frequency of pressure ulcers. To provide the best overall patient care, clinicians must assure that patients receive adequate nutrition. Understanding the basic concepts of metabolism and methods of providing nutrition is crucial to quality hospital care.

PATHOPHYSIOLOGY

Adequate nutrition consists of several different components: energy (calories) to support normal function and repair tissues, protein to provide the

463

essential amino acids, carbohydrates to prevent ketosis, fat to provide the essential fatty acids, and vitamins and minerals to support cellular functions. Basic metabolism requires energy obtained from carbohydrates (4 kcal/g), lipids (9.1 kcal/g), and proteins (3.7 kcal/g). In general, the daily required calories should be provided by carbohydrates and lipids. Approximately 100 g of carbohydrates must be supplied daily to prevent ketosis. **If sufficient carbohydrates are not provided, protein will be broken down via gluconeogenesis to form glucose**, producing ketone bodies as a byproduct. Protein is essential for adequate growth, wound healing, and immune function. Protein intake should supply the nitrogen necessary for protein synthesis and provide the nine essential amino acids which the body cannot manufacture. Protein and energy supplies are closely linked to one another. If energy supplies are inadequate, body proteins will be metabolized for energy. Thus, negative nitrogen balance requires higher protein intake in order to prevent catabolism. The remainder of nutritional supplementation consists of supplying essential vitamins, minerals, and fatty acids. Table 63-1 lists the essential vitamins and disorders of vitamin metabolism. Single vitamin deficiencies are seldom encountered; **if a diet is deficient in one vitamin, it is usually deficient in multiple**. The major minerals are supplied by most diets; however, trace minerals must also be considered in individuals with malnutrition (Table 63-2). Essential fatty acid deficiency causes dermatitis, hair loss, and impaired wound healing. For most patients, approximately 5 g of linoleic acid per day (1–2% of total calories) is required to prevent essential fatty acid deficiency.

The goals of nutrition in the hospitalized patient are:

1. Provide enough nonprotein calories to meet overall caloric needs
2. Provide enough nitrogen to replace amount of protein catabolized daily
3. Provide essential nutrients which the body cannot manufacture
   a. Amino acids—histidine, isoleucine, leucine, lysine, methionine, phenylalanine, threonine, tryptophan, and valine
   b. Vitamins
   c. Minerals—calcium, chloride, sodium, phosphorous, potassium, magnesium, and trace elements
   d. Fatty acids—linoleic acid, linolenic acid

CLINICAL PRESENTATION

On admission to the hospital, patients should be evaluated for existing malnutrition. No single finding confirms malnutrition; however, the history and physical can identify patients at high risk. A dietary history should be obtained to identify patterns of intake as well as possible deficiencies of required nutrients. Historic factors which are suggestive of malnutrition include a 10%

Table 63-1 **Essential Vitamins, Recommended Daily Requirements, and Results of Deficiency**

Vitamin	Deficiency
Vitamin A 5000 IU	Night blindness, xerophthalmia, xerosis, hyperkeratosis of skin, loss of taste
Thiamine (B_1) 1.0–1.5 mg	Early—anorexia, muscle cramps, paresthesias Late—high output heart failure, sensory neuropathy, Wernicke's encephalopathy
Riboflavin (B_2) 1.1–1.8 mg	Cheilosis, angular stomatitis, glossitis, seborrheic dermatitis, anemia
Niacin (B_3) 14-18 mg	Early—anorexia, weakness, irritability, glossitis, stomatitis Late—pellagra (dermatitis, dementia, and diarrhea)
Pyridoxine (B_6) 1–2 mg	Early—cheilosis, glossitis, weakness, irritability Late—hypochromic anemia, peripheral neuropathy, seizures
Folate (B_9) 400 µg	Megaloblastic anemia, glossitis, anorexia, diarrhea
Cobalamin (B_{12}) 3 µg	Megaloblastic anemia, glossitis, anorexia, diarrhea, peripheral neuropathy, red, sore tongue or smooth tongue
Ascorbic acid (C) 60 mg	Scurvy—mucosal bleeding, slow-healing wounds, atraumatic hemarthroses, petechiae, purpura
Vitamin D 400 IU	Rickets, osteomalacia, hypocalcemia, bone pain
Vitamin E 10–15 IU	Areflexia, gait disturbances, ophthalmoplegia, hemolysis, retinopathy, neuropathy
Vitamin K 50–100 µg	Easy bruising, mucosal bleeding, melena, hematuria

weight loss over the prior 3 months, anorexia, chronic vomiting or diarrhea, and the presence of a chronic illness, particularly renal or hepatic disease. On physical examination, signs of malnutrition include muscle wasting particularly of the temporal and proximal extremity muscles, loss of subcutaneous fat, pressure ulcers, petechiae or ecchymoses, and a body mass index <19. (Note, many obese patients also have poor diets and can also be malnourished.) The examination should also look for signs of vitamin or mineral deficiencies, particularly of the skin, hair, nails, and mouth (Tables 63-1 and 63-2).

Patients who are at risk for malnutrition should have basic laboratory evaluation to determine their nutritional stores. **Prealbumin** is the most clinically useful laboratory measure of nutritional status. Its short half-life of

Table 63-2 **Trace Elements**

Element	Deficiency
Iron	Fatigue, anemia, headache, glossitis, nail changes
Selenium	Keshan's dilated cardiomyopathy, myalgia, myositis
Chromium	Hyperglycemia, hyperlipidemia, metabolic encephalopathy, peripheral neuropathy
Copper	Hypochromic, microcytic anemia, neutropenia, psychomotor retardation, decreased visual activity
Iodine	Goiter, somnolence, bradycardia, constipation, high blood pressure
Zinc	Delayed wound healing, decreased sense of taste and smell, night blindness
Manganese	Hypercholesterolemia, dementia, dermatitis

2 days makes it useful in the acute setting and it is a good predictor of outcome. A prealbumin of <15 indicates a mild protein deficiency and has been associated with a greater risk of complications; a patient with a prealbumin of <11 requires aggressive nutritional support. Albumin is the most widely used measure of nutritional status; however, it can be affected by nonnutritional problems, particularly liver disease and systemic illness. An albumin <3.4 g/dL generally indicates malnutrition and <2.2 g/dL is severe malnutrition.

Other laboratory tests suggestive of malnutrition include transferrin (<200 mg/dL), lymphocyte count (<1500/mm³), and total cholesterol (<160 mg/dL) if not on a cholesterol-lowering medication.

MANAGEMENT

Any patient with suspected malnutrition on admission or with risks for developing malnutrition (elderly, diabetes, hypertension, renal disease, nutrient losses, not eating >5 days) should receive a nutrition consult on admission. In general, to determine an appropriate diet, several factors must be taken into consideration. The first step is to consider the amount of energy and protein required. A way to estimate daily kcal requirements is to calculate the total energy expenditure (TEE) by multiplying the patient's weight in kg by 25. This will provide a rough estimate, recognizing that the TEE will be higher when metabolic demands are higher (i.e., stress due to trauma or infection). The required protein intake in a normal individual is approximately 1 g/kg/day; however, patients who are postoperative or critically ill can require over 2 g/kg/day of protein.

A second consideration is the consistency of the diet. A clear liquid diet is often provided to patients with intestinal ileus, gastroenteritis, or who are transitioning from a prolonged period of not eating. A clear liquid diet typically provides only 500–1000 kcal/day in simple carbohydrates with basic electrolytes. It is sufficient to prevent ketosis, but does not supply most essential nutrients. A full liquid diet can be used in similar situations as well as for patients with difficulty swallowing or chewing. Its caloric value varies, but it can supply a patient's caloric needs. Unless specially designed, full liquid diets are often deficient in vitamins and trace minerals. Soft diets are designed primarily for patients with difficulty swallowing or chewing and are typically nutritionally adequate.

A third consideration is whether a patient requires a restricted diet. Patients with diabetes should receive a diabetic diet which restricts carbohydrates, is low fat, and controls the number of calories. A sodium-restricted diet is typically ordered for patients with cirrhosis, heart failure, or renal failure to control edema. Many sodium-restricted diets also involve a fluid restriction. Protein-restricted diets may be ordered for patients with cirrhosis or renal failure to limit production of nitrogenous wastes. These diets typically provide the minimum required protein 0.6 g/kg/day but they are controversial as these patients also frequently have a baseline poor nutritional status and increased nutritional needs during an acute hospitalization. Many commonly ordered diets combine multiple restrictions. For example, a cardiac diet typically limits cholesterol, fat, and calories. A renal diet typically restricts fluid, protein, sodium, potassium, and phosphorus.

Last, the mode of delivery must be selected. Most patients will be able to meet nutritional requirements by oral intake alone; however, some patients may either not be able to take an oral diet or not be able to meet nutritional needs with oral diet alone. Initially, patients should be given nutritional supplements between meals to meet their requirements. However, in patients not able to meet nutritional requirements by oral intake, enteral feeding should be considered. Well-nourished patients with mild to moderate illness tolerate up to 7 days of fasting with little or no adverse consequences. However, patients with documented malnutrition on admission as well as those patients with complex critical illness/injury clearly benefit from early enteral nutrition. Enteral feeding consists of liquid nutrition provided to the gastrointestinal (GI) tract via a tube placed into the stomach (prepyloric) or small bowel (postpyloric). A postpyloric feeding tube is preferred in patients with greater risks for aspiration.

Total parenteral nutrition (TPN) is used when enteral feeding is not possible or when nutritional needs are not met by enteral feeding alone. Typical conditions requiring TPN include feeding tube intolerance (diarrhea, abdominal distention, and vomiting), bowel obstruction, inadequate bowel surface area (short gut), or high output GI fistula. Central venous access is required for administration of TPN. Nutritional requirements are met with dextrose (carbohydrate), amino acids (protein), and lipids along with additional elec-trolytes, vitamins, and trace elements. TPN is only used when other options have been exhausted because it bestows numerous complications. Obvious problems exist with the central venous lines, such as sepsis, thrombosis, and problems with insertion (pneumothorax). However, TPN is also associated with fatty liver (due to excess carbohydrate calories), oxidation-induced cell injury (due to lipids), and mucosal atrophy (due to bowel rest).

SUICIDE

Bruce L. Houghton

KEY POINTS

- Approximately one-third of people will have suicidal ideation at some point in their lives.
- In depressed patients, the lifetime risk of suicide is approximately 10%.
- Rates of suicide are markedly higher in Whites and Native Americans compared to African Americans, Hispanics, or Asians.
- Physical illness and substance abuse are risk factors for suicide, both obviously prevalent in patients on inpatient medicine services.

INTRODUCTION

The topic of suicide may seem out of place in the Internal Medicine Clerkship. However, in practice, internists frequently care for patients who have diagnoses of depression and other psychiatric conditions (specifically bipolar disorder and schizophrenia) that carry an increased risk of suicide. Indeed, in the United States in the year 2000, suicide was the third leading cause of death among people aged 15–24 years, the 8th leading cause of death for men of all ages, and the 11th leading cause of death among all Americans. In addition, internists often are involved with the care of patients who are hospitalized following an attempted suicide.

PATHOPHYSIOLOGY

Studies have identified many factors that may affect the likelihood of a patient attempting suicide. As with many aspects of medicine, suicide involves complex interactions among environmental, psychosocial, and biological factors (Table 64-1).

Table 64-1 **Evaluation of Suicide Risk in Adults and Adolescents**

Demographic and Social Profile	High Risk	Lower Risk
Gender	Male	Female
Marital status	Separated, divorced, or widowed	Married
Family history	Chaotic, conflictual Family history of suicide	Stable
Job	Unemployed	Employed
Relationships	Recent conflict or loss of a relationship	Stable relationships
School	In disciplinary trouble	No disciplinary problems
Religion	Weak or no suicide taboo	Strong taboo against suicide
Health		
Physical	Acute or chronic illness	Good health
	Excessive drug or alcohol use	Little or no drug or alcohol use
Mental	Depression	No depression
	Schizophrenia or bipolar history	No psychosis
	Panic disorder	Minimal anxiety
	Disruptive behavior	Directable, oriented
	Feelings of helplessness or hopelessness	Has hope
Suicide ideation	Frequent, intense, prolonged	Infrequent, low intensity, transient
Suicide attempts	Repeated attempts	No prior attempts
	Realistic plan	No plan
	High risk	High likelihood of rescue
	Guilt	Embarrassment about suicide ideation
	Continuing wish to die	No continuing wish to die
Other	Lack of concern	Good insight
	Unsupportive family	Concerned family
	Socially isolated	Socially integrated

Source: Adapted with permission from Tintinalli JE, Kelen GD, Stapczynski JS, et al. *Tintinalli's Emergency Medicine: A Comprehensive Study Guide,* 6th ed. New York: McGraw-Hill, 2004, Table 289-2.

Although the genetic factors that may contribute to suicide are still unknown, it has been shown that patients who attempt or commit suicide have a higher rate of suicide reported in their families; this relationship has borne out when correlated with studies of twins' and adopted children's suicide risk. Women attempt suicide more often than men, but men are four times more likely to die from suicide. Furthermore, of those patients who complete suicide, more than 90% have a diagnosable psychiatric illness at the time of death, generally depression, alcohol abuse, or both.

One model that attempts to predict suicide is the "stress-diathesis" model. An acute stressor (such as a psychosocial problem or worsening psychiatric condition) acts on the diathesis or predisposing condition (e.g., genetic factors, support system, and childhood experiences) to precipitate a suicide attempt. Another controversial view is that the media contributes to some suicide cases. For example, the airing of a German television series showing a young person jumping in front of a train to commit suicide was followed by an increase in German youth suicides involving high-speed trains.

CLINICAL PRESENTATION

Patients who attempt suicide by overdose or toxic exposure are often admitted to a general medicine team for medical stabilization prior to discharge or transfer to an inpatient psychiatric facility. Patients who attempt suicide by more traumatic means (e.g., gun shot, stabbing, and hanging) are typically followed on a surgical team and are beyond the scope of this text. The care and management of patients who overdose or attempt other poisonings (e.g., carbon monoxide) is individualized according to the substance(s) or toxin. Frequently, the history must be obtained from a friend or family member and police reports as patients are lethargic or even comatose. Pill bottles can be helpful in identifying the types of drugs and number of pills ingested. It is common for patients to ingest more than one drug or substance. Thus, in addition to looking at the vital signs, skin, pupils, and the neurologic system for signs of specific toxidromes (clinical syndromes associated with particular drug overdoses; see Chap. 61), you also should look for signs of drugs of abuse (track marks, alcohol on the breath) and violence.

Many patients with chronic medical conditions have a concurrent diagnosis of depression that may lead to suicidal ideation and attempted suicide. Internists commonly treat patients with depression and need to be aware of the signs and symptoms of severe depression and suicide risk.

EVALUATION

There are opportunities for prevention as approximately 50% of patients who complete suicide have sought professional help within the month preceding.

Despite these numbers, the U.S. Preventive Services Task Force (USPSTF) was unable to find good evidence to recommend a generalized suicide screening program for all patients. This does not apply, however, to patients who are deemed to be a higher risk for suicide by the physician. Focused questioning of at-risk patients is effective. The physician must assess the patient's risk of suicide by evaluating the patient's medical and psychiatric condition, psychosocial stressors, and support system. Previous suicide attempts weigh heavily in the risk stratification for suicide. However, physical illness itself is a risk for suicide and thus it is reasonable to screen inpatients on a medical service for suicide.

Physicians may fear "suggesting" suicide to the patient and therefore not ask depressed patients about suicidal thoughts or plans. There is no evidence in the literature to support this reason for concern. This myth may be more related to the physician's own reluctance to discuss the topic than fear of harming the patient. In practice, the patient is often very willing to discuss his or her thoughts when given the opportunity, yet is reluctant to seek help or bring it up on his or her own.

Asking patients if they have suicidal thoughts or plans can be difficult, especially for the medical student. The student should be aware of his or her own beliefs about and reaction to suicide as it may affect the interaction with the patient. It is important to remain empathetic and nonjudgmental when interacting with suicidal patients as they are often extremely vulnerable. Any patient who expresses suicidal ideation should be brought to the attention of a supervising physician.

MANAGEMENT

The acute management of a patient who has attempted suicide is performed in the Emergency Department and the method of suicide attempt determines the specific therapy. The subsequent management of the suicidal patient encompasses assessing the risk for suicide, diagnosing and treating the underlying psychiatric disorders, and removing the means for suicide. It is extremely important to convey to the patient your commitment to help. The stigma associated with suicide cannot be overemphasized. Clinicians involved with the care of the suicidal patient must be cognizant that this can affect their care of the patient. Physicians should recognize that their own beliefs and feelings about suicide can affect their response to the suicidal patient.

When alcohol or substance abuse is involved, it is important that referrals to treatment programs be made as part of the plan of care. Depression is frequently a facet of the suicidal patient and requires vigorous treatment on the part of the physician. Unfortunately, fewer than one in six patients with a major depressive episode who complete suicide are receiving adequate doses of antidepressant medication.

The physician often must collaborate with psychiatry, social work, pastoral care, substance abuse counselors, and other services in the care of the suicidal patient. Awareness of local resources and medicolegal responsibilities is also an integral factor in this process. Caring for the suicidal patient can be one of the more difficult challenges for the medical student, but one that can be quite rewarding.

END-OF-LIFE CARE

ISSUES

Eric I. Rosenberg

KEY POINTS

- The physician who knows the patient best should take the initiative in obtaining specific advance directives from their patients, which may be a gradual process requiring several discussions.
- Discussion of advance directives should be initiated with any patient suffering from a chronic, debilitating illness such as metastatic cancer, end-stage renal disease, severe COPD or heart failure, or Alzheimer's disease.
- Intercultural differences can be problematic; in certain communities there is a legacy of mistrust toward physicians. Silence from patients or family members is a particularly ominous sign.
- The end point of these discussions should not simply be a "DNR" order, but a clear understanding and appreciation for the patient's overall expectations for treatment and care.
- Patients have the right to refuse medical interventions that they believe are not in their best interest.

INTRODUCTION

It's 2 a.m. and the emergency department pages your team to admit an 87-year-old woman with pneumonia. On your arrival, you encounter a cachectic woman who is alert but tachypneic on oxygen. In addition to her history of acute-onset dyspnea, fever, and productive cough, you discover she has a history of stage III non-small-cell lung cancer diagnosed a year ago. Her chest x-ray shows a large infiltrate in her left lower lobe with multiple opacities suspicious for metastatic disease. She is exhausted from a sleepless night amidst the busy emergency department and her only family, a son and daughter, are at the bedside. Her primary physician is unavailable. How can you best integrate a discussion of advance directives into your history taking? Is this an appropriate time and setting to review the patient's "code status"? Who should be present during this discussion? Should you wait to consult with the patient's primary physician before doing so? What do you feel should be the goals of this hospitalization?

Situations such as these are frequently encountered by medical students and residents on inpatient rotations. This chapter will focus on some of the specific problems that arise when attempting to clarify a terminally ill patient's preferences for end-of-life care, and will provide a practical six-part framework for better structuring these discussions.

CLINICAL DISCUSSION

Patients have the right to refuse medical interventions that they believe are not in their best interest—this includes cardiopulmonary resuscitation (CPR), hemodialysis, transfusions, chemotherapy, and diagnostic studies. In addition, patients can withdraw from therapies even after they are initiated, at any time. This includes mechanical ventilation, artificial nutrition, and fluids, even if it means hastening death.

The principles of autonomy, respect for persons, beneficence ("doing good"), and nonmaleficence ("preventing harm") are especially relevant when considering the best course of action for a patient who is terminally ill. Conventional advance directive statements can be vague (e.g., "no heroic or extraordinary measures"). Many advance directives do not address specific preferences in specific situations, with regard to CPR, advanced cardiac life support (ACLS) interventions, and other optional therapies noted above. For example, some patients with end-stage chronic obstructive pulmonary disease (COPD) would desire mechanical ventilation for a "reversible" and perhaps temporary condition such as pneumonia, but would not want intubation for the irreversible decline in their lung function from COPD.

In the case described above, input from the family and the patient's primary care physician is invaluable. However, hospitalists and physicians-in-training must frequently initiate discussions of end-of-life preferences despite not having had a close prior relationship with the patient. Medical students and residents often struggle with how best to begin these conversations due to fears of overstepping boundaries or concerns about being perceived as frightening or uncaring. Nevertheless, physicians need to take the initiative in obtaining specific end-of-life preferences from their patients. This can be a gradual process of discussion that can provide the physician with valuable insight into not only the patients' immediate preferences and concerns regarding medical treatment, but also the depth of the patients' overall understanding of their illness. It is helpful to structure the discussion of advance directives into six familiar steps: "Who, What, Where, When, Why, and How."

Who should be responsible for initiating a discussion regarding advance directives? It should be the physician who knows the patient best—perhaps a primary care doctor or a subspecialist who has been closely associated with a patient's care. Personal interaction between the doctor and patient is critically important. In certain circumstances, the most appropriate physician is a resident caring for the patient, as these individuals often spend many hours at the patient's bedside, getting to know the patient and his or her family even better than the attending physician. Students are not experienced enough to lead such discussions without direct supervision, but students can provide valuable insights into the patient's and family's preferences, as they too spend many hours at these patients' bedsides. Nurses and social workers may also be helpful in alerting physicians to when patients are ready to discuss these issues.

Who should be present for this discussion? The patient should be encouraged to have family members, friends, and supportive individuals present to assist with asking questions and witness his/her stated preferences. If the patient is incapacitated, next-of-kin should be identified, although this can be challenging with institutionalized or elderly individuals with deceased or uninvolved family. **Who** are appropriate patients for this discussion? In addition to patients with known imminently terminal illnesses, discussion of advance directives should be initiated with any inpatient suffering from a chronic, debilitating illness such as end-stage renal disease, severe COPD or heart failure, or Alzheimer's disease. (While all patients should discuss this with their personal doctor, discussing advanced directives with a 20-year-old admitted for cellulitis may cause unnecessary anxiety.)

What should be discussed and **How** should it be done? A common mistake is overly persistent questioning or insistence on a "DNR" or hospice order on first meeting a patient or the family. Some patients and families have never seriously discussed these issues with their physicians. It may be sufficient simply to raise the issue of advance directives and encourage the patient to talk with his/her family regarding specific wishes. The physician can follow-up later to determine what decisions have or have not been made. It may take days of gentle revisiting of this topic to answer new questions, discuss prognosis, and involve specialists before specific preferences are expressed.

Patients with complex or terminal illnesses fear being abandoned, and they may fear that expressing a clear desire to be made a "DNR" will lead to inappropriate withholding of aggressive medical care. Although preferences regarding CPR are important to determine, far more helpful is an idea of what the patient's overall philosophy and goals are as they approach the end of life. A specific wish, rather than vague legalistic language, is what is needed. It may be best to start with a summation or update from a medical perspective as to the patient's current health status. A common mistake is for the physician to provide this initial summarization. It is far more useful to first ask THE PATIENT to describe his or her understanding of their condition. This will alert the physician very quickly to whether the patient is prepared for the discussion and whether he or she has a realistic grasp of the situation. The same approach can be made with family. For example, in our earlier scenario, the resident physician might say the following:

> I understand that you were diagnosed with lung cancer a year ago... can you tell me your understanding of how your lung cancer is doing?

The patient is often very aware of his or her terminal condition. Once there is an understanding of the patient's beliefs regarding the condition, summarize for the patient what your recommendations are regarding further treatment plans. This will often lead naturally into a discussion of specific advance directives. For example:

> You have pneumonia, which I plan to treat with antibiotics, oxygen, and breathing treatments here in the hospital. I am concerned that your condition may make it more difficult to treat the infection. Have you thought about or discussed with your family what type of treatments you would want were you to get sicker?

These discussions need to be done with a great degree of sensitivity and awareness of how the physician is being perceived by the patient and family, especially when attempting to educate patients or families who don't have an accurate understanding of their condition. In addition, many patients and families have unrealistic expectations of the efficacy of CPR and ACLS. For example, about 15% of all patients who require resuscitation will survive to hospital discharge, and this percentage is much less (approaching 1% or less) for patients with end-stage medical conditions, such as terminal cancer. However, studies suggest that the general public thinks about 65% of patients survive resuscitations, perhaps influenced by the near-universal resuscitation success on purportedly realistic television shows. Therefore, it may be helpful to present ACLS measures as medical treatments that are optional. Further, it may be necessary to point out clearly that should the patient's condition deteriorate to the point where respiratory or cardiac arrest occurred, resuscitative measures have considerable likelihood of causing suffering without long-term benefit. The common goal to emphasize is preventing suffering, which may indeed entail no resuscitation, but that doesn't mean no therapy. Many patients fear the "undiscovered country" of death, especially fears of pain or abandonment. Often patients interpret DNR to equal "do not treat." Focusing on preventing suffering, one can point out specific therapies that will be offered to the patient, such as oxygen, morphine, and anxiolytics, all powerfully helpful means of treating patients near the end of life. Using phrases like transitioning from aggressive curative treatment to aggressive pain and suffering treatment can help reinforce the notion that you will be actively involved in treating the patient; it is only the treatment goal that has changed.

The patient's perception of quality of life is an important consideration; many patients, despite a terminal diagnosis, will hope for as much time with family as possible and will direct you to pursue aggressive treatment regardless of the poor likelihood of success. Others may defer to your professional judgment; "If you don't think I'm getting better, I wouldn't want to live hooked up to machines." The key, again, is understanding and documenting patient-specific preferences and wishes.

Intercultural differences can be problematic; in certain communities there is a legacy of mistrust toward physicians. Doctors may misinterpret silence or disagreement as a denial of the severity of illness. Some societies have taboos regarding speaking about death; they believe that this may increase the probability that their family member will die and may explain their reluctance to discuss advance directives. Our culture in the United States has been described as highly verbal; other cultures rely more on unspoken gestures and facial expressions and the amount of distance between individuals to communicate on sensitive topics. Physicians may be perceived as offensive if they attempt to discuss sensitive issues. Religious beliefs are also critically important, particularly in situations where family or patients are perceived by medical staff as requesting inappropriately aggressive treatment. In reality, the family may simply need more time to come to terms with a loved one's impending death. Social workers, psychologists, clergy, and family members can be of invaluable assistance in overcoming these obstacles. The most difficult situations occur when one concludes a discussion with a patient and is greeted with silence. This is invariably a sign of discontent. If this happens, stop and specifically inquire, "Is something wrong? Have I offended you?" This is essential to preserve trust and indicate that you are trying your best to communicate medical information and understand the family and patient's perspective.

Where and **When** should these discussions take place? In the outpatient setting, due to time limitations and because patients usually present with unrelated, acute issues, the discussion of advance directives often does not take place or, if it does, is not clearly documented for ready reference by other physicians. In the inpatient setting, the patient may be too acutely ill for the discussion to take place, and again we are faced with the dilemma of finding out "who" knows the patient best. If a patient or family member initiates this discussion, it's the "right time." For outpatients receiving hospice care, this discussion needs to occur at the very next clinic visit. And in any hospitalized patient with a terminal diagnosis, a physician should discuss this issue at the next office visit or prior to discharge. It should be made a part of the discharge summary that should be forwarded to all treating physicians. The discussion should not be rushed; the patient should be given time to comprehend and absorb the diagnosis of the terminal illness. **It is usually not appropriate to ascertain the patient's feelings regarding resuscitative preferences at the same time as giving a diagnosis**. Patients need time to understand their treatment options. In the hospital, the specific time of day is also a consideration. Early morning rounds when the physician is rushed and the patient is barely conscious are not optimal for such discussions. The ED is a poor location as well, unless the patient is in imminent danger of requiring ACLS. The patient or family may misinterpret a premature or rushed discussion as a sign that you are not prepared to offer appropriate care. Body language is also critically important. Aside from not appearing rushed, one should speak to the patient at eye level, not standing up and towering above them as they lie in bed. This may entail pulling up a chair to sit next to the bed, or even kneeling. Touch is important; a gentle holding of hands or a touch on the shoulder can offer great reassurance. In addition, for patients who are not conscious, one should not assume they cannot hear on some level what is being said, so speak into their ear, talk to them, and reassure them as if they are awake. Some families are scared to touch patients who are unconscious and near death. Emphasizing to them the importance of touch, stroking their cheek, or holding their hands, may on some level comfort the patient as death quietly approaches.

Physicians can take the lead in discussing specific advanced directives with their patients. It can be an amazing experience for housestaff and students, as patients reveal their most intimate goals and expectations, their hopes, and their darkest fears. It is important to initiate these talks whenever it becomes evident that treatment options are increasingly limited or palliative. However, only the team members actively caring for the patient should be present. This is not the time for the entire team to be standing around staring at the patient and family. Remember, the end point should not simply be a "DNR" order, but rather the avoidance of pain, suffering, and a clear understanding and appreciation for the patient's overall expectations for treatment and care. This empathetic and humanistic approach begins with these discussions before any end-of life decisions are made.

INDEX

NOTE: Page numbers followed by *f* or *t* indicate figures or tables, respectively.